KU-780-424

Health Visiting
and the Elderly

Health Visiting and the Elderly

Mary McClymont MSc SRN SCM HV QN HVT RNT
Formerly Principal Lecturer in Health Studies,
Stevenage College, Stevenage, Herts

Silvea Thomas BA MPH SRN HV HVT RNT
Formerly Senior Lecturer in Health Studies,
Stevenage College, Stevenage, Herts

Michael J. Denham MA FRCP MD
Consultant Physician in Geriatric Medicine,
Northwick Park Hospital, Harrow, Middlesex

Foreword by
Margaret Thwaites
Professional Officer, Health Visitor Education and
Training, English National Board for Nursing Midwifery
and Health Visiting, London

Churchill Livingstone ▦

EDINBURGH LONDON MELBOURNE AND NEW YORK 1986

CHURCHILL LIVINGSTONE
Medical Division of Longman Group UK Limited

Distributed in the United States of America by Churchill Livingstone Inc., 1560 Broadway, New York, N.Y. 10036, and by associated companies, branches and representatives throughout the world.

© Longman Group UK Limited 1986

All rights reserved. No part of this publication may be reproduced, stored in a retrieval system, or transmitted in any form or by any means, electronic, mechanical, photocopying, recording or otherwise, without the prior permission of the publishers (Churchill Livingstone, Robert Stevenson House, 1–3 Baxter's Place, Leith Walk, Edinburgh EH1 3AF).

First published 1986
Reprinted 1988

ISBN 0-443-03167-3

British Library Cataloguing in Publication Data
McClymont, Mary
    Health visiting and the elderly.
    1. Aged — Home care — Great Britain
    2. Visiting nurses — Great Britain
    I. Title   II. Thomas, Silvea
    III. Denham, Michael J.
    362.6′3   HV1481.G52

Library of Congress Cataloging in Publication Data
McClymont, Mary.
    Health visiting and the elderly.
    Includes index.
    1. Community health nursing.   2. Geriatric nursing.
I. Thomas, Silvea.   II. Denham, Michael J. (Michael John)
III. Title. [DNLM: 1. Community Health Nursing.
2. Geriatric Nursing. WY 152 M478h]
RT98.M29   1986   610.73′43   86–4188

Produced by Longman Singapore Publishers (Pte) Ltd.
Printed in Singapore

Foreword

Health for all by the year 2000 is the policy of the World Health Organization.

'Adding life to years not just years to life' has also been used as a slogan in recent years.

A similarly positive and constructive approach is taken by the authors of this book: they urge us to combat ageism.

Mary McClymont, herself recently retired from innovative health visitor course leadership, demonstrates three important attributes in health care: firstly, recognition and identification of health needs; secondly, planning and implementing care and support; and, thirdly, team work with her colleagues, Silvea Thomas and Michael Denham.

Historical factors such as the maternal and child health movement and the development of the school health service have tended to focus the work of the health visitor on the needs of the child-rearing family. However, although this emphasis continues to be prevalent, changes are beginning.

Health authority policies show increasing awareness of the health needs of the elderly, and health visitor caseloads of children under 5 years old are generally lower, enabling adjustments in patterns of work. Some health visitors have developed excellent group activities for older adults and others participate in pre-retirement activities. Links with colleagues in occupational health nursing at pre-retirement phases and with community psychiatric nurse colleagues for care of the elderly mentally frail, are adding new dimensions to team work already existing with district nursing and social work colleagues. The provision of age/sex registers in all general medical practices should have been a pre-requisite for 'attachment' policies and the lack of such a facility has seriously impaired the development of primary preventive services at 'neighbourhood' level. New patterns of co-operative planning between district health authorities and family practitioner committees should facilitate provision of such essential tools for team work in primary health care.

It is essential to ensure the provision of adequate practical experience for student health visitors to enable them to gain appropriate skills. Competent practice also depends upon health visitor courses having a greater regard for the knowledge base needed to meet the health needs of older age ranges.

The publication of this book is therefore timely. The 1980s provide a new opportunity for health visitors and other health professionals to reassess priorities, redistribute resources, restructure organisational frameworks, redetermine educational goals, reinforce competencies and regenerate a health focused service. The authors are to be congratulated on providing such a positive influence to aid this process.

Margaret Thwaites

Preface

The idea for this book was born as a result of the involvement of the authors in health visiting and related education. We particularly became aware of a lack of material specifically related to the health visiting care of older people. However, although its target audience is health visitors of all grades, together with intending health visitor practitioners, we believe that others who work with, or are interested in the care of older people, will find its contents useful. Whilst the theoretical aspects of such care are examined, a variety of vignettes are given which relate these to practical situations.

Chapter 1 discusses demographic and social trends, highlighting the claims of an ageing population on the caring services and stressing the contribution older people make to society and the need to combat ageism. It traces the historical involvement of the health visiting profession in the care of the elderly and examines some possible reasons for current under-development of that role. Chapters 2 and 3 examine the ageing process, from biological and psycho-social-spiritual angles respectively, drawing inferences for care and pointing out that whilst physical decline may inevitably occur, the potential for development in other planes is high.

Chapter 4 focuses particularly on what health visiting is and what it can offer older people; it is complemented by

Chapter 5, which sets out some ways in which health visiting care may be given. Case studies, set in the context of differing conceptual frameworks, give practical examples of such care. Some elements in these two chapters may prove controversial, but they are intended to provoke thought and discussion, as is Chapter 6, which examines the settings in which health visiting may be practised. Whilst the team concept in the care of the elderly is emphasised, the necessity for maintaining a primary preventive and community orientation to the health visiting role, is stressed.

This latter thrust is particularly evident in Chapter 7, where the concept of retirement is explored in three different ways, with the emphasis placed particularly on health education in later life. Recognition of the incidence and prevalence of disease and/or disability amongst older people is reflected in Chapter 8, which discusses their medical needs and care, and in Chapter 9, which considers the specific and non-medical needs of some vulnerable groups, including the carers of elderly dependants.

The tenor of the book is towards fostering optimum functional ability amongst older people, maintaining their well-being and improving their quality of life. Whilst maintaining that health visiting has an important, and at times possibly a unique contribution to make in achieving these aims, it is not intended to detract from the important multi-disciplinary facets of care, nor to disregard the essential input of other professionals and informal carers. Chapter 10, therefore, reinforces the need for mutual co-operation, and recognises that current constraints in manpower provisions and resources may make it difficult for health visitors to deliver care to the level they consider necessary or desirable. However, it also asserts the continuing need to develop the role. The book does not pretend to be completely comprehensive in coverage: its selections and omissions reflect the thinking of its authors, who do, however, believe that it will serve to fill part of the gap currently existing in the literature on the care of older people.

Stevenage 1986   M. McC.
S. T.
M. J. D.

Acknowledgements

Many individuals have contributed to the ideas expressed in this book — older friends and acquaintances; client-families with whom we have worked; professional colleagues from differing disciplines; and former students who have challenged us often and thus contributed to our role as educators. However, special recognition must be given to the following people who have significantly helped us in its preparation: Dr Lisbeth Hockey OBE, who reviewed the manuscript, made important suggestions for change and offered much encouragement; Sandra Betterton, Kate Brettell, Valerie Houchin, Margaret Illing, Beryl Munns, Doreen Norton, Edith Price, Ida Roberts, Geraldine Swain and Olive Wimble, who discussed ideas and gave us much food for thought. Liane Buob and Jean McGregor-Cheers gave time and attention to the preparation of chapter outlines and Vicki Reed and Sheila Selves were amongst those who read parts of the manuscript and offered useful critical comment. Esther Millar, Gillian Smith and Jennifer Wakefield provided much support and sometimes practical help during the writing process.

Our particular thanks are accorded the Earl of Stockton, for so graciously allowing us to use his photograph and derive benefit from his example.

We are indebted also to many writers for creative thought

Barber and Miss Joan Wallis for providing material and giving
us permission to quote from it, as did June Clark, Louise
Davies, Katie Herbst, Scott Kerr and Professor James
Williamson. The Office of Population, Censuses and Surveys,
through the courtesy of Her Majesty's Stationery Office, were
generous in granting us the use of much data, and some
illustrations. In this connection we record our appreciation to
Amelia Harris and her colleagues and to Audrey Hunt, for their
work which forms the basis of tables and illustrative figures,
in Chapters 9 and 1 respectively. Similarly we acknowledge
the data and help received from Age Concern, the Centre
for Policy on Aging, the Disability Alliance, The Equal
Opportunities Commission and the Royal Society for the
Prevention of Accidents, as well as those many organisations
and self-help groups whose publications we have studied. We
drew heavily on the work of such writers as June Clark, Priscilla
Ebersole and Patricia Hess; Jack Hall, Karen Luker, Ruth Murray
and her co-authors; Nancy Roper, Winifred Logan and Alison
Tierney; and Betty Neuman. We are grateful to them all for
generating ideas, as well as those many authors from whom we
have benefited but may have failed to specify.

Inevitably we have needed much literature and
consequently have received great help from a number of
librarians, most particularly from Sally Knight and her
colleagues at The Lister Hospital Library, Stevenage. We also
thank those at the Department of Health and Social Security,
particularly Mrs Stodulski, The Index of Nursing Research, and
staffs in the Royal College of Nursing Library and Northwick
Park Hospital Library and Stevenage College Library, for their
assistance.

We have benefited much from the informed counsel of Liz
Day, author and chairperson of the Health Visitors'
Association, Special Interest Group in the care of the elderly;
Linda Thomas (Nursing Adviser to the Geriatric Nursing
Society) and Ainna Fawcett-Hennessy (Nursing Adviser to the
Society of Primary Health Care Nursing), both of The Royal
College of Nursing; Avis Hutt and other members of the
Research Society, the Royal College of Nursing. To all of these
we tender our thanks.

We also thank the staff of Churchill Livingstone, Edinburgh

for their patience and guidance during the production of the text. Lastly but by no means least our grateful thanks are extended to all the long-suffering members of our families, who have tolerated our living with the book for so many months.

M. McC.
S. T.
M. J. D.

Contents

1

Setting the scene

The United Kingdom population is ageing. This trend has been growing for many years, but the 1981 census results revealed that there had been a 10% increase in the population of pensionable age in a decade. Even more marked was the 24% increase in the population aged 75 years and over. By contrast the rest of the population declined by 1%. Figure 1.1 shows this graphically, using absolute numbers.

Thus the country is faced with increasing numbers of very old people and at the same time a decreasing number available to care for them. Although many will continue to lead active lives outside institutions, able to give younger generations the benefit of their companionship and experience, some will rely upon community support to enable them to maintain their independence. This is likely to have considerable social, economic and political repercussions, and requires a realistic appraisal of facts and matching resource allocation. The continuing development of the health visiting service will, therefore, need to take account of these issues.

WHO ARE THE ELDERLY?

In 1981 attention centred on the death of Mr Harry Shoerats,

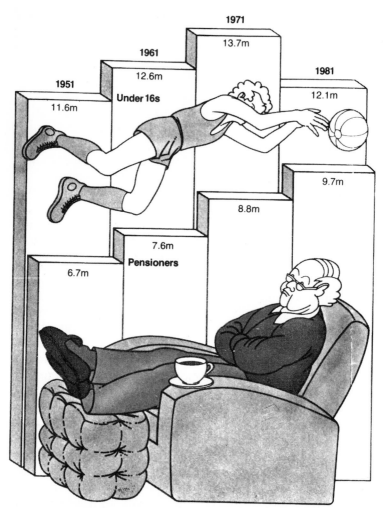

1951
11.6m

1961
12.6m
Under 16s

1971
13.7m

1981
12.1m

6.7m

7.6m
Pensioners

8.8m

9.7m

Fig. 1.1 The population is ageing. (OPCS 1983 'People in Britain' Poster)

who at 111 years of age was thought to be Britain's oldest
inhabitant. He was one of an increasing number of centenarians who have attracted interest (Thatcher 1981). Like
several of his peers, he attributed his long life to hard work
and self- discipline. The possibility of such longevity prompts
the question, at what point in a person's life cycle does he
or she become elderly? There is no simple answer. Ageing is
a gradual process, with biological, psychological and social

characteristics varying so broadly that they do not necessarily synchronise with chronological age. Traditionally the official retirement age has been arbitarily taken as the demarcation line. In the United Kingdom this is 60 for women and 65 for men, but this is now questioned and liable to alteration. Most current international documents use 65 years as the base line for describing the elderly of both sexes, so it is important to note which age is being used when comparing data.

The Concise Oxford Dictionary defines the term elderly as 'getting old', thus conveying the notion of process and continuity. 'Old' is in turn regarded as 'having existed for a long period, or being advanced in years'. Whilst this emphasises relativity, it may hint at value. Old wine, old gold, old furniture are often highly prized. Old people sometimes share their status. These definitions thus outline a period of time which begins with being elderly and culminates in old age. Murray et al (1980) prefer the phrase 'later maturity' to cover this last developmental period. Possibly this term captures the idea of continuity and experience bound up with this period and may, therefore, prove a more acceptable one for many people.

The elderly population, however, should not be regarded as an homogenous entity, particularly as the period from retirement to death can cover more than 30 years, a far larger era than most other sections of the life-span. A person of 95 may differ from a person of 65 more dramatically than does a person of 35. For this reason many researchers and statisticians are increasingly differentiating between the '*young-elderly*' (those aged 60/65–74 years) and the '*old elderly*' (those aged 75 years and above). A further distinction is sometimes made which categorises those aged 85 years and over as '*the very old*'.

DEMOGRAPHIC TRENDS

It should not be assumed that the ageing of the population is confined only to the United Kingdom, nor even to the Western world. Statistics show that the world population of persons aged 65 years or more will virtually treble in the period 1950–2000 AD growing from 200 million to 585 million.

Furthermore, by the turn of the century 60% of those aged 60 years and 46% of those aged 80 years within the world population will be living in the less developed countries. This is because although these trends are characteristic of both more and less developed nations, the relative rate of increase is higher in the latter (Skeet 1981). The enormous socio-economic impact that such trends will create demands urgent strategic plans.

It is difficult to grasp such vast figures, but perhaps even more importantly it is necessary to comprehend that population shape is most affected by the proportion of older persons within it. Thus in parts of South-East Asia the percentage of persons aged 65 years and over is below 3%, whereas in parts of Europe, Japan and the United States it is 20%. However it is the ratio of younger to older people which indicates the nature of a nation's likely problems and the type of services it may require. Thus in parts of South-East Asia there are 15 children to every elderly person, whereas in Europe, Japan and the United States the ratio is 1.5 children to 1 senior citizen respectively.

Some of the reasons for these great differences are found in the continuing high birth rates in the developing countries, compared to the falling rates in other parts of the world. Also the differential mortality rates, which although very disparate between less and more developed countries, still favour the young in each population. Thus those children now being born, who manage to overcome the stresses of life's earliest years, are likely to experience considerably enhanced chances of survival to late maturity.

It will be realised that the care of dependent young and elderly rests on the intervening adult population. Concern is expressed in several countries that this caring sector is being depleted, either through lower birth rates, or the migration of economically active persons aged between 20 and 50. Whilst it is valid to recognise this difficulty and to realise that it may affect a country's ability to sustain adequate care for its dependents, the issue must be looked at in the context of human ingenuity and the great capacity people have for adaptation and change. There is great scope for the harnessing of technology for social benefit.

Turning from this glance at the world perspective, we now

consider in greater detail the position within the United Kingdom.

UNITED KINGDOM POPULATION

Age structure

The age and sex structure of the United Kingdom population, for the period 1901 to 2000 is illustrated in Figure 1.2. From the shape of the population profile during this time, it is clear that it has, and will, become less steeply pyramidal. This is because during the 20th century the overall population has risen by 52%, but those aged 60 years or more, of both sexes, have increased by 300%. Thus in the United Kingdom at present, 2 in 9 females and 1 in 6 males are aged 60 years or more.

Nevertheless, in spite of these large changes, and the fact that those of 65 years and more within the population form 15% and will continue to do so until the turn of the century, the rate of increase has now stabilised. This means the absolute numbers of older people are not expected to rise appreciably in the forseeable future, unless very striking changes occur in the mortality experience of those in earlier and middle life.

The most significant fact to grasp, however, is the relative increase in the proportion of the elderly population aged 75 years or more, particularly those aged 85 years or more (Fig. 1.3). This is likely to continue. It is this fastest growing segment which many policy makers believe poses the greatest challenge to the nation in general and the caring professions in particular. Acheson (1981) points out that this is the age group which suffers from the greatest physical and mental disability. He estimates that this group requires more than 6 times the resources from the health services and 26 times the resources from the personal social services, than the average for the rest of the population. To date such a demand has not been matched by resources, and there is concern that this gap will widen in the future. Furthermore, this rapid growth in the proportion of the population aged 75 years and more must be viewed in relation to the slowly falling section aged 60–74 years. It is this latter group of active 'younger-elderly' who so often care for the very old. Additionally this increase

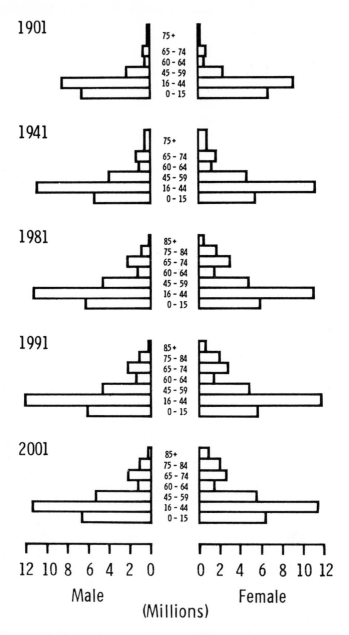

Fig. 1.2 Sex and age structure of the population of the United Kingdom for selected years between 1901 and 2001. (Social Trends 1984 HMSO, London)

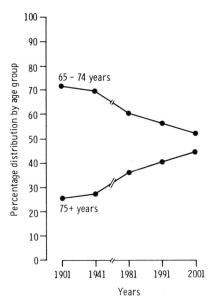

Fig. 1.3 Comparison of the proportion of the elderly population aged 60/65–74 years with those aged 75 years and upwards. (Social Trends 1984 HMSO, London)

in the percentage of 'old elderly' and the 'very old' must be related to the reduced numbers of non-employed women, who traditionally have been family carers and who have frequently staffed voluntary organisations as well.

Nevertheless, while it is prudent to note all these implications, it would be wrong to assume that all the very old are frail dependants. Figure 1.4 gives some indication of the average pattern of activity amongst two 'reference groups', one aged 65 years and the other aged 85 years. Although there is declining independence with advancing years, a significant number cope well. We can all cite examples of active octogenarians and nonogenarians, who continue to live full and autonomous lives until shortly before death. This is the level of independence and participation which those who offer preventive health care seek to encourage.

Sex disparity

Another significant demographic feature is the disparity

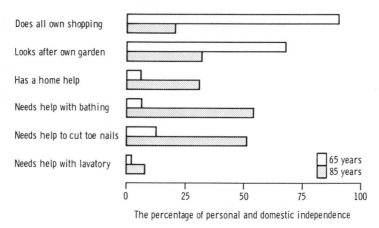

Fig. 1.4 Average pattern of activity amongst two reference groups of elderly people, one aged 65 years and one aged 85 years. (Derived from data in Hunt 1978 and OPCS 1982.)

between the sexes, which favours females and reflects world-wide trends. This sex difference is emphasised in each age group over 60 years, but reached a peak ratio of approximately 1 male to 5 females aged 85 years and over in 1981. The reason for this imbalance lies not in the birth of fewer males, but in their greater mortality experience at almost every age. The average life expectancy rates have shown general improvement for both sexes at birth; nevertheless the average male infant can currently only expect a further 70 years of life, compared to 76 years for the average female infant. There has been comparatively little gain in life-chances for either sex after 65 years: even so, males can only

Table 1.1 Marital status of the population of the United Kingdom aged 60 years and over shown by percentage, sex and age for 1981 (Census year)

Age	Single	Married	Widowed	Divorced
Males				
60–64	8.5	83.6	5.2	2.7
65+	8.1	72.9	17.4	1.6
Females				
60–64	8.1	67.7	20.7	3.5
65+	12.1	37.1	48.9	1.9

Based upon data supplied by the Office of Population, Censuses and Surveys and The General Registrar's Office, (Scotland) in: Social Trends 1984.

anticipate on average a further 12 years, whereas females can expect an additional 16.

Why women live longer than men is a complex matter. Tinker (1981) suggests it is because women have less stressful or dangerous occupations; smoke and drink less and have a biological advantage, possibly hormonal. Certainly high male death rates due to two world wars in this century have skewed the picture. It remains to be seen if there will be any reversal of the prevailing trend now that women play a far greater part in the labour market, travel more widely and smoke, drink and drive more frequently. Meantime the implications of an older population, heavily weighted to females, must be borne in mind.

PATTERNS OF LIVING AMONG THE ELDERLY

Although four out of five men and two out of three women aged 60–64 years are married and living with their spouse, there is a marked change after 65 years, due to the high percentage of women now aged 65 years and over who have either never married, or are widowed (Table 1.1). In fact women of this age group account for almost half the widows in the total population. This is an important feature as grief, loneliness, lack of physical and psycho-social support in the home result from the loss of a spouse. Elderly widows often experience great financial hardship, becoming dependent on widows' benefit. Although at present only 2% of the elderly population are divorced, this is likely to rise more steeply in future in line with general trends in society.

Analysis of the latest census data shows that 30% of people of pensionable age in Great Britain, lived alone in 1981, compared with 19% in 1961. Women were twice as likely to do so as men (OPCS 1984). Conversely the number of households with three or more people, in which the elderly would probably be living with a family, has fallen by one-third. Detailed scrutiny shows that 43% live with one other pensioner, mostly a spouse, and the majority of others with one younger person, often a son or daughter. Only 3% overall are in communal establishments, although there is a wide range from less than 1 for the under 75s, to 18% for those aged 85 years and more. Thus, at a time when due to earlier marriage, younger-age child-bearing and increased longevity we are seeing more 4 and 5 generation families, the traditional picture of the 3 generation family living together is rapidly diminishing.

Although some people may choose to live alone it is worth noting that persons in later maturity tend to do so at least three times more often than people of non-pensionable age. Living alone does not necessarily equate with loneliness, but those who are suddenly confronted with the loss of a spouse, relative or companion may be profoundly lonely. If they are also isolated, their vulnerability is increased, compounding their 'high risk' so that greater professional surveillance is required.

Hunt (1978) found in her survey of the elderly at home, that is was helpful to compare two groups: those aged 65 years and those aged 85 years. She found a much higher proportion (30%) of the older age group were living with their families. A great deal has been said and written about the lack of family involvement in the care of their older members, but both Hunt and Abrams (1978) found much evidence to refute this. Abrams showed three-quarters of the 75-year-old persons in his survey, who had surviving children, had seen them weekly during the preceeding month. However, this must be seen in the context of the 35% of older persons who have no children, and the 16% who claim 'no family at all'. One striking and poignant feature, revealed by these studies, concerns the most vulnerable group of all, the elderly bedfast or housebound. They constitute just under 5% of all elderly persons, and approx 2% of them never receive visits from relatives or friends — an important point to be borne in mind by those aiming to work within the caring services for elderly people.

Hunt (1978) made a helpful study of the lifestyle of those living in private households, and Figures 1.4 and 1.5 illustrate some of the patterns found. When the two 'average reference groups' are compared, people aged 65 years not unexpectedly appear more independent in daily living. They have more amenities and are more likely to hold a current driving licence. A sizeable majority of those aged 85 years appears to depend on public transport, public telephones, launderettes or less sophisticated forms of household washing, and prob-

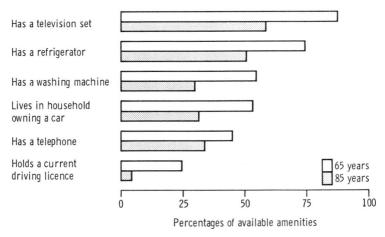

Percentages of available amenities

Fig. 1.5 Average pattern of activity and use of amenities amongst two reference groups of elderly people, one aged 65 years and one aged 85 years. (Derived from data in Hunt 1978 and OPCS 1982.)

ably have less adequate forms of food storage. Without making undue assumptions, such factors should be considered, when first visiting the older elderly and 'very old'.

Whilst the trend is increasingly to encourage older people to remain in their own homes, some inevitably require communal care. Surprise is often expressed that this is only around 4%.

Approximately two-thirds of these require hospital or nursing home services and increasingly these are from the 'very old' group. Although many of those in hospital are found in Geriatric Units, the nature of illness in old age means that many occupy beds in general medical, surgical, orthopaedic, ophthalmological and psychiatric wards. The emphasis of care must be towards rehabilitation and restoration, but for those elderly patients who fail to respond to such programmes long-term care will be required. Their quality of life and high dependency needs are issues currently receiving much attention (Denham 1983).

Of the remaining one-third who require communal residential care, half are currently found in local authority homes, approximately one-third are in privately run establishments and the rest are in the care of voluntary organisations. Over the past decade the average age of such residents has risen, so that many are now quite highly dependent. Consequently the training needs of care staff dealing with these residents must be greater. Recently there have been trends to encourage more privately-run nursing homes and boarding-out schemes. This is intended both to reduce NHS costs and prevent 'institutionalisation'. Ideally this should mean older people receive more personalised care but there are also increased risks of exploitation. There is thus greater need for supervision, support and education of carers. This is an area of activity which directly impinges on health visiting. Practitioners can help to assess education and training needs, and can run courses, seminars and workshops for the staff and lay-carers. Within these group establishments they can also help to encourage residents to form exercise and fitness groups; take up creative diversional activities and participate where possible in their own care. Such action will help to prevent the all too-familiar scene of bored, apathetic old people, lounging badly in chairs set round the periphery of rooms, failing to interact with each other or the staff and possibly becoming over-querulous.

ATTITUDES TO AGEING

Attitudes towards ageing have always been ambivalent. In spite of a keen interest in longevity, shared by almost all societies, few individuals have looked forward, unreservedly, to the realities of old age. This may be due to the association of the period with declining physical and psychological capacity as well as the heightening of awareness about personal mortality. Self- image may be threatened, especially when a person's belief system does not include an appreciation of the phase of later maturity as the rounding-off of the cycle of temporal life.

Historically this equivocalness is well demonstrated. In pre-literate societies, where survival was the overriding issue, the knowledge and experience of older people were valued highly. However, when they became physically or economically dependent, they were often abandoned, neglected, ritualistically killed or encouraged to commit 'altruistic suicide'. It is as much a false assumption to believe that all old people held high prestige or were cherished by their kin in the past, as it is to claim that they are more often abandoned in our present more mobile society.

Positive attitudes towards ageing were displayed by the Taoists and by the early Chinese, who regarded long life as 'a crown of development', doubtless greatly enhanced by its rarity. The Hebrews too revered longevity. They considered it a reward for godly living, which led them to call for great respect towards the elderly and encouragement to aspirants to keep the Mosaic Law. Paradoxically, however, the most graphic lament on old age is found in Ecclesiastes, Chapter 12. In 55 BC Cicero wrote in De Senectute one of the most spirited and lengthy defences of old age ever recorded. Translated by Falconer (1923) it well repays reading. One excerpt may serve to indicate the tenor of his work:

> Those, therefore, who allege that old age is devoid of useful activity are like those who would say that the pilot does nothing in the sailing of the ship, because, while others are climbing masts, running about gangways, or working at the pumps, he sits quietly in the stern and simply holds the tiller. He may not be doing what younger members of the crew are doing, but what he does is better and much more important. It is not by muscle, speed or physical dexterity that great things are achieved, but by reflection, force of character and judgement: in these qualities old age is usually not only not poorer, but often even richer.

More recently Norton (1982), the pioneer gerontological nurse-researcher, offered another heartening view, declaring:

> Old age is the fulfilment of every individual's birthright, which many more people will achieve over the next two decades.

Conversely negative attitudes were shown by the early Egyptians, who feared the physical decline of old age. They sought to defer its ravages by eating the glands of young animals — a rejuvenation theory which has had more modern resurgence within monkey-gland therapy!

The Greeks held contradictory notions. Their mythology is shot through with accounts of their quest for eternal youth, which often led to inter-generational conflict. Nevertheless Plato, who died over 80 years old, with pen in hand, and his fellow-philosopher, Aristotle, asserted the value of a gerontocracy. Both of them emphasised the experience and wisdom brought by many seniors to political and civic life. Whilst many of these examples were valid, it is necessary to realise that the accounts of several old worthies are the stories of the privileged few. For many people of their time, life was brutish and short. The average expectation of life was below 30 years and even those who achieved the sixth decade were sometimes sick, often disabled, and especially if they were of the poorer classes, had experienced great deprivation.

Shakespeare immortalised much of this ambivalence when he created his classic character, King Lear. Elsewhere, in his satirical poem on the seven ages of man, he wrote his well-known, melancholic and rather cruel comments on the sixth age:

> The sixth age shifts into the lean and slippered pantaloon, with spectacles on nose and pouch on side. His youthful hose well sav'd, a world too wide for his shrunk shank: and his big manly voice, turning again towards childish treble, pipes and whistles in his sound.
>
> *As You Like It*

Unfortunately, what often is intended to be humorous, or possibly provocative, is accepted; it may then be used to fuel ageism, that subtle denigration of the elderly, which it is so difficult to nail.

Personal attitudes

Personal attitudes towards ageing are often equally ambivalent. Whether old age is regarded as a blessing, a burden, or a birthright seems to depend as much on an individual's present age, his personal values, his life experiences, personal health levels and self-concept, as much as it does on the nature and frequency of his contact with old people. Nevertheless no individual can really be in two minds about the challenge currently presented, for that is singularly clear. If more individuals are achieving longer life, should not the aim of any caring person or society necessarily be directed towards helping them add quality to those latter years?

Social attitudes

The attitudes of society towards the elderly are often encapsulated in legislation, and the Poor Laws (1601–1948) demonstrate the slow, often chequered move towards more humane and dignified treatment of older people, especially the elderly poor. It is true that even as recently as the 19th century many feared the harsh routines of the workhouse. The anguish of many old people was captured by Dickens and epitomised in his character, Betsy Higden:

> Oh master! ... master!' returned Betsy, '... I've fought against the Parish and fled from it (the workhouse), all my life, ... and I want to die free of it.'
>
> *Our Mutual Friend*

Nevertheless, the principle of collective responsibility for vulnerable members of society has gradually emerged. Philanthropy, patronage and reactive concern are all shown in the different voluntary organisations formed to care for elderly people in the past, as well as in the statutory and voluntary services being established in the present. However, whilst it is clear that older people have benefited from the more humane social and personal attitudes which prevail, there is no room for complacency. Revelations over the last three decades affecting many different aspects of the care of the elderly, show not only a lack of empathy, accountability and respect for old people, but also the gross under-resourcing of essential services for the aged.

Children are seen to have needs, whereas the elderly are often regarded only as having problems. With limited bargaining power, except at elections (and so often unable to be exercised by the most needy section), the elderly have themselves often been unable to redress policies which apparently receive mass support. There is, however, now some evidence of a collective raising of consciousness. There are pointers indicating that many now retiring will prove more articulate and politically active than earlier generations of elderly. Federations are being formed to fight for improved conditions for pensioners and there are signs that if the elderly were united in a common cause they could, numerically, wield considerable socio-political influence. However, in spite of some assertive actions, both for and by older people, ageism continues to adopt many guises. Some forms of subtle denigration can be as hurtful, or more so, than overt physical neglect. For example, compare the great prestige which is currently attached to youth, beauty, sexual attractiveness, speed, competitiveness, aggressiveness, productivity and rapid adaptation, with that afforded contemplation, wisdom and experience. Stress on the use of sophisticated technological machinery; concern with materialism and an emphasis on planned obsolescence can all enhance the pain some older people feel at enforced social relegation following retirement.

Such approaches ignore the many older people who remain fully independent; run their own households; maintain recognised roles with their children, grandchildren and sometimes their great grandchildren, and still play a prominent part in their local neighbourhood, and sometimes in wider community and political life (Fig. 1.6). Similarly, there is often a tendency to overlook the many unifying values, which enable younger and older people to find affinity in common concerns.

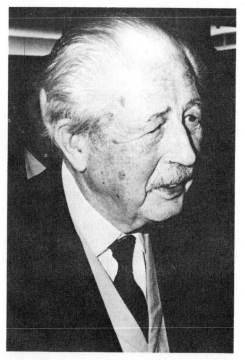

Fig. 1.6 The Rt Hon. The Earl of Stockton OM PC, an active member of the House of Lords in his 90s (photograph taken at a Distinguished Company Luncheon and reproduced by permission of the Foundation for Age Research).

Myths and stereotypes

Myths and stereotypes often heighten our expectations of the behaviour of older people, causing us to act towards them in pre-determined ways, or react sharply when they differ from our pre-conceived notions. Hendricks & Hendricks (1977) discuss this, pointing out the common 'ideal types' of the elderly which we often create. One such is as follows:

> The ideal old person is white-haired, inactive, unemployed and enjoys passivity. . . . Makes no demands; is docile, accepting loneliness, boredom, and other constraints without murmur. Can live cheerfully on a pittance, having few needs. Is often slightly deficient in intelligence: tiresome in talk,—usually asexual, and if not unseemly! ... Main occupations are religion, reminiscing and attending the funerals of friends ...

Although this description may be regarded as a blatant caricature, there are other stereotypes which are equally demeaning. Comfort (1977) discusses these, pointing out that assumptions are often made that the elderly can no longer exercise rational choices; should not be allowed to take personal risks; will always wish to conform; are unlikely to hold relevant views. Terms used towards older people, or about them, are often patronising or depriving of dignity. Even compassionate behaviour can create over-protection and under-estimation. Simone de Beauvoir (1970) argues that in spite of better education and the dissemination of research findings over a period of time, duplicity is still a hallmark of the adult's attitude to the aged.

> Whilst bowing to the ethic of respect, subtle under-mining of their authority can occur, leading to their abdication of autonomy and their adoption of passive roles.

At this point it may be salutary for us to review our own personal perceptions of, and values about, old age. Murray et al (1980) suggest that such an exercise is an essential prelude to effective work with older people. However, even those of us who work regularly with seniors need to re-appraise our attitudes, to discover if 'hidden ageism' is under-lying our work. It is only by appreciating the uniqueness of each individual, the distinctiveness of their life patterns and coping mechanisms, and hence of their needs, we can go some way towards offering improved personalised care.

The development of health visiting services for the elderly

Although some forms of medical care have always been available to older people, the specialty of Geriatric Medicine, which concerns the treatment of disease in the elderly, is of comparatively recent origin. Similarly, the geriatric nursing services have undergone marked changes in the past half century, as reviewed by Evers (1981). However, gerontology, which is the scientific study of ageing, and the application of derived knowledge to the promotion and maintenance of well-being in later life, is a distinct field, involving multi-disciplinary perspectives. It is in the gerontological field, therefore, that health visiting finds its affinity.

Florence Nightingale (1893) appreciated the contrast between sick nursing and the education, surveillance and supportive care of the apparently well. As a result she urged the nascent health visiting profession to 'develop this new work of home health-bringing'. In recognising the need to work with the community, for the development of the community, she was appreciating the essence of the early service, and encouraging health visitors in their educative thrust towards health.

Health visiting was born in the middle of the last century in the period of rapid industrialisation, with its accompanying socio-economic changes, marked inequalities, poverty, deprivation and degradation, rampant infectious disease, malnutrition, and premature death. Influenced by the Sanitary Reform Movement, and closely associated with feminist groups, the early practitioners sought to visit all age-groups and to 'elevate the people, physically, mentally, morally and spiritually'. They co-operated closely with lay workers, often spearheading teams of volunteers, and much of their work was conducted in self-help groups, and through mutual aid societies. However, they were deflected somewhat from their comprehensive ideals and universal approach, by the prevailing socio-political influences.

The latter part of the 19th century saw the struggle between the dominant medical profession and the emerging professions of midwifery, nursing and social work. Caught up in the politically popular, and rapidly expanding maternity and child welfare movement, the limited numbers of trained health visitors found themselves under the administrative sway of the powerful but benign Medical Officers of Health and channelled into a concentration of effort on child health and sanitation (MacQueen 1962; Owen 1983). Nevertheless, the claims of the elderly were pressed very firmly by Beatrice and Sidney Webb (Royal Commission on The Poor Law 1909). With two other members they wrote a Minority Report, setting out proposals for a national health visiting service for the aged. They were particularly impressed by three main features of health visiting and these they wished to see applied to the care of older people. They were:

1. the humanising and educational character of the service.
2. the stimulus it gave to personal responsibility.
3. the active strengthening of recipient self-respect, personal willpower, participation and self-help.

The Webbs advocated:

> Just as the Public Health Authority exercises general supervision over the health of infants, so it must exercise similar guardianship over its older citizens. Through these health visitors going their daily rounds, the Authority will become aware of the aged *before* they are sick, neglected or lack care.

Whilst some may feel that this approach smacks of paternalism and interference in personal liberty, others may place it in its historical context and perceive it as a genuine concern to improve the lot of a then, very deprived group.

Health visitors will be interested to note that the role of the health visitor as a case-finder was clearly seen. However, although the goals of such a proposed service were clearly within the remit and original aims of health visiting, in the event the recommendations of the Minority Report were not accepted and the care of the older person was left to the policies of individual local authorities. One may speculate how far the health care of older people suffered in consequence.

In spite of some role extension for health visitors as a result of the Local Government Act 1929, there was little national encouragement to enlarge the scope of the work, and no efforts were made to expand the work force between the two world wars. Nevertheless, because of the statutorily perscribed duties in the maternity and child health, school health and child life protection fields, together with the responsibility for care and after-care services, mainly for those suffering from prescribed infectious disease, or mental subnormality, the demands for the service continued to outstrip the supply. Consequently few local authorities, or practitioners, were able to exercise a preventive health function for other age groups, including the elderly. Services remained both curative and custodial. There were, however, a few pioneers who managed to keep a corner of their case-load for preventive work with the seniors in their community.

Lamont (1954) considered that the National Health Service Act, 1946 was the gateway of opportunity for the health visitor, since it provided the legislative base for widening and enriching her work with all age groups, including the elderly. It not only gave greater scope for home visiting and liaison activities, but opportunity as well for work in other settings. Statutory duties included the promotion of health, the prevention of disease, and care and after-care, especially for those suffering from chronic infectious disease such as tuberculosis; the aged and the mentally disordered. The subsequent National Assistance Act 1948, which brought an end to the old Poor Law, gave additional chance for innovatory care to be given, through visiting the elderly in residential accommodation, as well as participating in their health promotion through the new provisions for recreational, diversional and social welfare facilities. Unfortunately, the depressed levels of recruitment to health visiting during the war, meant establishments were not always filled, and low staffing levels meant that many practitioners were unable to seize the opportunities which the new legislation offered them. Furthermore local authority policies were not always conducive to greater development, as there were many financial claims on different services in post-war Britain. Nevertheless, in some areas, a few practitioners were encouraged to develop initiatives in care, and a number forged links with voluntary committees such as those for Old People's Welfare, and offered health education programmes in the newly developing Old People's Clubs. A few were involved in health advisory clinics for the middle-aged and elderly, and some, together with community medical officers and health education officers, ran community programmes designed to prepare people for retirement; prevent accidents in later life, or assist carers to meet the needs of their ageing friends or relatives.

During the 1950s and early 1960s further diversification took place, as Ministry of Health Circulars re-emphasised the all-purpose family health care role of the health visitor. Certain Medical Officers of Health and nursing managers encouraged policies of attachment of nursing staff to general medical practice, and in some instances to hospitals and university departments. Such changes were often hotly debated. Hitherto health visitors had been perceived as related to defined geographic communities with their major thrust towards primary prevention. This is defined as all those efforts taken to promote health and increase human resistance to disease. Thus it includes maintaining sound nutrition and healthy life-styles; fostering optimum development; encouraging social well-being; teaching about specific protection and helping to make the environment safe and less favourable to human-disease-agent interaction.

There were those who feared that attachment schemes would divert practitioners from primary to secondary and tertiary prevention. Although health visitors had always played a part at these levels they had not formed major functions. Secondary prevention is defined as all action taken to identify deviation from the normal; thus it includes early diagnosis and prompt referral for treatment, so that the period of disorder may be shortened. Activities comprise individual and mass care-finding measures; screening surveys and selective examinations of the population. Tertiary prevention on the other hand occurs at a later stage in the disease process. At this level the goal is to reduce the effects of disorder, prevent complications, aid restoration, and prepare the community to support and use the rehabilitated person where possible. Exponents of attachment schemes argued that they were but extensions of earlier activities and that they would facilitate access to other vulnerable groups in the community, especially the elderly and handicapped. The three levels of prevention were seen by them as inter-related and complementary.

Some clarification was provided by the Jameson Committee, (Ministry of Health 1956). In their Report they reiterated the main functions of the health visitor as 'health education and social advice' and itemised the duties they felt this family worker should undertake. Functions referring to the care of the elderly are listed below:

- health education to individuals groups and communities
- supportive visiting to older people to facilitate independence and mobilise necessary services
- ascertainment and supervision of specific health problems
- assessment of psycho-social and economic need
- liaison with, and assistance to, voluntary bodies working with the aged
- supportive help to the staff of Welfare Departments
- special attention to the elderly sick, infirm or needy, in collaboration with the General Practitioner and/or District Nurse (This however, excludes specific curative duties.)

In arguing that the major role for health visitors should be health education and social advice, the Committee stressed that the care of the elderly must begin in earlier years and be intensified in middle-age to avoid a disease-orientated approach to ageing. Modifications of some of the welfare-directed services may have occurred with the expansion of Social Services Departments since 1970, but other duties have remained substantially the same, being elaborated in the Mayston Report (DHSS 1971) (see Appendix 1).

Changes in the preparation of health visitors as a result of the Health Visiting and Social Work Act 1962, led to a broadening of the curriculum. More theory was included on gerontological principles, the physical and psycho-social aspects of ageing; current health problems and policies affecting care. Written examination questions on the elderly were included in all sections of the syllabus (Appendix 2b), and at least one of the 3/4 health visiting studies presented for the qualifying oral examination had to cover the care of an elderly client. Thus the next decade saw some advances in health visiting contact with elderly people, as field work teachers helped students to obtain comprehensive preparation, and as qualified practitioners put their new skills into practice.

Reorganisation of the NHS in 1974 brought about greater integration of hospital and community nursing services. Consequently more liaison schemes developed, and in several areas the number of health visitors, working mainly in the field of the elderly, increased. Several innovatory schemes involving health visitors were developed. For example, Griffiths & Eastwood, (1974) describe a psycho-geriatric follow-up service. Thursfield (1979) outlines one type of hospital after-care for the elderly, and Halladay (1981) gives details of a Manchester-based geriatric team, led by a health visitor who liaises between hospitals, community health and social services. Day & Mogridge (1981) describe a joint-funded experimental scheme, whereby an health visitor was seconded to the Social Services Department of a London borough, with responsibility for health education and liaison between health and social services staff working with elderly and handicapped people. There are accounts of other health visitors who are running bereavement counselling groups for older persons and supporting elderly people in high-rise flats or large impersonal housing estates. Some act in conjunction with the voluntary organisation **Extend** to run exercise and keep fit classes for older people, whilst others participate in community self-help projects for seniors, or workshops on retirement. Frequently these efforts are unrecognised, either because practitioners fail to publish them, or because the present pattern of statistical collection takes no account of them.

The publication of a number of Reports has further endorsed the health visiting role with the elderly. These include such documents as the Committee on Nursing (DHSS 1972), DHSS (1976a, 1976b, 1977, 1978), The Royal Commission on the National Health Service (1979) and The Black Report (1980). Specific Government policies about the care of the elderly (DHSS 1981) and the Reorganisation of the NHS again in 1982 have further emphasised community care. They presage even greater demands on the community nursing services, including health visiting. Although to date some promised resources have yet to be switched towards the community, there is hope that these will be forthcoming to enable much needed projects to develop.

Nevertheless, in spite of all this emphasis on health visiting the elderly, Dunnell & Dobbs (1982) found that health visitors spent only 9% of their time with those aged 65 years and over, whilst Taylor et al (1983) in their study estimated that an

Table 1.2 Number of health visitors, student health visitors and numbers of persons visited by health visitors 1976–1981 for England only

Year	1976	1977	1978	1979	1980	1981
Numbers of health visitors	7090	7602	7807	8111	8797	*****
Numbers of student health visitors	947	882	898	919	1027	
Total number of persons visited at home (thousands)	3509.1	3486.9	3542.7	3684.3	3757.5	3730.4
Children 0–16 years	2512.8	2442	2457.9	2503.5	2554.4	2514.0
Adults aged 65+ years	531.0	520.4	504.6	506.4	480.6	465.0
Others	465.3	524.5	580.2	674.4	722.5	751.4
Rate of visiting of adults aged 65+ years per 1000 of the population aged 65+ years	79.9	77.3	73.9	73.3	68.7	****

Based upon data derived from OPCS Social Trends 1982 and Health and Personal Social Services Statistics for England, 1982 p. 91.

average of 17% of health visits within the United Kingdom are paid to the elderly. This is further confirmed in Table 1.2, which shows that fewer elderly persons in England currently receive visits than do children, the latter still claiming approx 70% of health visiting time. Students may wish to question this apparent inequitable distribution of health care, at a time when demographic trends show falling birth rates and rising numbers of very old people.

Various reasons for this disparity have been given, including the following:

- historical developments within health visiting
- policy decisions and constraints from employing authorities
- low staff establishments, leading to high case-loads and

insufficient time for health visitors to cope with competing demands
- traditional low priority-rating for the elderly throughout all the health and social services
- personal inclination/disinclination
- greater job satisfaction from work with younger people.

Dingwall (1977) considered the length of time needed for a visit to the elderly acted as a disincentive, but Luker (1982) refuted this from her research. Instead she postulated that health visitors adopted an avoidance strategy with the elderly, because they lacked an appropriate frame of reference for dealing with this group. Using a more focused, goal-directed intervention she was able to demonstrate improvements in care. By contrast, Fitton (1980) argued from her study that health visitors *do* have a distinct agenda and do set goals when working with the elderly. Another viewpoint, advanced by Taylor et al, (1983) is that health visitors find the thought of visiting all the elderly in a practice population so impracticable and daunting, that this acts as a major disincentive. They suggest the remedy lies in adopting a more selective approach, given present staffing levels, and concentrating on those elderly whom research shows are at particular risk (see Ch. 6). Others assert that whilst this approach has advantages for secondary and tertiary prevention, it could limit primary preventive activity which is the health visitor's raison d'être.

Little attention has so far been directed towards studying how far the present low levels of involvement with the elderly may be related to practitioner frustration at the intractable nature of certain client problems with which they are presented. Many of these difficulties are of a socio-environmental nature, and remediable only through socio-economic and political measures. A few relate to medical causes and in such cases, perhaps closer involvement of specialists in geriatric medicine, both in health visitor education and in-service training, might have a beneficial effect.

DILEMMAS AND OPPORTUNITIES

Within their work with the elderly, health visitors face both dilemmas and opportunities. One such dilemma concerns the effective deployment of professional skills and resources, particularly time. For whilst acknowledging the demands created by increasing longevity and changing demographic trends, practitioners have to balance the needs of the elderly with the competing claims of other vulnerable groups, often ably presented (DHSS 1976c). This can create much ambivalence, as Dunnell & Dobbs found (1982). Although over half of their respondents rated the elderly as a high priority group, urgently requiring more care, fewer expressed their readiness to give this, citing 'insufficient time' and 'lack of support from nursing management', as some reasons for their apparent reluctance.

A second dilemma has already been mentioned and concerns the delicate balance to be achieved between the three levels of preventive care. Health visitors are very aware that the nature of their preparation fits them particularly for primary prevention. Moreover, they know that few other workers can make this their primary concern. At present many of the referrals of the elderly are of a crisis nature: accepting and meeting these, whilst enhancing health visitor acceptability with colleagues, and providing an immediate response for clients and their carers, leads to a reactive service which negates true health visiting practice. Only corporate professional debate will decide how far other workers should exercise secondary and tertiary preventive functions, so that health visitors are freer to concentrate in their main field of work (McClymont 1976).

A third dilemma concerns the question of specialist versus generic workers. There is broad acceptance in the profession that the strength of health visiting lies in its generalist approach. However, the specific needs of the elderly often call for depth knowledge and expertise that comes through concentration with the one age-group. The development of clinical consultants in nursing may point to ways in which a small cadre of health visitors, specialising in the care of the elderly, can provide a back-up advisory service for those engaged in generic duties. In this way there is no abdication of interest in all age-groups, but scope for some practitioners to extend their skills. Using an epidemiological approach enables practitioners to identify the various health problems present within their elderly population; it is then that flexible forms of care are required to meet the needs of disparate localities.

A further dilemma relates to how far the health visiting profession is prepared to specify its own role with the elderly, or how far it will allow others to impose their ideas and expectations upon the service. There are many different views from outside the profession about the direction health visiting should take. Lobbying for health visiting skills is becoming more apparent. In the past the profession may sometimes have allowed itself to be channelled into specific areas. Today professional autonomy is more zealously guarded. That there are urgent and crucial matters to discuss and resolve cannot be denied. In coming to a decision about the care of the elderly one important point cannot be disregarded. Our health visitor predecessors fought hard to reduce premature death in earlier life: they thus helped many citizens to achieve greater longevity. In so doing they presented their professional successors with both an opportunity and a socio-moral responsibility to continue to offer comprehensive care, so that those who have reached later maturity may experience quality of life in those added years.

SUMMARY

In this chapter we have sketched in the background to the rest of the book. The claims of the elderly for our attention and care have been outlined in the context of world-wide increases in their numbers and changing proportions and ratios within different populations. The implications of these demographic trends have been discussed, particularly as they affect health and social services. However, the emphasis has been on the resources older people represent and the contribution they can and do make. Whilst recognising that there are many who offer care to older people and pointing out the importance of multi-disciplinary approaches, the focus has been on the relationship between elderly clients and health visitors. Factors affecting professional attitudes and issues regarding priorities in care have been examined, as a prelude to subsequent and more detailed discussions about specific aspects of care.

REFERENCES

Abrams M 1978 Beyond three score years and ten. A first report on a survey of the elderly. Age Concern, Mitcham

Acheson E D 1981 Introduction. In: Shegog R F A (ed) The impending crisis of old age. Oxford University Press, for Nuffield Provincial Hospital Trust, Oxford p 7

Comfort A 1977 A good age. Mitchell Beazley, London

Day L, Mogridge J 1981 Health visitor who stayed. Health and Social Services Journal 91: 1114–1115

de Beauvoirs 1970 Old age. Penguin, Harmondsworth

Denham M 1983 (ed) The care of the long-stay elderly patient. Croom Helm, London

DHSS, Scottish Home and Health Department, Welsh Office 1971 Report of a working party on management structure in the local authority nursing services (Mayston Report). HMSO, London

DHSS 1972 Report of the committee on nursing. Cmnd 5155. HMSO, London

DHSS 1976a Prevention and health: Everybody's business. HMSO, London

DHSS 1976b Priorities for health and personal social services in England. A consultative document. HMSO, London

DHSS 1976c Fit for the future: Report of the committee on the child health services. Cmnd 6684. Chairman: Court D. HMSO, London

DHSS 1977 Priorities in the health and social services. The way forward. HMSO, London

DHSS 1978 A happier old age. A discussion document. HMSO, London

DHSS 1980 Inequalities in health. Report of a research working group. Chairman: Black, Sir D. HMSO, London

DHSS 1981 Growing older. HMSO, London

Dingwall R 1977 The social organisation of health visitor training. Croom Helm, London

Dunnell K, Dobbs J 1982 Nurses working in the community. Office of Population, Censuses and Surveys, Social Survey Division, HMSO, London

Evers H K 1981 Tender loving care? In: Copp L A (ed) Care of the aging. Recent Advances In Nursing. Churchill Livingstone, Edinburgh

Falconer W A 1923 Translation of Cicero. De Senectute, De Amcita, De Divinatione. Heinnemann, London, p 27

Fitton J 1980 Health visiting the aged. Health Visitor 53(12): 521–525

Griffiths A, Eastwood H 1974 Psycho-geriatric liaison health visitor. Nursing Times 70: 152–153

Halladay H 1981 A geriatric team within the health visiting service. Nursing Times 77: 1039–1040

Hendricks J, Hendricks C D 1977 Ageing in mass society, 2nd edn. Winthrop, Cambridge, Massachusetts, p 20–28

HMSO 1972 Report of the committee on nursing. Cmnd 5115. HMSO, London, para 164, 547

Hunt A 1978 The elderly at home. Office Of Population Censuses And Surveys, Social Survey Division. HMSO, London

Lamont D J 1954 The role of the health visitor in the care of the elderly. The Medical Officer 92: 162–163

Luker K A 1982 Evaluating health visiting practice: An experimental study to evaluate the effects of focused health visitor intervention on elderly women living alone at home. Royal College of Nursing, London

MacQueen I A G 1962 From carbolic powder to social counsel. Health Visiting Centenary Lecture. Nursing Times 58:866

McClymont M E 1976 Some quandaries facing the health visitor in these times of change. In: Health Care in A Changing Setting: The UK Experience. Ciba Foundation, Symposium 43 New Series, Elsvier Amsterdam, p 76–79

Ministry of Health, Department Of Health For Scotland, Ministry Of Education 1956 Working party on the field of work, training and recruitment of health visitors. Chairman: Jameson Sir W. HMSO, London

Murray R B, Huelskoetter M M, O'Driscoll D 1980 The nursing process in later maturity. Prentice Hall, Englewood Cliffs, New Jersey

Nightingale F 1893 Sick nursing and health nursing. In: Nightingale F 1954 Selected writings. Compiled by Seymer L R Macmillan, New York, p 353–376

Norton D 1982 Foreword, In: Anderson Sir W F, Caird F L, Kennedy R W, Schwartz D (eds) Gerontology and geriatric nursing. Modern Nursing Series. Hodder and Stoughton, Sevenoaks, Kent

Office of Population, Censuses and Surveys 1982 The general household survey. HMSO, London

Office Of Population, Censuses And Surveys, Central Statistical Office 1984 Social Trends No 14. HMSO, London, p 30

Owen G (ed) 1983 Health visiting, 2nd edn. Bailliere Tindall, London

Royal Commission On The Poor Law, Minority Report. 1909 Webb B S, Webb S. HMSO, London, p 793–795, 919–943

Royal Commission on The Health Service, 1979 Chairman: Merrison Sir. A. Cmnd 7615. HMSO, London

Skeet M 1981 Nursing care of the elderly. WHO/Age 81.1 6158 B. World Health Organization, Geneva

Taylor R, Ford G, Barber H 1983 Research perspectives on ageing: The elderly at risk. Age Concern Unit Mitcham

Thatcher A 1981 Centenarians. In: Population Trends Autumn 1981. HMSO, London, p 11–13

Thursfield P J 1979 The hospital that does not say goodbye. Nursing Mirror 150(6): 50–52

Tinker A 1981 The elderly in modern society. Longman, London

FURTHER READING

Gray M, Wilcocks G 1981 Our elders. Oxford University Press, Oxford

Hobman D 1981 The impact of ageing: strategies for care. Croom Helm, London

2

Biophysical aspects of ageing

Ageing is a complex process, involving biological, psychological, social and spiritual, as well as environmental components, so that it is necessary to adopt an holistic perspective, appreciating that while structures age, it is people who grow old. Biological changes, which are progressive, decremental and cumulative in effect, constitute the basis of ageing, and in turn modify psychological and social functioning. With increasing age there is a change from growth and evolution, towards atrophy and involution, although the rate varies due to the interplay of heredity and environment. This heterogeneity explains why some elderly people look young and full of mental vigour, whilst others appear 'old' before their years. What seems to be important is how people feel and look in old age, and their abilities to carry out the activities of daily life, rather than their chronological age. A summary of these changes is given at the end of the chapter, in tabular form, and is intended to provoke thought and discussion, as a basis for determining goal-related professional activity. However, it must be appreciated that this does not represent a comprehensive range of health visiting duties with the elderly.

BIOLOGICAL THEORIES OF AGEING

Adams (1981) says that there are more theories than facts about ageing, largely because research in this field is so complex. As the process begins at birth, and continues gradually throughout life, all age groups have to be studied. However, since the longitudinal studies, so essential to scientific understanding, have to be conducted over such a long time span, few researchers can offer continuity. Animal studies are useful, but cannot supply all the answers appropriate to humans, and many experiments involving them and people were unsuitable on ethical grounds. Furthermore, some earlier studies are conducted on older people in institutions, so a somewhat distorted view emerged.

The normal model of ageing is time-related, involutional, irreversible, and eventually damaging (Fig. 2.1) with the unique components of heredity and environment acting on cellular activity, immune mechanisms and body chemistry to produce this differential yet inevitable process. By contrast the pathological model assumes that the changes of age, although equally damaging, are potentially preventable, or at least reversible or controllable, given prompt effective action. (Fig. 2.2). Thus improvements in socio-economic circumstances, personal health measures and specific protection (such as via prophylaxis) can help to stop the normal, but

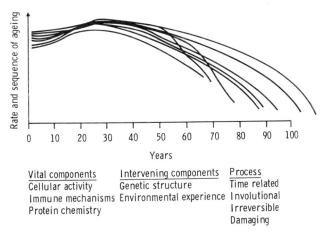

Vital components	Intervening components	Process
Cellular activity	Genetic structure	Time related
Immune mechanisms	Environmental experience	Involutional
Protein chemistry		Irreversible
		Damaging

Fig. 2.1 Elements in the normal model of ageing.

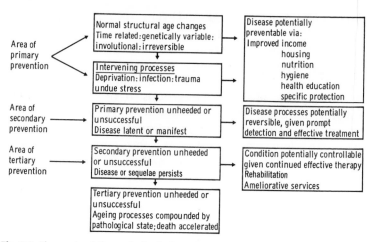

Fig. 2.2 Elements of the pathological model of ageing.

inevitable, structural age changes from being affected by disease.

Gerontological research, therefore, is aimed at reducing the rate and ravages of normal ageing, so that health and vigour can be preserved for as long as possible. This is an entirely different approach from that of geriatric research, which seeks to identify more effective diagnostic and therapeutic measures related to disease in later life. Whilst both approaches are necessary, neither are concerned with the prolongation of life in a grossly diseased state, what has been called 'medicated survival'. Health visitors, as stated in Chapter 1, are more likely to be concerned with gerontological activities.

CURRENT THEORIES OF AGEING

Current theories of ageing are based mostly on research in the fields of immunology, molecular biology and protein chemistry. They have been classified as mainly genetic programme theories, or environmental insult theories. To date there is no objective proof available to support either of these views so that the multifactorial stance is probably to be favoured. Students should bear in mind that since there are no core theories, each provides some clue to the ageing process. They should also note the apparent interrelationship between the different theories.

Auto-immune theory

Under this view ageing is thought to relate to a decline in cellular immunity and an increase in the amount of auto-anti-bodies, so that active self-destruction occurs (Walford 1981). These changes are attributed to alterations in the secretion of thymosin, together with faulty interaction between the thymus-mediated lymphocytes (known as T cells), which are concerned with cell resistance, and the B-lymphocytes, which produce antibodies. This auto-immune mechanism is thought also to increase the risk of neoplastic changes in later life, as well as maturity-onset diabetes and senile amyloidosis. If this theory holds, it is postulated that manipulation of the immune system could slow the rate of ageing.

'Biological clock' theory

Protagonists of this theory contend that each of us has an 'internal clock', which governs the *rate* of cell activity, especially mitosis replication. Hayflick (1976) considers this clock to be located in the cell nucleus and that eventually it may be possible to control environmental influences, thus modifying the mechanism and so slowing down senescence. Variants of the theory exist. One is that embryo-genesis and cell differentiation are genetically controlled. At a certain point in the life-span it is thought the usual 'regulator genes' are replaced by 'ageing genes', which produce a repressor, thus effectively stopping the essential transcription of messenger RNA. As a result subsequent protein synthesis is affected. This process has been likened to the running out of a tape on a tape-recorder, except that rewind is not possible!

Cross-linkage theory

This theory supports the view that chemically active, unwanted, migrant molecules link together co-valently, creating strong bonds between molecular structures that are normally separate. Lipid, protein, nucleic acid and carbohydrate are major body chemicals which are capable of cross-linkage. Damage is caused, particularly within the bonds of the DNA double helix, so that eventually cell mutation or cell death occurs. Cross-linkage in collagen leads to insoluble, rigid, less resilient connective tissue, whilst affected elastin becomes brittle and frayed. Since all materials that pass between cell and vessels must go through connective tissue, the cross-link impact on body ageing is profound. Research suggests that certain chemicals known as lathyrogens, calorific restriction and the action of penicillamine, each *inhibit* cross-linkage formation (Sacher 1977). If the process could be prevented it might be possible to add years to life, but at present it is difficult to determine how far it is a cause or an effect of ageing.

Error-accumulation theory

The basic proposition is that genetic mutations are caused by external factors like viruses, toxins or radiation. Successive generations of faulty cells thus develop. When mitochondria are attacked, cellular energy is affected. If ribosomes are damaged protein synthesis becomes disorganised. If lysosomes are harmed enzymes become defective, with consequent misselection of amino acids and disruption of cell life. Cumulative errors can eventually interfere with the ability to maintain biologic function. Comfort (1977) describes the process as either faults in the original blue-print, or in the copying process, or in the tools used. In each case imperfect reproduction affects ageing adversely.

Free radical theory

It is postulated that unpaired molecular fragments attach themselves to other molecules, damaging, or altering, their original structure or function, through oxidization. Such fragments can be generated from chemicals such as petrol, by-products of plastics and certain paints, atmospheric ozone, tobacco smoke and rapidly oxidising foods. They can cause chromosomal aberrations and intra-cellular havoc. Some researchers suggest that free radical scavengers, named mercaptans, provide protection from rapid oxidization. These include vitamins A, C and niacin. The anti-oxidizing action of vitamin E is also thought to retard ageing, through inhibiting free radical behaviour. If this theory is as important as its proponents suggest, then environmental control of pollution and the monitoring of nutrition should lead to healthier ageing.

Hormonal and enzyme theories

These theories link ageing to centralized endocrine control in the hypothalamus and pituitary glands, although some researchers consider the thyroid gland has a critical role. Cerebral metabolism and the action of monoamine neuro-transmitters are important features, as through their action retardation of ageing may be possible (Kent 1976).

Wear and tear theory

This view argues that repeated injury or overuse of body structures causes them to wear out, and hence cease to function. It is closely linked to the stress adaptation theory of ageing.

Stress adaptation theory

The constant bombardment of the individual by internal and external stressors is thought to lead to cumulative residual damage, so that the body is eventually unable to resist and thus dies.

Whilst some theorists, like Comfort (1977), feel the prospects for age retardation are bright and quite imminent, others are concerned about the implications of research, especially their possible socio-political repercussions. Although a knowledge of the different biological theories of ageing is helpful in understanding the physiological manifestations which can affect the aged client, health visitors need to think about the benefits and problems which might be involved in age retardation. It is important to consider the ethical issues of such intervention, in order to safeguard the rights, dignity and integrity of persons in later maturity (Davis 1981).

PHYSICAL ASPECTS OF AGEING

> It is important to distinguish between ageing as a long-term biological process and 'old age' as a natural and inevitable stage of individual development.
>
> Skeet 1983

It is these natural changes, resulting from molecular and cell inactivity, which result in impaired functioning in later maturity. Some of these normal physiological features have a significant effect upon the diagnosis and treatment of co-existing pathological states. Thus impairment of homeostatic mechanisms, which can occur with age, can affect postural control of blood pressure. Many drugs can potentiate this effect and thus can result in falls, due to hypotension. Changes in hepatic and renal function can alter the speed with which drugs are excreted, so affecting drug reactions. For this reason it is important to monitor medications and to ensure appropriate drug compliance, which may sometimes be difficult with some older people.

External signs

Skin changes

Due to atrophy of the epidermis, sweat glands and hair follicles, and loss of subcutaneous fat, which reduces body insulation, skin becomes thinned, wrinkled, dry, fragile and discoloured. The hair becomes sparser, grey or white and some recession of the hair line occurs at the temples. Facial skin-folds develop which can cause considerable distress for some people, who may be helped by advice on cosmetic management. Pruritus may prove troublesome, especially in those living in over-heated dwellings. Advising against the use of strong soaps and alkalis, and recommending the use of moisturising agents can be helpful. Of course it is necessary to determine that there are no underlying pathological reasons for such skin irritation.

Height

Normally the height of the young person equals the span between the tips of the outstretched fingers, but in the elderly loss of height results in the span eventually exceeding the height. This is partly due to narrowing of the intervertebral discs, with collapse of vertebrae due to osteoporosis, and partly due to a tendency to walk with a stoop. Consequently health visitors must encourage older people to adopt a healthy posture and should check the physical environment of older persons to see whether they have difficulty in reaching curtains, hooks, or cupboards, or even seeing out of windows, which formerly were accessible. These difficulties increase accident risks. Some older people experience difficulty in adjusting to chair and table heights which hitherto were manageable. They may therefore need advice.

Weight

Weight tends to remain constant until the late 70s, but the proportion of fat to muscle changes; muscle is lost whilst fat is gained. However fat is often lost from the face, whilst remaining more marked over hips and abdomen. Establishing wise eating patterns in earlier life is the most effective measure for weight control in later years. Nevertheless some obese older people benefit from supervised dieting, and extra exercise.

Sensory changes

Vision

This vital function deteriorates with age. The lens becomes less elastic and degenerative changes occur in the muscles of accommodation, which make it more difficult to focus for close work (presbyopia). Visual acuity, i.e. ability to distinguish objects, diminishes, whilst depth perception becomes impaired and visual fields may contract. The light-dark adaptation mechanism is reduced for elderly people, which can be a factor in accidents. Consequently some older people may need advice about night driving, or the use of photo-chromic lens. Increased intraocular pressure can cause simple glaucoma, with a gradual loss of peripheral vision. A white line (arus senilis) develops in the outer aspects of the iris, due to lipid deposits in the cornea. Loss of orbital fat sometimes causes the eyes to appear rather sunken, and there may be ptosis of the lids. Sensitivity to glare and flicker may increase and colour discrimination may deteriorate. Health visitors must, therefore, take the initiative in advising about the wise use of lighting, television watching and general eye care.

Hearing

It is well known that hearing is impaired with age. Tests show hearing loss over all sound frequencies, especially high tones. This is usually due to degeneration of the organ of Corti and/or loss of neurones in the cochlea. Rigidity of the ossicles and impaired elasticity of the basilar membrane, affecting vibration, can also increase difficulties in sound discrimination. Degeneration of hair cells in the semi-circular canals contributes to uncertainty of balance, especially during darkness or on other occasions when visual input is reduced. Hardness of hearing can lead to difficulties in communication, sometimes generating distress, suspicion and social isolation. Such situations call for empathic and supportive intervention. Health visitors need to emphasise that it will help to face the client and to make sure that speakers enunciate their words clearly and slowly to older people. Much can be achieved without shouting. Older persons need to receive regular auditory screening and to be taught how to use any supplied aids correctly. The annoying sounds which are experienced with many hearing aids are due to background noise being reflected back into the receiver. Unfortunately it is difficult to control this, but future research may result in improved hearing aids.

Nose, throat and tongue

Atrophy of the mucosa and reduction in the number of taste buds result in an impaired sense of taste and smell, which can affect appetite, enjoyment and sometimes safety. Loss of elasticity in the laryngeal muscles and cartilage reduces the responsiveness of the cough and swallowing reflexes, as well as altering the power, range and pitch of the vocal cords.

Advice on suitable diet can help to prevent the unpleasant gagging sensations which some older persons experience.

Touch and sensation

Temperature and pressure responses are reduced as a result of skin, vascular and neuro-endocrine changes. Diminished touch perception may increase accident risks. Thus older persons may burn themselves during cooking and fail to notice the lesions, which can become sore and infected. They and their carers need to be warned to guard against such happenings. Pain thresholds rise in some old people, therefore pain, such as from a fractured neck of femur may be reduced. Sensitive awareness to subjective pain reaction is an important health visiting skill. The kinaesthetic sense, i.e. awareness of body position and movement, may also degenerate; thus some elderly people may adopt very inappropriate posture, which can increase their discomfort, through alteration of body alignment. Advice on this matter may be particularly needed, where older people have experienced problems such as a cerebrovascular accident. Teaching older people to exercise in front of mirrors can help.

Musculoskeletal changes

Ageing is associated with progressive bone density loss from the skeleton and continuous re-modelling. Bone becomes more porous and demineralised with bone mass being lost from about 45 years onwards, especially in women, hence the disparity in fractures between the sexes. Genetic factors explain why osteoporosis occurs more frequently in certain ethnic groups, such as Northern Europeans and Asians. For these reasons older persons should be cautioned about excessive weight gain and should take special care to avoid accidents. There are also other changes: cartilage tends to calcify, especially in the ribs; synovial membranes of joints thicken; articular cartilage becomes damaged, hence pain may occur and mobility be affected; degenerate ligaments decrease in elasticity. Nevertheless regulated exercise and careful positioning, together with weight control, help joint protection.

Muscle power peaks between 20–30 years and thereafter declines. Thus older people may be unable to manage dexterous tasks as easily as when young. Progressive atrophy occurs and the strength of the left hand is usually less than the right in both sexes, although power is greater in men. Whilst decreasing power can be regarded as inevitable in ageing, keeping fit through balanced exercise undoubtedly helps to maintain strength and the sense of well-being. Incorrect use of muscles can generate tension and soreness; hence correct posture, movement and relaxation are important. Since the centre of gravity is changed in age, problems of balance can arise. Adaptive mechanisms for stability include wearing well-fitting, low-heeled shoes, adopting a wider-based gait, taking shorter steps with toes pointed out and using a stick, or other walking aid. It should also be remembered that postural changes in turn compress body cavities, often altering cardiac, respiratory and digestive function; so prolonged sitting and shallow breathing can be hazardous in the old.

Cardiovascular system

This system shows ageing changes quite separate from pathological processes like atheroma. The heart becomes smaller, with an increase in fibrous tissue, which can affect the conducting system. The ability to elevate the pulse rate falls with increasing age and, therefore, there is reduced exercise capacity. Thus an older person can walk up a hill, but not run for a bus. Heart rhythm is essentially unchanged and the capacity for hypertrophy is retained, in sensitive response to extra loading.

Blood pressure rises in many older people living in Western societies. This is probably a pathological process, but whether hypertension should be treated in the elderly is debatable. Care needs to be exercised when monitoring blood pressure readings in the elderly, because of their sensitivity to emotional and physical stress. Inappropriate treatment can lead to the prescribing of large doses of anti-hypertensive drugs and the consequent risks of fatigue, dizziness and postural hypotension.

Inefficiency in venous valves, coupled with poorer muscle

tone, can lead to pooling, stasis, dependent oedema, organ hypoxia and thrombus formation. However, exercise and appropriate positioning can do much to reduce such hazards. Changes in capillary permeability can cause poorer tissue oxygenation and nourishment, so care is needed to reduce tissue injury.

Blood constituents

Generally ageing has little effect on blood constituents. The haemoglobin in the elderly is the same as in younger persons. Red cell life-span is unaltered. The erythrocyte sedimentation rate may rise slightly and platelets may show some diminished clotting power. There might be a slight fall in the total number of white cells. However, anaemia in the elderly is usually the result of disease.

Respiratory system

The total lung volume remains unchanged, but calcification of the costal cartilage, kyphosis and demineralisation of the rib cage impedes respiratory efficiency. The lung itself becomes less elastic and the chest muscles less strong. Total lung capacity is not significantly altered but residual capacity increases and vital capacity decreases due to the diminished strength of the muscles of respiration. Peak expiratory volume is also reduced. Alteration in the size and number of alveoli, sclerosis of bronchi and supporting tissue, and degeneration of bronchial epithelium can lead to diminished oxygen diffusion, less effective cough reflexes, faulty clearance of secretions and lowered resistance to infection. It is therefore important to assess these by objective means, such as the use of a peak flow meter. However, encouraging appropriate maximum activity, correct breathing, as well as encouraging suitable posture can considerably improve respiratory performance in many older people.

Digestive system

The ageing changes in the alimentary tract are well documented, but they often cause little symptomatic change. In addition to the blunting of the sense of taste, changes occur in the gingival tissue and cement. Dentine formation and pulp are also affected, caries and tooth loss being common, although it is debatable if this represents normal ageing. Changes in the shape of the mouth due to reabsorption of maxilla and jaw, can affect chewing. In edentulous states, properly fitting dentures are needed for adequate mastication and for cosmetic reasons. Loss and thickening of saliva, coupled with atrophic tongue changes, can lead to mouth dryness and burning sensations. These may cause considerable discomfort and distress to some older people and may lead to anorexia. Adequate hydration is essential, particularly if the older person is taking anti-depressants, anti-spasmodics, anti-histamines, or other drugs causing dry mouth. Regular assessment of mouth state is a guide to general well-being.

Changes in oesophageal motility and mucosal atrophy contribute to swallowing difficulties in ageing. Reduced absorption of nutrients may occur due to atrophy of gastric and intestinal mucosa, achlorhydria, decreased digestive enzymes and altered blood flow. This can particularly affect the absorption of vitamins and iron, which can lead to energy loss, malnutrition and/or anaemia, especially where there is a reduction in intrinsic factors. Health visitors can do much to help promote appetite through the improvement of visual presentation of the diet, can advise on different ways of safely flavouring foods, and can also guide on the appropriate consistency of items, where swallowing difficulties are present.

Elimination may also be affected, as poor colonic muscle tone and decreased peristalsis lead to delayed transit time, constipation, sometimes faecal impaction, considerable discomfort and possibly faecal incontinence. Dietary advice regarding adequate intakes of high-fibre foods and fluids, together with unobtrusive supervision, are therefore fundamental for older people.

The liver decreases in size and hepatic blood flow diminishes, which has some impact on drug detoxification. Decreased weight, glycogen storage and protein synthesis can also affect function. Avoidance of high-fat diets and the intake of glucose drinks may then prove helpful.

Genito-urinary system

Renal function deteriorates significantly with age. This may be exacerbated by dehydration, infection and impaired cardiac output. Thickening of the membrane of Bowman's capsule, together with impaired permeability and degenerative changes in the tubules, results in a reduction of the life-span of nephrons. Tests of glomerular filtration show a 50% reduction in rate in a fit 80-year-old man, compared to his 20-year-old counterpart. A two-thirds reduction occurs in the sick elderly, which has important implications for drug excretion.

Although incontinence is pathological, frequency, nocturia and stress incontinence are common with ageing, it being estimated that 1 in 10 women are so affected. Many clients are too embarrassed to seek help, yet they welcome factual objective advice. Health visitors can help to promote continence in older people by modification of the environment where necessary and encouraging voiding habits in relation to body rhythms. Advising on the use of appropriate aids and protective garments, when required, can help to reduce social embarrassment.

Changes affecting sexual functioning

Shaw (1984) deals sensitively with this aspect, showing how ageing can modify activity, but stressing the importance of continuing creative, health-giving relationships. Sexual activity is more common among the elderly than is popularly assumed, varying as much as any other characteristic.

In women the production of oestrogen, progesterone and follicle-stimulating hormones changes with menopause, resulting in gradual atrophy of the ovaries and uterus, with involution of the vagina, labia and clitoris. The vagina decreases in expansive ability, the epithelium thinning and drying so that dyspareunia and vaginal burning may result from coitus. Regular lubrication and/or oestrogen replacement therapy may help. Whilst breast engorgement and orgasm is of shorter duration in later maturity, it should be remembered that sexual pleasure is more than a physiological response.

In men, lessened androgen production causes the testes to diminish in size and firmness. The seminiferous tubules thicken and seminal fluid is reduced and also thins. Both erection and ejaculation are slower and scrotal vaso-congestion and muscle tone decrease. Sperm production and viability are inhibited, with some reduction in male fertility. Sexual functioning can, therefore, be maintained throughout life. Health visitors may often be called upon to advise regarding sexual activities in later life and should be aware both of the inhibitions and prejudices which exist, and the techniques which may be helpful to older people (Butler & Lewis 1976, Masters & Johnson 1970, Steffl 1978, Wood 1979).

Central nervous system

Neurones are lost, although there is controversy over the rate at which this happens. Changes in the basal ganglia and deposits of lipofuscin occur, with peripherally some thinning of the myelin sheaths and atrophy of fibres. The significant change is in reaction time. Performance is slower and time must be allowed for response. Reflex action is also diminished, which, together with reduced vibration responses and proprioceptive ability, causes balancing problems and thus increases accident risks. However, it must be remembered that wisdom and experience have led older people to adapt, and that they are still able to develop new neural patterns, although less likely to do so. The effect of nervous system changes on mental and emotional states are mentioned in the next chapter.

Endocrine system

There seems little difference in endocrine function with age, apart from the loss of secondary sex characteristics, and alteration in thyroid and cortisol levels, already mentioned. However, there is difficulty in differentiating normal age changes and disease. Pancreatic changes, with modifications in insulin production and in utilisation, lead to impaired glucose tolerance. Renal threshold for glucose rises, which means persons with hyperglycaemia may not show glycosuria. Hence the need to test blood, rather than urine, when screening for diabetes in the elderly.

Temperature control

This becomes less effective with age, causing body temperature to fall and increasing the risk of hypothermia. This is potentiated by diminished shivering response and impaired appreciation of changes in environmental temperature. Some elderly people with a body temperature of less than 35° C do not appear ill, but are clearly at risk.

SUMMARY

Normal biological age changes are thus seen to be complex, plural, often cumulative, and eventually damaging. They vary in rate from system to system and from person to person, and are often compounded by associated disease. Gerontological research aims to define the causes and course of normal ageing, in order to delay its progress, thus hoping that vigour and activity may be increased for more older people for a longer time. However, this raises profound ethical and social issues, affecting clients, professional workers and policy-makers. Health visitors, therefore, share with others the responsibility to observe, assess and monitor biological age changes, advising on how to deal with them, helping to alleviate their effects and preventing complications as far as possible. These changes begin with birth and continue throughout life, but such intervention should be greatly intensified in middle and later years. It is in this health education role, which aims to teach people earlier in life how to act positively and thus help control their own ageing, that the greatest strength of the health visiting role is demonstrated. Furthermore it is the continuity over the life-span which confers such an advantage for health visitors.

DETAILS OF AGE CHANGES

Lists of symptoms and tables such as that presented in Table 2.1, though important, are abstract, and therefore tend to be perceived as lifeless and lacking reality. The following case study of an elderly person is intended to provide the balance. It demonstrates the inevitable marks of biological ageing with

Table 2.1 The ageing process showing system, normal age changes, the pathological associations and the implications for health visitors caring for clients

System	Normal age changes	Pathological associations	Caring for clients: implications for health visitors
Skin			
Decreases in strength	Wrinkling and thinning	Skin abrasions Pressure sores	Careful skin handling Teach skin care and relief of pressure
Atrophy of epidermis and sweat glands	Fragility and dryness Greater irritation	Infections Intertrigo	Use less soap but more moisturising creams Reduce exposure to extremes of heat or cold Encourage use of humidifiers if central heating used
Reduction in subcutaneous fat	Laxity of skin Less body warmth	Greater risk of hypothermia	Maintain level of personal appearance to cope with altered contours Monitor body and environmental temperature
Pigmentary changes	Greying hair Less body and more facial hair	Lentigo Keratosis	Explain skin changes and teach appropriate cosmetic care
Nails			
Reduced peripheral circulation	Thickening, ridging and brittleness	Onychogryphosis Paronychia Fungal infection	Teach suitable nail care including need for regular chiropody Check for infections and ensure treatment
Height			
Decreases inversely to span	Thinning of intervertebral discs leading to trunk shortening, postural changes and stoop	Backache, kyphosis, locomotor and balance disturbance	Assess and then modify environment to bodily changes Teach postural exercises Reduce accident risks

Eyes			
Loss of orbital fat	Sunken ocular appearance, ptosis of eyelids	Entropion Ectropion	Teach eye care and ensure ophthalmic examination when necessary
Changes in shape of cornea, lipid deposits	Astigmatism Arcus senilis Increased visual sensitivity	Myopia Corneal ulcer	Encourage regular visual screening and the use of corrective lens as prescribed Ensure correct lighting and caution against glare, flicker, or the use of sharp objects near eyes.
Stenosing of lacrimal duct	Reduced tears	Lacrimal abscess	Advise against effect of sudden cold or use of volatile substances near eyes
Reduced elasticity and some sclerosing of lens	Presbyopia Decreased colour awareness	Cataract	Monitor degree of blurred vision and poor colour perception. Explain need for preoperative waiting period and support before and after surgery (lens extraction) whilst adjustments made. Maximise colour contrasts and teach safety measures. Supervise personal hygiene
Shallowing of anterior chamber and reduced absorption of ocular fluid	Increase in intraocular pressure	Glaucoma	Encourage annual tenometry for all high risk clients Monitor installation of eye-drops and supervise prescribed drug regimes which aim to reduce intraocular pressure and so prevent blindness Check that close relatives know associated risks
Degeneration of — choroid	Decreased blood supply	Reduced visual efficiency	Ensure adequate general nutrition and monitor general health
— ciliary body	Presbyopia	Refractive errors	Teach use of and care of any prescribed aids
— iris	Contracted pupils and slowed reflexes	Pupillary change may indicate systemic disease	Monitor reactions and co-ordination and teach safety measures

Table 2.1 Contd.

System	Normal age changes	Pathological associations	Caring for clients: implications for health visitors

— retina
— reduced visual neurones
	Poorer light-dark adaptation, visio-spatial and depth perception	Retinopathy and/or retinal detachment
		Occlusive or cortical blindness
			Caution against sudden changes from light to dark, advise on the wise use of sunglasses and care during night driving
			Encourage
			  — orientation
			  — safety
			  — use of resources for the visually impaired

Macular degeneration	Blurring and fading of vision	Loss of central vision	Re-assure will not usually cause total blindness Teach to use aids and view eccentrically

Ears
Degeneration of organ of Corti
	Impaired sensitivity to high tone frequencies	Degrees of deafness with risk of
		  — isolation
		  — suspicion
		  — depression
			Teach auditory protection for clients of all ages
			Advise on regular auditory testing for elderly
			Teach correct use of aids, both personal and environmental.
			Encourage lip-reading and communication.
			Support research for improved aids

Impaired endolymph production	Alterations in balance	Meniere's syndrome	Teach compensating posture and balancing techniques
			Teach management during episodic attacks and preventive measures in effort to reduce frequency
			  — low sodium diet
			  — diuretic therapy
			Monitor correct use of vasodilators if prescribed to reduce formation of endolymph

Excess secretion of wax	Impacted cerumen due to narrowing of canal and dryness of skin	Pressure Tinnitus	Monitor aural hygiene Refer for removal of wax by irrigation
Diminished vibratory power	Decreased hearing acuity	Conductive deafness	Teach compensating communication techniques for hard of hearing and promote understanding of needs of elderly deaf clients amongst others

Nose, throat and tongue

General mucosal atrophy	Impaired sense of — smell — taste	Increased risk of — fire — gas poisoning — food poisoning	Advise on oral hygiene. Explain risks and work out safety measures with client
		Anorexia	Review diet and improve visual presentation of food whenever possible
Neural degeneration	Diminished cough and swallowing reflexes	Increased risk of aspiration or choking	Teach emergency measures in event of choking. Help client eliminate foodstuffs which create undue gagging or swallowing difficulties
Muscular in-elasticity	Alteration in the power, range and pitch of voice	Aphonia	Refer for general medical check. Encourage general muscular relaxation

Sensation and temperature control

Degenerative changes	Impaired awareness of — heat — pain — cold — touch — position and balance	Defective localisation of pain. Risk of burns, hypothermia and other accidents	Monitor sensory reactions via unobtrusive measures. Carry out regular checks of skin state to reduce risk of infection from unrecognised lesions, especially in existing neuropathies. Alert to risks of accident and hypothermia and check regularly on environmental temperature. Teach compensating balancing techniques

Skeletal
Bone

— porosity — demineralisation — reduced mass	Loss of strength. Brittleness	Fractures. Osteitis deformans. Osteo-malacia	Check diet and advise on adequate intakes of calcium and vitamin D. Reduce hazards in home and outer environment. Teach general safety measures and gait adaptation

Table 2.1 Contd.

System	Normal age changes	Pathological associations	Caring for clients: implications for health visitors
Osteoporosis	Calcification of cartilage Reduction in size of rib cage and in shoulder width Compression of body cavities	Increased bone pain and fragility Impaired respiratory, cardiac and digestive functions	Advise on posture and movement, especially lifting techniques Teach suitable breathing exercises and measures to reduce risk of respiratory infections Advise on modifying diet to facilitate digestion Encourage appropriate exercise to strengthen cardiac reserves Advise on suitable sleeping positions
Muscles Loss of bulk	Decreased power for muscular activities	Increased accident risks and greater fatigue	Safety measures Teach food-related exercise to improve stamina and strength. Avoid over-fatigue through balanced activity and sleep and rest
Atrophy of fibres	Less flexibility, poorer co-ordination, limitation in range and speed. Tremor	Personal and environmental accidents Myopathies	Teach muscle relaxation techniques Encourage full range of movement daily Re-arrange environment to improve safety and encourage use of modified equipment for clumsier handling
Joints Thickening of synovial membrane and cartilage degeneration	Loss of elasticity and resistance Aching and stiffness	Greater risk of trauma. Osteo-arthrosis, rheumatoid arthritis and gout	Encourage suitable posture and movement as well as a daily full range of exercises Monitor weight control and supervise prescribed drug regimes. Advise re dangers of self-medication Recognise potential threat to independence and take positive steps to increase diversional interests whilst maintaining optimum self-help

Cardiovascular			
Reduced elasticity in blood vessels	Increased systolic pressure	Aortic dilatation and incompetence. Hypertension	Support through waiting period and post-operatively if surgery is indicated. Teach correct use of aids and appliances if used. Encourage weight control, non-smoking and general relaxation, balanced by optimum physical exercise related to capacity
Increased deposits of lipofuscin — fibrous tissue — sclerosing	Decline in cardiac 'stroke volume'. Reduced capacity for physical work	Atheroma. Ischaemic heart disease and cerebral-vascular accidents	Encourage regular health checks and monitor blood pressure readings. Monitor compliance in, and reaction to all prescribed treatment, reporting as necessary. Supervise management and correct elimination. Inculcate a positive psychological outlook, especially towards any rehabilitative measures
Other vascular changes			
Reduced blood flow and vascular efficiency	Peripheral stasis with venous 'pooling'	Venous obstruction leading to varicose veins	Teach correct use of shoes and supportive hose. Encourage regular calf-muscle exercises. Compliance with prescribed therapy
Reduced tissue oxygenation	Dependency oedema	Tissue hypoxia. Gravitational ulcers	Caution against excessive sitting and prolonged standing, or sudden changes of position
Altered capillary permeability	Poor peripheral circulation	Risk of chilblains, thrombo-peripheral disease and orthostatic hypotension	Raise resistance to infection via good diet and sound hygiene measures with regulated exercise. Advise on suitable footwear and hosiery and how to keep warm in cold weather
Respiratory			
Alteration in size and number of alveoli	Decreased vital capacity	Lowered efficiency. Increased risk of infection	Maintain optimum but regulated activity. Encourage sound ventilation. Encourage to stop or reduce smoking and control weight. Maintain optimum nutrition

Table 2.1 Contd.

System	Normal age changes	Pathological associations	Caring for clients: implications for health visitors
Sclerosing of bronchi and degeneration of mucosa Reduced muscle power	Impaired tissue oxygenation and self-cleansing mechanisms Decreased reserves	Chronic obstructive disease	Strengthen muscles of respiration through suitable exercises. Teach appropriate posture and measures to facilitate expectoration Maintain general health through sound personal hygiene, adequate sleep and diet designed to increase resistance to infection
Cell alteration	Increased risk of 'wild' cells	Neoplastic disease	General ameliorative care and psycho-spiritual support Pre and post-operative care when surgery is undertaken
Digestive and excretory Jaw atrophy and tooth changes	Altered bite, worse if wearing ill-fitting dentures	Jaw pain Dental caries and periodontal disease	Teach sound oral hygiene and checck denture fit if applicable
Waning muscle power leading to altered mouth shape	Mastication problems	Restricted diet leading to malnutrition Oral ulcers and stomatitis	Advise on modifications to diet which preserve nutritional elements but facilitate mastication Maintain oral hygiene Monitor adherence to prescribed regimes if therapy given
Reduced swallowing reflex and thickened saliva	Sensitivity in swallowing Dry mouth	Parotitis Dysphagia Reflux	Check diet and oral hygiene Ensure adequate fluid intake Advise on sucking ice or using sugarless chewing gum Monitor drug therapy which may contribute to mouth dryness

Reduced oesophageal motility	Choking tendencies	Hiatus hernia Oesophageal cancer	Teach correct positioning and movement and offer symptomatic care as indicated
Atrophy of mucosa and reduced enzyme action	Decreased digestion of fat, vitamins and iron	Malabsorption syndrome Iron deficiency anaemia. Peptic ulcer	Monitor energy levels. Reduce fat and increase fibre content of diet. Encourage social eating. Supervise remedial therapy. Maintain exercise and general relaxation techniques
Liver Decreased weight and impaired efficiency	Decreased detoxification ability	Nausea and lethargy Drug accumulation and toxicity	Advise ameliorative measures and increase glucose fluids Modify activity Ensure adequate nutrition, modifying fat intake Monitor drug actions and reactions and report same
Elimination Prolonged intestinal transit time	Slowed peristalsis Constipation Formation of diverticula	Faecal impaction Diverticulitis Increased risk of colonic cancer	Ensure adequate bulk in diet Encourage regularity of meals and adequate fluid intake Supervise management of remedial regimes
Poorer colonic and sphincter tone	Reduced bowel control	Greater risk of faecal incontinence	Teach remedial pelvic exercises and the avoidance of injurious laxatives. Advise on personal hygiene measures
Genito-urinary Membranous thickening Impaired filtration Lowered renal blood flow	Limited renal efficiency Lower specific gravity Stasis	Lessened homeostasis Electrolyte imbalance Greater risk of — infection — calculi — prostatic disease in males	Encourage high fluid intake — at least 2000 ml daily Modify salt intake and check diet Promote perianal hygiene to prevent infection Monitor compliance with any prescribed regime for urinary infection, or diuretic therapy Check to avoid potassium depletion

Table 2.1 Contd.

System	Normal age changes	Pathological associations	Caring for clients: implications for health visitors
Reduced muscle tone in bladder wall	Frequency, nocturia and stress incontinence	Frank incontinence	Provide bladder training related to circadian rhythms and encourage pelvic floor exercises to improve tone Modify environment to promote continence and advise on suitable aids if required Teach appropriate skin protective care and deodorant measures where necessary.
Sexual functioning Alterations in hormonal levels	Females: labia and clitoris shrink and ovaries atrophy Fertility ceases	Irritation after coitus with dyspareunia Increased risk of cystitis	Advise on modifying sexual techniques Use of lubricating cream Vulval toileting, use of non-occlusive hosiery, avoidance of potentially irritating substances such as bath foam, and care when taking hot baths Encourage sound nutrition and high fluid intake
	Males: genital organs decrease in size and elasticity Seminal fluid and sperm production diminish, but fertility is retained	Scrotal irritation Prostatic enlargement with risk of urinary retention.	Advise on suitable scrotal support and use of protective cream Refer for medical aid: support client during pre and post operative phase where applicable Offer symptomatic advice and reassurance during period of readjustment
Endocrine functioning Reduction in levels of activity Increased catabolism	Modified fat distribution	Increased auto-immune responses	Monitor metabolic responsiveness Encourage weight and dietary controls Raise general resistance

Nervous system			
Reduction in levels of nerve activity	Slowed reaction time	Poorer co-ordination	Adjust pace of interaction. Allow time for sensori-motor responses
Reduced brain weight and blood flow	Poorer cerebral oxygenation	Vertigo and transient ischaemia. Stroke	Teach suitable posture and movement, avoiding rapid changes of position, especially from horizontal to vertical state
Some neurones lost. Fibres and impulses degenerate leading to weaker reflexes	Reduced proprioceptive ability	Confusion. Increase liability to falls	Teach gait adaptation and improve environment to facilitate safe locomotion. Reinforce safety education. Monitor rehabilitation after accidents
Neuro-chemical changes	Impaired thermal control with diminished shivering	Liability to burns, cold and other injury. Misleading presentation of symptoms	Protect against extremes of temperature. Observe closely for any disregarded symptoms

which health visitors are commonly confronted. Whilst the physical aspects of ageing are deliberately emphasised in this example, it is essential to recognise the inter-dependence of the physical, psychological, social and spiritual facets of a person's personality. This close and inseparable relationship between all parts of a 'whole' person and the environment are illustrated in the case study that concludes Chapter 3.

Case study

Alice, who is 79, lives with her 62-year-old son. Measuring 1.4 m in height and weighing 31 kg, she epitomises the title of 'little old lady '. However, her seeming frailty belies her vitality. Her marked loss of height often causes her distress, as she can now no longer easily see out of her kitchen window to watch the birds in her garden; cannot reach her larder shelves without difficulty and has to resort to ingenious ways of obtaining jars and tins via butterfly nets and similar means; and must have a cushion on her chair to allow her to reach the dining-room table. This causes her to feel childish, and increases her frustration, but she jokes away her sense of shame by amplifying the ridiculous.

Her formerly glossy black hair is now silver-white and thinning, but is still well-styled and groomed. Her skin is dry, wrinkling and pigmented in places, with laughter lines apparent at the corner of her eyes and over her rosy cheeks. At times she says she is plagued by pruritus, which she attributes to the drying effects of her central heating, but she is aware of the wise use of moisturising lotion and applies her make-up with discretion and to good effect.

She bemoans the loss of the speed and dexterity which she formerly enjoyed. The sequel to a fractured wrist is poorer fine movement and painful arthritis. She is ataxic at times, being prone to fall. Although she still manages to do most of her own housework and cooking, and has a washing machine for her laundry, she frequently experiences fatigue and so indulges in short naps whenever she relaxes. In spite of well-fitting dentures she often complains of sore gums and an ulcerated mouth. Her mastication problems, due to waning power in her masseter muscles, tend to restrict her menu choices, so she goes for softer-textured food, although still retaining a strong liking for steak and kidney pie. Alas, she often finds this aggravates her hiatus hernia and causes her great discomfort.

Since cataract surgery 5 years ago, Alice has some difficulty coping with stereoscopic vision, and has some diplopia. She thus frequently fails to see surface dust, wash plates cleanly, or cope with objects immediately under her feet. These instances thus sometimes cause her social embarrassment and distress.

Although her appetite is small, she eats regularly, preparing meals for her son who is not yet retired. Since she can no longer manage the walk into town, and is too unsteady to cope with buses, she must shop at the small neighbourhood shops, where choice is limited and the prices often higher. As her son is unskilled and has little income, they cannot afford a car. Alice, however, is very content. She prefers a routine life and still rises at 7 a.m. and retires by 10.30 p.m. Frequently she sleeps in the upright sitting position to afford her greater comfort, but she is a light sleeper and often spends hours awake, thinking of the past, and wondering about the future. She appreciates the use of a commode at night, and experiences some stress incontinence by day, which did cause her some social embarrassment, but now she wears protective clothing and copes well.

Alice is very clothes conscious, but has difficulty finding smart suitable garments which cater for her small size, high waist, sloping shoulders, mild kyphosis, and yet allow sufficient room for a rather disproportionately large abdomen to be accomodated comfortably. Her mild hypertension and osteoarthritis are controlled by drug therapy, and she benefits greatly from regular chiropody. In spite of a recent episode of thrombophlebitis and occasional bouts of bronchitis, Alice considers she enjoys good health. Marked hearing loss caused her to seek advice, but she rarely uses the prescribed aid, since it hurts her ear, and reflects background noise, of which she is very intolerant. In consequence her son is provoked and often frustrated by their difficulties in communication.

Alice manages to bath herself, with minimal assistance to reduce accidents; she also follows body exercises on breakfast television programmes. Although fine motor movement is less sensitive, she still crochets, knits, sews and cooks for her family, her church and the many friends she still has. Sadly her network of contemporaries is narrowing through death, and she often reminds visitors that she is the sole survivor of her nine siblings. Her days are full, nights 'tolerable'; as she says, she has learned to know and respect her body over the years and considers it has served her well.

REFERENCES

Adams G F 1981 Essentials of geriatic medicine. Oxford Medical Publications, Oxford
Butler R N, Lewis M I 1976 The later years: a guide to sexual and emotional adjustment. Sun Books, Melbourne
Comfort A 1977 To be continued. In: Barry J R, Wingrove G, (eds) Let's learn about ageing. John Wiley, Chichester, p 99–110
Davis A J 1981 Ethical issues in gerontological nursing. In: Copp L A (ed) Care of the aging. Churchill Livingstone, Edinburgh, p 38–45
Hayflick L 1976 The cell biology of human ageing. New England Journal of Medicine 295: 1302–1308
Kent S 1976 Why do we grow old? Geriatrics 31(2): 135–136
Masters W H, Johnson V E 1970 Human sexual inadequacy. Little Brown, Boston
Sacher G A 1977 Life table modifications and life prolongation. In: Finch C E, Hayflick L (eds) Handbook of the biology of ageing. Van Nostrand Reinhold, New York
Shaw M W 1984 (ed) The challenge of ageing. Churchill Livingstone, Melbourne p 14–15, 29
Skeet M 1983 Protecting the health of the elderly. Public Health in Europe No 8. WHO, Copenhagen
Steffl B M 1978 Sexuality and ageing: implications for nurses and other helping professions. The Ethel Percy Andrews Gerontology Centre, University of Southern California, quoted in Ebersole P, Hess P 1981 Towards healthy ageing. Mosby, St Louis, p 323–341
Walford R L 1981 Immuno-regulatory systems in ageing. In: Danon D, Shock N W, (eds) Ageing: a challenge to science and society, Vol 1, Biology. Oxford University Press, Oxford
Wood N F 1979 Human sexuality in health and illness. Mosby, St Louis

FURTHER READING

Danon D, Shock N W (eds) 1981 Ageing: a challenge to science and society, vol 1. Biology. Oxford University Press, Oxford
Wilcock G K, Gray J A M, Pritchard P M M 1982 Geriatric problems in general practice. Oxford Medical Publications, Oxford.

3

Psycho-social and spiritual aspects of ageing

The study of the biological aspects of ageing, with its evidence of decline and loss, may induce a sense of bleakness about old age. Not so, however, when we come to study the psycho-social and spiritual aspects, for although some faculties may wane, current studies show that later maturity has the potential to be a time of enrichment and development (Fig. 3.1). One recurring theme throughout recent literature on the elderly is the continuity of growth and the process of adaptation, although the risk of maladaptation is present as for any age group. Integrating experiences and reflecting on them can move one forward to greater understanding, but

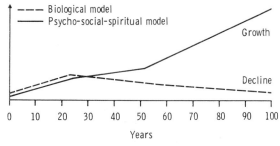

Fig. 3.1 Comparison of biological and psycho-social-spiritual models of ageing.

it is important to appreciate that for older as well as for younger people, full living requires a present orientation, 'an appreciation both of being and becoming' (Ebersole & Hess 1981).

As in the biological realm, there is a great variation in the rate and manifestations of ageing in psycho-social and spiritual planes. This is partly because every old person is constitutionally unque, with potential still present which can be maximised, and partly because the force of different life-events, and the availability of solutions, produce highly individual responses. For these reasons health visitors need to be flexible in their approaches and to apply their interventions creatively, in order to meet the different needs of older people.

THEORIES OF PSYCHO-SOCIAL AGEING

Theories attempt to explain and predict events and behaviour met with in practice. However, the psycho-social theories of ageing are at present as debatable as the biological ones, so an eclectic approach is probably preferable.

Psychological theories

Psycho-analytic theories

Freud was one of the first theorists to consider the components of personality development. He postulated that developments in later life depend on processes in childhood, hence his emphasis on sound psychological management in the early years. His contemporary, Jung, who stressed the varied developmental patterns shown by introverts and extroverts, asserted the importance of the last half of life in its own right. Defining its purpose as inner discovery through reflective activity, he thought that those who search for personal meaning and the spiritual self are less likely to experience restlessness or disorientation in old age.

Erikson (1963) introduced epigenetic theory, based on Freudian dynamics. He described the life-span as having eight specific developmental phases, each with developmental tasks to be achieved. The last stage he considered was a vantage point, from which one could view one's life, with either integrity or despair. He stressed that good health, sound socio-economic circumstances, regular and satisfying social contacts, and the presence of at least one reference figure, could assist people in achieving integrity.

Peck (1968) also stressed the need for the establishment of ego-integrity, but believed that to achieve this persons must let go of their occupational identity, rise above any bodily discomforts, and perceive meaning in their experiences. Such ideas have been criticised as failing to appreciate that not all people have the capacity to rise above their circumstances.

Humanistic theories

Buhler (1964) carried out considerable research in this field and identified three types of developmental progress, which eventually affect those in later life:

1. development dominated by bio-physical performance
2. development concerned with achievement and production
3. development characterised by contemplative activity.

Each of these stages is important to the full rounding of the personality. Stage 3 may be considered to have particular relevance to the old.

Continuity theory

This is one of the most recent postulations which emphasises the complex interrelationships between the biological, psychological and social influences which make for change or stability in individuals. It stresses the importance of the continuing nature of skills, preferences and experiences, as components of successful ageing (Ruff 1982). Health visitors should, therefore, look at their clients in terms not only of their present, but also of their past. Building on skills and experiences and helping clients to select from their repertoire, in order to solve problems in the here and now, is a technique of value with older people.

Sociological theories

Disengagement theory

This theory was propounded by Cumming & Henry (1961). They developed their ideas, following a 5-year study of 275 fit, financially secure old people aged 50–90, living in Kansas City, USA. They contended that as individuals age they relinquish certain roles, either on their own initiative, or through pressures from society. Inevitably and universally, mutual withdrawal or disengagement occurs between ageing persons and the social systems to which they belong. This disengagement varies within groups, paving the way for the ultimate withdrawal — death. Societies retract because of the need for continuity, with younger persons filling the roles vacated by older persons, whilst ageing individuals retreat because of awareness of diminishing capacities. Problems arise if societies force withdrawal when individuals are not ready for such disengagement. However, the authors of this theory did concede that whilst disengagement might take place in one area of life, re-engagement was possible within new settings and using new skills. Testing of this theory has led to contradictory findings; the major criticisms are that it is over-simplistic, assumes inevitability, fails to take account of differing personality factors, leads to damaging restrictions, and disregards the many older people who do not disengage, and thereby thrive.

Further research by Cumming, after several years, led to the amendment of some of her earlier views. She acknowledges the effect of individual differences, although she found disengagement was more likely to occur early in those who customarily react to stress by turning inwards and insulating themselves from society (Cumming 1975). Present consensus seems to support disengagement as just one of several life-styles which are manifest in later maturity (Crandall 1980). Health visitors, cognizant of this theory, would recognise the right of individuals who wish to disengage, and would support them, whilst discouraging blatant withdrawal and consequent social isolation.

Activity theory

Maddox (1963), Havighurst (1968), Neugarten (1972) and

Bromley (1976) are the major advocates of this theory, which is the opposite of disengagement. It asserts that older people institute compensatory activities to offset role loss, narrowing of their social radius and threats to their self-esteem. By developing alternative role options and maintaining an active lifestyle, they sustain their morale and well-being. However, merely busying oneself with meaningless activities is not thought to contribute to adjustment. Both longitudinal and cross-cultural studies have shown a positive, although not incontrovertible, association between personal adjustment, morale and activity levels in later maturity.

Sub-culture theory

Rose (1965) proposed that the elderly increasingly live within the context of an aged sub-culture; thus they interact within a group composed of persons of the same age or social background. Sharing similar interests, values and friendships, they tend to develop strong group identity, which may then be linked to recreational or political activity. Status is conferred by good physical and/or mental health, as well as by levels of social activity. Examples of this phenomenon are multipurpose senior citizens clubs, or holiday schemes for the over-60s. Harris (1983) discusses the advantages and disadvantages of such peer groups, comparing them somewhat unfavourably with the extension of social relationships which can be brought about by associational participation on grounds other than age.

Social exchange theory

Under this idea successful ageing is perceived as involving a rebalancing of exchange relationships. The theory assumes that individuals offer certain inputs to society, in order to gain certain rewards. The level of social interaction is determined by the benefits received, in relation to the costs involved. However, with less influence over their environment, together with shrinking social networks, older people have fewer commodities with which to bargain. In consequence some assert that they use compliance as a means of winning support and acceptance from others. An example of social exchange theory in action is seen where older people have been used as sources of local history for school children. The children are then encouraged to contact seniors and ask them questions relating to their earlier life. Tape-recordings of such interviews enhance the children's learning, whilst the older people are able to barter their knowledge and experience in exchange for increased social contact and prestige-rating. Possibly at present society undervalues its older citizens and does not exploit this theory sufficiently.

Social breakdown theory

Linked to the notion of social exchange, the proponents of social breakdown theory systematically underline the inter-dependence between older people and their social world. They argue that older persons affected by unfamiliar circum-stances, role loss or dramatic changes in lifestyle reach out for clues to guide their reactions. However, this act of reaching out for help is regarded as evidence of their incom-petence. Concern is then generated in those around them, which gives negative feedback to the seniors. In turn they, somewhat bewildered, adopt the negative characteristics ascribed to them, thus deepening their dependent status. Kuypers & Bengston (1973) thus describe this process as the 'social break-down cycle in old age'. The theory has much in common with the concept of 'labelling', which has been seen to apply to other age groups. Enabling persons to function competently within more structured environments and emphasising their personal strengths can help to replace the cycle of breakdown with one of reconstruction.

Age stratification theory

This theory is based on the belief that all societies arrange themselves in age strata, with rights and obligations linked to the social roles considered to be appropriate to each age band. The matching role-behaviours are, however, influenced by a number of factors. One major interpreting force is thought to be the unique social conditions with which history presents each biological cohort. Prevailing social and econ-omic conditions produce overriding values, which dominate outlook and shape social roles. Thus behaviour is related to socio-historic context.

Riley et al (1972) liken their theory to persons stepping on to an escalator at birth and moving up in a collective, though not an identical, fashion. Various external factors influence their ride, and determine the manner and point at which they get off. However, as successive cohorts move up, they alter the conditions to such a degree, that subsequent cohorts *never* experience the same ride. Thus the general reaction towards ageing of those now aged 85 years, in our society, might be expected to be different from those now aged 60 years. This is because they grew up before the First World War, when the work ethic predominated and the welfare state did not exist. Their thinking was often dominated by fear of 'the workhouse', and their reactions led to values of thrift, self-sufficiency, and mutual aid. Similarly the reactions of those who grew up in the affluent 1960s might be expected to differ considerably, when they become old, from those of people who experienced the grinding poverty that accompanied the economic depression in the 1930s.

What is the practical consequence of these various theories for health visitors? Clearly it is important for them to recognise individual differences in the motivations and personality characteristics of older people. They will also need to take account of socio-historic contexts and interpret behaviour in the light of these. Health visitors must encourage older people to identify and make the best use of their abilities, take up new activities, keep their minds active and foster their independence. They should support and utilise peer-group activities but also encourage older people to associate with other age groups, and should encourage communities to recognise and utilise the contribution which the wide-ranging skills of their senior members can offer. In addition practitioners should press for improved social and educational provisions to be made for older people, which will enable them to continue to develop and participate.

PSYCHOLOGICAL ASPECTS OF AGEING

Distinct from the theories of ageing, which are at times

tentative and debatable, the psychological and social aspects of ageing have been relatively well documented. The components of psychological ageing are both cognitive and emotional. Cognitive elements include intelligence, perception, memory, reasoning; the capacity to assess, analyse and interpret situations, to process, store, recall and utilise information, to orientate oneself in time and space, to respond to stimuli, and to organise complex data. As with biological ageing, chronological age is a poor indicator of cognitive state. Some old people are alert, mentally active and successfully hold down positions of great financial or political responsibility, whilst others become less able at a much earlier age.

Intelligence

Until recently, much of the research indicated that maximal intellectual performance occurred about 30 years of age, those aged 60 years having three-quarters of the intellectual acuity of younger persons. However, the rate of deterioration varied, with those showing poorer intellectual performance in earlier life demonstrating greater decline than those with high IQs in childhood, given the absence of disease. Now, recent evidence suggests that the research methodology used, which was mainly cross-sectional studies, has impeded a proper understanding of the relationship between ageing and cognitive competence. Schaie (1975) using 'sequential designs', which involve a combination of cross-sectional and longitudinal studies, showed a very different trajectory for the course of intellectual development in later life. Consequently, he and his associates advocate the use of a 'plasticity model' for studying the relationship between chronological ageing and intellectual potential. He makes the point, already acknowledged with much younger age groups, that the growth of intelligence of an adult may have much to do with the complexity of his environment (Schaie 1975, Labouvie-Vief 1977).

A recent British study supports this view, finding that those elderly people who remain in good health and keep active may be just as efficient as young people in carrying out mental tasks (Huppert 1982). Those, therefore, who are mentally creative appear better able to cope with the cognitive effects of old age. This is a significar.t point for health visitors to note; already they are involved in encouraging young persons to be mentally active; now they have to apply thier energies to stimulating older people as well.

Intelligence is of particular importance for older people, to assist them in assessing, manipulating and organising their environment. Where measurable cognitive decline exists, there is a tendency to deal with the environment in non-intellectual ways. Experience and routine may compensate, but response patterns appear rigid, especially if there is an increasing sensory deficit. While spatial perception and decoding ability do decline with advancing age, intelligence decreases appear to be mostly associated with loneliness, isolation and poor social relations. Thus, encouraging older people to be involved with and accepted by others would seem to be a very worthwhile health visiting activity.

Reaction time does slow in later life, owing to diminished conduction time, alterations in the perceived strength of signals, or lower levels of interest and motivation. This is exacerbated in those suffering from cerebral ischaemia or depressive states. Speed is sacrificed to greater accuracy, but comprehension and verbal fluency are preserved into extreme old age, particularly amongst women. Although old people are less likely to develop new classifications, or find novel answers, they retain the capacity to solve problems. Creative works, such as compositions by Handel, Haydn, Verdi and Goethe, have been produced after the age of 70 years. Grandma Moses, the great American painter, is also a classic example of latent ability surfacing in old age.

Memory

Short-term memory is generally thought to be blunted in old age, though Craik (1977) disputes this. Some loss of brain cells in the hippocampal region, which is associated with memory, may account for this, although it may also be partly due to a lack of concentration, or limited interest in recent events. How far long-term memory is affected in later life is a controversial issue, with research producing some contra-dictory findings (Hultsch 1977, Labouvie-Vief 1980, Zelinski et al 1979).

Learning

Contrary to popular belief, older persons do continue to learn and to respond to new situations, given time and motivation. This indicates the value of educational opportunity at all stages of the life-span.

> If our ultimate aims are to increase the quality of life in the later years, and to eradicate our negative social construction of ageing, then we must seek to make learning as visible an avocation of older people, as gardening or grandparenting, currently are. This goal will never be real-ised if education continues to be defined in terms which are irrelevant to the vast majority of older people.
>
> Allman (1983)

Whilst Allman's comments indicate that highly academic learning may not, necessarily, be appropriate for all older people, it is worth noting that older students on Open University Courses are getting better academic results than younger students (Sunday Telegraph 30.12.84). There is also a considerable response to the activities of the University of the Third Age (address given in Appendix 6).

There are, however, hints in the research literature that fear of failure, or lessened concern with success, may inhibit learning responses in some older people. Material given must therefore, be relevant, strong and logical; it should be presented in well-defined stages, and with opportunity for spaced repetition. Most of all older people should be encour-aged to discuss it freely and relate it to their own experience. These features are significant for health visitors, because of their involvement with health education for the elderly (Strehlow 1983).

Exercising judgment and making decisions about their lives are also crucial activities for the elderly. Thus all that is already known about these complex mental activities can be related to people in later life. Nevertheless, it must be recog-nised that impairment from organic brain syndrome is not uncommon, and can affect memory, comprehension, judg-ment, orientation and affect. Functional disorders arising from loss, bereavement, and/or social isolation may lead to apparent cognitive deterioration, which is usually reversible. Thus, as with biological ageing, it is important to distinguish pathology from the inevitable developmental changes. In this way what can be prevented, treated, possibly reversed, or at least controlled and ameliorated, can be identified.

EMOTIONAL ASPECTS OF AGEING

The personality structure and characteristics displayed in earlier life become crucial to emotional well-being in later maturity. There is a tendency for individuals to become more what they are, i.e. their personality traits are exaggerated. Sound self-esteem in earlier years, together with well-practised coping strategies, can help individuals to weather the stresses of ageing. Positive influences include a realistic appreciation of body-image changes; identification with various groups; and unobtrusive support from family, friends, lay and professional carers. Adaptive mechanisms frequently used to counteract the anxieties and frustration accompanying bodily limitation include rationalisation and over-compensation. Many old people use denial selectively, as in a certain disregard of disabilities or depriving circumstances. Some level of regression may be helpful in enabling a senior to tolerate increasing dependency. Sublimation may sometimes be used to enable older persons to channel their energies into socially acceptable activities, sometimes being experienced through younger people. Some seniors cultivate detachment whilst others convert their emotional reactions into physical symptoms — somatisation.

Learning to accept altered goals, reduced levels of activity and increasing dependency, whilst maintaining self-identity and ego-integrity, is a formidable task, comparable to the developmental tasks which must be accomplished in earlier years, and to which we direct so much attention. Thus older people, too, require all the understanding and help that can be given them. However, because of their role-relationships and the emotional reactions which these sometimes evoke, other people may be reluctant to offer seniors overt support. Like all other groups, the emotional reactions of older people will differ between them, but recognising that there is a general tendency towards greater lability will help health visitors to offer empathic, objective care. It may be necessary to fill many different roles towards them: such as interpreter, teacher, confidante, enabler or advocate. A willingness to listen, realistically re-assure, comfort and/or activate, can assist older persons and their carers and families to make the necessary adjustments.

SOCIAL ASPECTS OF AGEING

As we have already seen, ageing, to a certain extent, is socio-culturally determined. Although there are some universal institutions and values, there may be considerable variation in conventions and customs associated with growing old. In a pluralist society ethnic minority groups may show very diverse reactions towards ageing. Elderly migrants may be particularly lonely and isolated, especially when there are language barriers. A key element in deciding whether ageing can be termed successful is the interaction between the individual and his or her environment, and several recent studies emphasise the threats to self-identity and adapative behaviour which can arise from unsuitable, intrusive, demanding or limiting environments (Lawton 1980). Levels of interaction are frequently affected by states of health, and there is evidence to show that ethnic minority groups, particularly West Indians and Asians, are disadvantaged as far as enjoyment of good health is concerned (Blakemore 1982; 1983). Additionally housing conditions may be poor and transport lacking, or there may be unfavourable comparisons between expectations and realities of care (Pyke-Lees & Gardiner 1974; AFFOR 1981). It is necessary for health visitors to discover the social norms and values of the different ethnic and cultural groups in their communities, in order to adapt their approach to such older people. For example Blacher (1983) points out the particular needs of elderly vagrants, whilst Hennessey (1976) and Alford (1978) highlight the discrimination and difficulties sometimes attending the affluent elderly.

The social aspects of ageing also involve families and significant others, so health visitors may sometimes find there are three or even four generations to consider. Not infrequently late middle-aged persons may have two sets of ageing parents to care for, to say nothing of the possibility of other elderly relatives. Recognising and helping to meet the needs of each generation, therefore, becomes an integral part of each health visitor's work in social ageing. This is where the identified function of the health visitor as a 'family visitor' is so relevant, and where the belief in continuity of care has such application.

MORAL AND SPIRITUAL ASPECTS OF AGEING

Just as people develop and change in other dimensions with ageing, so they do morally and spiritually. The older person may cling even more firmly to personal values and principles discovered through life-experiences, particularly if their biophysical or psycho-social world is shifting. Although spirituality is not necessarily synonymous with religious observance, many elderly people derive considerable strength and comfort from identification with a church group. They are also often helped by following through the practices and rituals of their specific religious body.

Assessment over a period of time will enable a health visitor to determine the level of spiritual interest displayed by an ageing person, so that liaison with appropriate carers can be made. Recognising the value of prayer, meditation and worship, and accepting one's own spiritual needs, will help health visitors to see that the spiritual needs of elderly people are met in personally satisfying ways. It will also help to ensure that prescribed regimes do not infringe client beliefs. Coleman & Coleman (1983) point out that spiritual care widens the definition of caring, since it introduces the concept of love into what may be a technical service. Thus the work of the professional carer, in enabling non-professional carers to function more effectively, may help to introduce that spiritual quality which is the vital ingredient in caring.

SUMMARY

This chapter had as its focus the psychological, social and

spiritual aspects of ageing and stressed the important influence of culture and environment, while the biological aspects of ageing were the subject of Chapter 2. However, the separation of the different aspects of ageing is at best artificial and undesirable and at worst, dangerous. In real-life situations they are inextricably linked and influence each other and must be respected accordingly. The following case study is intended to demonstrate this close inter-relationship, as it often presents itself.

Case study

Martha is 90 years old and still enjoying life to the full. Her personal history has spanned the later years of the industrial revolution, to the space age. She has learned to adapt from an era of gas lamps to one of micro-technology, and as she works in her kitchen or listens to her transistor radio, her seamed face and gnarled hands tell their own story. She regularly surprises her visitors by her quick insights, fund of anecdotes, rich humour and remarkable perspective. The oldest of seven children, she knew poverty and deprivation in a Scottish city in her childhood and, impelled by the need to help support her family, emigrated to the USA before she was 20.

No stranger to hard work, she quickly found a job, although she passed through a difficult time when tuberculosis was diagnosed and she required treatment. Her fiancé was killed in the First World War and subsequently she never married. Her social status as a domestic servant, though valued at a personal level, never allowed her to become affluent. However, habits of thrift and frugality, and a strong sense of filial duty, enabled her to provide on a postal basis for the care of her ageing parents during the economic depression of the 1930s.

Returning to Britain for the first time after the Second World War, to care for a recently widowed brother, she faced a culture from which she had grown away. The subsequent death of four of her siblings, and the years she spent caring for a brother with an organic brain syndrome, added to her personal stresses. She lost weight and became grossly fatigued, but her strong faith in God, and the belief that she must solve her own problems without undue reliance on others, have carried her through these various vicissitudes.

It is 5 years since she was reluctantly transferred to sheltered accommodation, as her general frailty rendered her highly vulnerable. However, she takes a fierce pride in her personal and domestic independence, and has only accepted limited home help since becoming a nonogenarian. She has been partially sighted since cataract surgery 6 years ago, and her environmental excursions and social networks have contracted with lowered mobility and the loss of many of her contemporaries. Nevertheless she is an avid television viewer and reads as much as her vision permits. Not for her the peer group activities of an over-60s club, or senior citizens' centre, although she acknowledges the benefits they may provide for others. She has strong views on life, is self-contained, monitors her own health assiduously and is often intolerant of weakness in others. Her dry, often philosophical manner endears her to her relatives and friends, who admire the fortitude with which she has coped with major abdominal surgery and the sequelae of a 'stroke'.

Which theory of ageing best applies in her case? Her biological decline is apparent in almost every system — is her 'biological clock' running down? Age stratification theory might seem to explain her interpretation of social roles, rights, responsibilities and behaviour. She 'knows her place', but is fiercely determined to remain in control. Does she demonstrate activity theory as she keeps abreast of current affairs, and pushes her frail body to the limits in managing her home? Or does disengagement theory explain her ability to tolerate social restriction and apparent community withdrawal? Genetic and environmental influences have played their part in enabling Martha to face old age with dignity, humour and equanimity.

Nevertheless she remains assertive, inquisitive and tenacious. She has seemingly accomplished the developmental tasks outlined by Erikson and Peck, achieving integrity. Like Jung, she has searched for meaning in her life and this belief and sense of purpose now sustain her. At times her psychological outlook is dominated by her biological needs, but mostly she over-rides such frailty, considering it 'weakness to give way'. She derives much comfort from the regular weekly visits from her minister, and from taking communion. She shares her wisdom with those who care to listen, yet never assumes that she has a monopoly on this commodity. In the matter of daily living Martha triumphs, and to that extent she transcends all theories.

REFERENCES

All Faiths for One Race (AFFOR) 1981 Elders of the Minority Ethnic Groups. AFFOR, Lozells, Birmingham

Alford D 1978 The affluent elderly: problems in nursing care. Journal of Gerontological Nursing 4 (44) March/April

Allman P 1983 The potential for learning in later life. In: Jerome D (ed) Ageing in modern society. Croom Helm, Beckenham, Kent, p 168–187

Blacher M 1983 Elderly vagrants. In: Jerome D (ed) Ageing in modern society. Croom Helm, Beckenham, Kent, p 61–80

Blakemore K 1982 Health and illness amongst the elderly of minority ethnic groups, living in Birmingham. Health Trends 14(2): 69–72

Blakemore K 1983 Ageing in the inner city: a comparison of old blacks and old whites. In: Jerome D (ed) Ageing in modern society. Croom Helm, Beckenham, Kent, p 81–103

Bromley D B 1976 Research in social and behavioural gerontology. in: Research in gerontology: problems and prospects. British Council for Ageing, London

Buhler C 1964 The human course of life: its goal aspects. Journal of Humanistic Psychology 4:1

Coleman P, Coleman M 1983 Spiritual care. In: Clark J, Henderson J (eds) Community health. Churchill Livingstone, Edinburgh, p 56–64

Craik F I M 1977 Age differences in human memory. In: Birren J E, Schaie K W (eds) Handbook of the psychology of ageing. Van Nostrand Reinhold, New York

Crandall R C 1980 Gerontology: a behavioural science approach. Readings. Addison Wesley, Massachusetts

Cumming E, Henry W 1961 Growing old: the process of disengagement. Basic Books, New York

Cumming E 1975 Engagement with an old theory. Ageing and Human Development vi (3): 187–91

Ebersole P, Hess P 1981 Towards healthy aging. Mosby, St Louis, p 527–530

Erikson E 1963 Childhood and society, 2nd edn. W. W Norton, New York

Harris C 1983 Associational participation in old age. In: Jerome D (ed) Ageing in modern society. Croom Helm, Beckenham, Kent

Havighurst R J 1968 Personality and patterns of aging. The Gerontologist 8: 20–23

Hennessey M J 1976 Group work with the economically independent aged. In: Burnside I (ed) Nursing and the aged. McGraw-Hill, New York

Hultsch D F 1977 Changing perspectives on basic research in adult learning and memory. Educational Gerontology 2: 367–382

Huppert F 1982 Does mental function decline with age? Geriatric Medicine January: 32–37

Jung C 1971 The stages of life. In: Campbell J (ed) The portable Jung. (Translated by Hull R F C), Viking Press, New York

Kuypers J A, Bengston V L 1973 Social breakdown and competence: a model of normal ageing. Human Development 16: 181–201

Labouvie-Vief G 1977 Adult cognitive development: in search of alternative interpretations. Merill-Palmer Quarterly

Labouvie-Vief G 1980 Adaptive dimensions of adult cognition. In: Datan, Lohman (eds) Transitions of ageing. Academic Press, London

Lawton M P 1980 Environment and ageing. Brooks/Cole, Monterey, California

Maddox G L A 1963 A longitudinal study of selected elderly subjects. Activity and morale. Social Forces 42: 195–204

Neugarten B L 1972 Personality and the ageing process. The Gerontologist 12: 9–15

Peck R 1968 Psychological developments in the second half of life. In: Neugarten B (ed) Middle-age and ageing. University of Chicago Press, Chicago

Pyke-Lees S, Gardiner S 1974 Elderly ethnic minorities. Age Concern, Mitcham

Riley M W, Johnson M, Foner A 1972 A sociology of age stratification. Ageing and Society 3:9

Rose A M 1965 The subcultures of the ageing. In: Rose A M, Peterson W A (eds) Older people and their social world. F A Davis, Philadelphia

Ruff C 1982 Successful ageing: a developmental approach. The Gerontologist 21: 209–214

Schaie K W 1975 Age changes in adult intelligence. In: Woodruff D S, Birren J E (eds) Ageing: Scientific perspectives and social issues. Van Nostrand, New York, p 111–127

Schaie L W 1976 Quasi-experimental research designs in the psychology of ageing. Van Nostrand, New York

Strehlow M S 1983 Education for health. Lippincott Nursing Series. Harper and Row, Cambridge

Zelinski E, Gilewski M J, Thompson L W 1979 Do laboratory tests relate to self-assessment of memory ability in the young and the old? In: Poon L W, Fozard J L, Cermak L et al (eds) New directions in memory and ageing. Laurence Erlbaum, New Jersey

FURTHER READING

Jerome D (ed) 1983 Ageing in modern society. Croom Helm, Kent

4

Health visiting and the elderly client

Health visitor students often raise questions about the care of persons in later life. Two such questions which frequently provoke animated discussion are:

What can health visiting offer older people?
Does such health visiting care differ from that offered to persons in other age groups; if so, how?

The issues that lie behind these questions are complex, since they are concerned with defining a specific and possibly unique contribution to care on the one hand, yet raise ethical points about discrimination on grounds of age on the other. Many students recognise, also, that what health visiting can offer seniors depends on a blend of factors, not all of which lie within professional jurisdiction. Thus care is influenced, not only by practitioner competence, but by the timing of the intervention, the expectation of clients, their particular needs and circumstances, and the policies of employing authorities. Some students and practitioners argue strongly that the particular developmental needs arising from the process of ageing, justify a modification of practice with the elderly. This stance is reinforced by those who feel that recognising differences, and exercising more positive discrimination in favour of vulnerable groups, allows resources to be concentrated on those in greatest need. A counter-view, however, is that labelling any group as 'different' increases the risk of stigma, in this case ageism. Furthermore, others claim that as the strength of health visiting lies in its universal application, selectivity undermines the essence of the service.

Whilst each of these viewpoints is relevant, answers to the questions posed above, can only be found if we examine what health visiting is, what it seeks to be, and what it aims to achieve, and then, through a comprehensive research programme, evaluate whether it attains its goals. In this chapter we can only concern ourselves with the intent of the professional activity, and so we will discuss the matter under the following headings:

- the nature of health visiting
- the nature of the professional commitment
- the nature of the professional relationship.

This approach is adopted as a prelude to Chapter 5 in which the frameworks and processes of health visiting care are considered.

THE NATURE OF HEALTH VISITING

> The nature of any human service is constantly challenged and changed by the goals of the social mileu in which it operates, and by the varying capabilities and commitments of those who provide the service.
> Freeman & Heinrich 1981

Clearly health visiting is no exception, since some of its distinctive features have arisen from earlier stages of professional development, having been moulded by the social and political influences then prevailing. Other characteristics stem from current definitions of the service, which not only indicate reality, but contain idealised elements, representing the service not only as it *is* but what and how practitioners perceive it or intend it to be. This is a significant point when considering the care of the elderly, because the health visiting role with this age group is currently underdeveloped.

Features of early health visiting practice

Traditional features indicate that early health visiting aimed to stimulate self-respect and personal-social responsibility, through education, encouragement and participation. As agents of social change, the early practitioners offered an unsolicited, non-coercive and non-stigmatising service, and these characteristics still mark present day practice. Such features appear relevant to the care of older people, who need to maintain their dignity, as well as their self-care and independence for as long as possible.

Offering an unsolicited service means that health visitors do not necessarily depend on referral before contacting potential clients; they can actively seek out those who need preventive or remedial help and proffer this. Such action is particularly useful for seniors who are less likely to seek help in the early stages of need, perhaps because they do not recognise the significance, or the severity of symptoms. Sometimes older people are less articulate than younger ones; they may lack awareness of sources of help, have greater difficulty contacting services, or have a cultural tradition of self-sufficiency and tolerance of circumstances, even when these are adverse, yet remediable. However, proffering an unsought service could be considered an intrusive action, so some elderly people may regard it as an invasion of privacy. This calls for great tact and sensitivity when making initial contact. Visiting by appointment, inviting older clients to express their views on the type of health care they require and respecting their idiosyncrasies, are ways of recognising rights and upholding dignity. However this nurturing of tenuous relationships until clients are ready and able to utilise care is not confined to the elderly (Robinson 1982).

Balancing the offer of an unsolicited, yet comprehensive service must be the assurance that it is non-coercive. Whilst most older people recognise this and therefore welcome health visiting contact, a few sometimes regard practitioners as representatives of a threatening bureaucracy, causing them to react negatively to overtures of care. Such reactions may be heightened if seniors are striving to retain independence in the face of fast-declining capacity. Care is therefore needed to ensure that the health visiting role is presented as enabling and non-authoritarian, with emphasis on client self-determination.

Because health visiting operates on a universal basis, without qualification of need, it is usually perceived by clients as non-stigmatising. However, Luker (1982) found a small number of elderly women who were *not* helped by health visiting intervention, because they regarded the service as 'intended for the ailing, the lonely or the disabled'. Consequently, when they became the focus of health visiting attention, they felt demoralised and their coping skills were undermined. It is important to admit the relevance of such findings, as workers are frequently unaware of their clients' perceptions of care, or of the unintended consequences of intervention.

Contemporary characteristics of the service

The traditional features of health visiting are also complemented by more recent characteristics. Whereas earlier practitioners came from several differing backgrounds, including medicine, the Council for the Education and Training of Health Visitors, soon after its inception, stipulated nursing as an essential pre-requisite for entry to health visitor training (CETHV 1969). This means that, although many professional workers share the perceptual, relational, teaching, and planning skills which are used in practice, the particular combination derived from basic nursing, obstetric nursing, possibly additional post-registration nursing experience and the health visitor course, constitutes a unique blend (RCN 1972, 1983).

Another characteristic, stressed by the Health Visitors' Association, is the independent nature of the activity, since practitioners initiate most of their care (HVA 1970, 1980). This does not mean that health visitors do not accept referrals, neither does it mean that they operate a solo practice, without recourse to others. It does mean that as qualified practitioners they have the right to make their own judgments about health visiting needs, and to arrive at decisions about how best to meet these. Of course professional awareness, education, competence, attitudes and values will clearly affect such discretionary decisions, for which practitioners are then held accountable (RCN 1984). Additionally, client views will have been fully taken into account. The position of health visiting within the caring occupations also indicates another characteristic, namely inter-dependence, since it occupies the inter-face between medicine, nursing, education and social work. This position is reflected in the independent and inter-dependent nature of the health visitor, within the health and social services team.

The most recent definition of practice, which highlights the features of the service, was however made following an intra-disciplinary participative exercise, held to re-appraise health visiting principles. It is reproduced here in full, because it encapsulates much of what can be offered to clients.

> The professional practice of health visiting consists of planned activi-ties, aimed at the promotion of health and the prevention of ill-health. It thereby contributes substantially to individual and social wellbeing by focusing attention at various times on either an individual, a social group, or a community. It has three unique functions:
>
> 1. Identifying and fulfilling self-declared and recognised, as well as unacknowledged and unrecognised, health needs of individuals and groups.
> 2. Providing a generalist health service in an era of increasing special-isation in the health care available to individuals and communities.
> 3. Contributing to the fulfilment of these needs and facilitating appro-priate care and service, by other professional groups.
>
> CETHV 1977

Similarities in this and other world-wide definitions of community health nursing can be noted (RCN 1983).

In addition to the definition, four reformulated principles were agreed, which predict and guide health visiting practice. Each of these has an application to the elderly client:

- the search for health needs
- the stimulation of awareness of health needs
- the influence on policies affecting health
- the facilitation of health-enhancing activities.

From the definition and the associated principles, certain characteristics can be extrapolated, which indicate what the professional practice of health visiting might represent for elderly people. These characteristics are embodied within:

planned activities
multi-focused practice
comprehensive, co-ordinating and facilitating service.

Planned activities

The health visiting service for the elderly is, as for other age groups, designed to be systematic and purposive, rather than random or reactive. Thus desirably it is seen as planned and continuing even when contact is intermittent. It operates on a long-term basis, from conception throughout life, on the premise that all activities designed to promote health and prevent ill-health in earlier years contribute to a healthier old age. Given opportunity it is intensified at periods of greater vulnerability, and most particularly would direct its attention to those in middle-age, where its educative thrust can enable people to control those behaviour-patterns and environmental hazards which build up problems for later life. It uses logical processes, identified conceptual frameworks and models of care, and aims to:

— maximise independence
— promote optimum well-being within the limits of ageing
— improve the quality of life
— assist in the achievement of a dignified and peaceful death.

Multi-focused practice

To be effective health visiting must also be multi-focused, operating at individual, group and community levels. This means practitioners are not only interested in caring for individual elderly persons, their families and the many groups in which seniors share experiences, but must also consider the general population, particularly the aggregate of elderly people within their area. This enables an epidemiological perspective to be adopted. For example, health visitors may find, through astute observation and scrutiny of statistics and patterns of consultation, that a certain segment of the elderly population appears exceptionally fit. Further study may show an association with behaviour patterns, calling for deeper investigation so that all may benefit. Such rigorous assessment of the status of the elderly within the community, which utilises the search principle, can equally well discover deprivation, disease, poverty, loneliness, contentment or fulfilment, and is an essential prelude to informing the community

about their elderly members, so that more imaginative participation can improve care. Unless clear statements about local
needs and progress are regularly made to the public, attitudes
towards, and policies about, the care of older people are
unlikely to change. Resources can often be wasted on low-
priority schemes, whilst more pressing elements are
neglected through ignorance. Through stimulating awareness
of the health needs of the elderly and influencing policies
affecting them, health visitors can help to enhance health.
However, such action calls for skilled, sophisticated
communication techniques. There is much scope for development in this sphere.

Comprehensive, co-ordinating and facilitating service

The health visiting service for the elderly should also be seen
as comprehensive, co-ordinating and facilitating. Because of
its generalist nature across all age groups, and within a variety
of settings, practitioners adopt a holistic approach and are
well placed to note family and community interrelationships,
observing the multifactorial influences which operate on
elderly clients. When they become aware of functional disability amongst old people they have a duty to make comprehensive assessment and report this to those who can give
remedial care. Similarly when health visitors, observe the
effects of prescribed regimes upon older clients and their
families, they have a responsibility to discuss outcomes with
those prescribing care. Beneficial effects confirm specialists
in their decision-making: detrimental effects can probably be
altered. This interpreting role is often necessary with older
clients, who may be too nervous or overawed to tell 'experts'
that they are not benefiting from their treatment. Of course
such advocacy, which is integral to the nature of health
visiting, calls for both courage and humility on the part of
practitioners.

Co-ordinating care becomes a particular challenge when
older persons, with their multi-pathology, receive multi-
specialist care. Discovering the ramifications of such care, and
maintaining contact with all the agencies involved, can be
very time-consuming, but is necessary to reduce the risk of
fragmented or depersonalising service. Elderly people often

become confused, anxious or frustrated about prescribed treatments and therefore, may require help to decipher prescribed programmes, or to understand multiple drug therapy. The educational nature of health visiting means that practitioners can offer such help. They can also contribute to discussion on ethical prescribing for the elderly; make prompt referral of elderly people to other workers whenever their special skills are needed, thus reducing avoidably deteriorating situations; and participate in case conferences. Other co-ordinating activities include attending intra- and inter-disciplinary meetings, consultations, and the provision of informative, succinct reports.

One aspect of facilitating activity lies in building up clients' confidence in the care they are receiving from other workers. The following example involving an elderly person demonstrates this.

Case study
An elderly widower was receiving care from a district dietician, as part treatment for his diabetes. When visited by the health visitor he expressed some anxiety about the inclusion in his diet of items he found unpalatable. He was assured the dietician would welcome a discussion. Contact was arranged and the client received a modified programme, which enabled him to comply with therapy and enjoy his meals, aware that his wishes were considered important.

Contributive, facilitating aspects are also shown when health visitors work with students from different disciplines. During field work practice they can help students identify the needs of old people and of their families, differentiate the roles of other workers, and correctly select agencies for referral. Teaching follow-up care of the elderly, and encouraging students to liaise with other workers, can foster respect for the respective roles and hence enhance multi-disciplinary care.

An example of the inter-linking of some of these features of health visiting was noted by a student who accompanied a health visitor to the family of a young baby, where the elderly grandparent was visiting, following partial recovery from a 'stroke'. Having reached a plateau in rehabilitative progress, this elderly woman was somewhat disheartened. Aware that her district nursing colleague was visiting, and having already discussed goals of care with her, the health visitor was able to reinforce the exercise programme instituted for this client. As she emphasised the many successful results such care by her colleague had produced for other similar clients, the student observed that even this small positive comment acted as a fillip for the family, probably enhancing their confidence and increasing their perseverance.

Thus the role of health visitors with elderly clients can be seen to be multi-faceted and dynamic. However, although these are the features which demonstrate the nature of the activity, the extent to which practice may reflect the ideals of the service varies considerably. Extraneous factors may foster or constrain development. Such influences include the pattern of health needs presented by the elderly in any particular locality. The type and extent of health visitor education, the number and types of other workers with the elderly, and the scope, format and aims of their care, as well as their expectations of, and attitudes towards, health visiting all produce modifications. The size of the available health visiting work force, the organisational and administrative settings which they work, and the national and local policies concerning the elderly also affect development. Likewise public expectations of, and attitudes towards, health visiting care of the elderly, and their financial and moral support of this, can develop or hamper care.

These factors suggest a political dimension to the health visiting role. It is no longer sufficient, if indeed it ever was, for health visitors to concern themselves only with the provision of a personalised service to clients and their carers, important though this is. Research has to be initiated to identify more fully the health visiting needs of the elderly and the most efficient and effective ways of meeting these. Role expectations and perceptions have to be tested against actual performance; consumers' views have to be sought. At times of fierce competition for scarce resources, claims for shares have to be justified. This requires health visitors to increase their own professional monitoring; to develop assertiveness in arguing their case; to stimulate public interest in, and recognition of their role with the elderly; and to improve their own education and training which fits them for such care. These activities are all embodied in the professional commitment.

THE NATURE OF THE PROFESSIONAL COMMITMENT

Chapman (1980), in discussing the rights and responsibilities of nurses and patients, emphasised the reciprocal nature of their contract. However in health visiting the elderly, practitioners may pledge themselves to offer safe and competent service, but the extent to which clients can fulfil their side of the contract by co-operating in care actions is likely to vary considerably. Although practitioners believe in the principle of client self-determination, so that each client exercises the right to decide what shall be done to help him and how such care shall be carried out, the client's cognitive impairment may prevent this being fully implemented. Action may sometimes have to be taken for the client's own (or others') safety. Workers then may have to accept a greater share of decision-making about care and may, therefore, be cast sometimes in the role of social control agents. Such situations increase the need for ethical and prudent behaviour, emphasising the importance of full consultation and collaboration with families, colleagues and nursing managers. However, it may be necessary sometimes to champion the client's rights in the face of other opinions. Elderly clients are frequently very vulnerable and often need a skilled advocate. Hasty decisions should not be made, and all aspects should be fully examined before confronting such issues.

Professional confidence

Studying the foregoing, and examining the many reports which advocate increasing health visiting involvement with the elderly, may lead students to consider the work highly demanding, consequently questioning their own readiness for such tasks. This is a mature and thoughtful response, injecting realism and showing awareness of accountability.

Professional confidence stems from professional ability.

This in turn rests on an adequate professional education, the acquisition and maintenance of a valid knowledge base, appropriate values and a repertoire of professional skills. Helpful steps have already been taken by the United Kingdom Central Council for Nurses, Midwives and Health Visitors, under Statutory Instrument No. 873, (1983) sections 18 to 24, to state rules concerning the competencies which are to be achieved at Registration, and moves are afoot to ensure continuing education. However, professional ability means more than professional competence; it includes being able to wield matching resources such as equipment, space, information, time, and access. In this way care is more likely to be commensurate with professional knowledge. This issue is well argued by Bergman (1981).

The ability of health visitors to care adequately for the old rests largely on their capacity to be aware of and have access to *all* the elderly persons within their practice population. Only in this way can they identify those most vulnerable. However, such action means using an administrative device, broad enough for representative measurement, yet sharp enough to detect susceptibility. In the case of young children this need has been recognised; it was met through the notification and registration of births. There is, at present, no such system for discovering the elderly, and indeed the issue of instituting one is highly debatable. Health visitors are therefore, forced to find alternative measures, since to rely solely on referral would be to negate the universalistic and preventive nature of their work. These alternatives include the use of age-sex registers, vulnerability indices and/or computerised records of practice populations. There are few devices for those working on a geographic basis, other than the electoral roll, which does not indicate age. However, even for those working within general practice settings, it is estimated that fewer than 40% have access to age-sex registers and less than 10% have the use of cross-referencing systems, which would increase efficiency and reduce frustration. Moreover, the provision of these vital tools lies outside health visiting jurisdiction.

There are also other examples of under-resourcing which affect the ability of health visitors adequately to care for elderly people. These include inadequate supplies of equipment for simple clinical assessment; lack of specific screening apparatus; insufficient space in which to conduct health advisory clinics; a paucity of tests for determining levels of dependence; and difficulties in obtaining comprehensive statistical data from which to compile health profiles. Furthermore, deficits in supportive social services can often render detection of need and referral for help meaningless. Another factor concerns low staff ratios to population, so that within busy generic work loads there are insufficient health visitors to meet the not inconsiderable needs of older people.

Part of the professional task is to point out such deficits and to call for remedial action. This may be particularly difficult at times of economic recession and financial stringency. Sometimes in the past practitioners may have accepted such under-resourcing as almost inevitable, and may not have pressed firmly enough for redress. It is now clear that such behaviour constitutes a violation of the professional commitment, and does gross disservice to elderly people. These points are now being aired by the profession (RCN 1984).

Professional responsibility

In addition to professional confidence and ability, health visitors also have professional responsibility. This is defined as 'a mandate or charge; a trust, for which if accepted one becomes answerable' (Batey & Lewis 1982a).

Responsibility as a charge should not be confused with 'being responsible' which is a personal attribute which all professional practitioners should demonstrate. Responsibility for the care of the elderly can only be accorded when practitioners have recognised the content and implications of the charges being assigned them, and have signified their willingness to accept these. Sometimes health visitors have accepted roles and functions assigned to them, without necessarily questioning whether these fell legitimately within their professional province or not, or if they had the ability adequately to fulfil them. Now there is a growing realisation that it is not a negation of the spirit of vocation to submit roles and functions to the 'reality test', since neither clients nor communities can benefit, and may even be harmed, if duties assigned are accepted and then cannot be fulfilled.

Moreover, effective responsibility requires authority, whether this derived from the power of position, knowledge or the situation (Batey & Lewis 1982b). Responsibility without authority undermines professional autonomy and creates great frustration, as many health visitors ruefully realise when they find themselves powerless to implement assignments. An incident, all too common, illustrates this:

Case study
Miss T., aged 70 years and severely arthritic, was sent home late one Friday afternoon from the local casualty department, having been treated for a fractured right wrist, and severe bruising of shoulders and legs. Follow-up care was requested and the health visitor asked to assess and to mobilise services.

Miss T., lived alone, and clearly was only marginally independent. Domestic assistance and facilitating aids were required, in addition to nursing care. This last was quickly arranged, but authority to provide assistance and aids is vested in another department (the Local Authority Social Services Department), and because of timing, help could not be obtained immediately. Miss T. had thus to depend on the goodwill and services of neighbours, until alternative arrangements could be made several days later.

Although such community help is to be encouraged, it is not always available, or appropriate.

Accountability: meanings and measurement

Another facet of the professional commitment concerns accountability. There are several definitions, including those of Bergman (1981), Batey & Lewis (1982a), and the RCN (1984). The one used here is given by Murray & Zentner (1975):

> Accountability is being responsible for one's own acts and being able to explain, define, or measure in some way, the results of one's own decision-making.

Accountability thus includes notions of purpose, disclosure, justification, evaluation and reckoning. It refers to acts of commission (what *is* done) and to acts of omission (what is *not* done). It may be direct or indirect. However, it should be appreciated that if accountability is delegated, this does *not* constitute abdication of responsibility.

Accountability is multiple. In health visiting the elderly, while the primary focus is towards the client, account must also be rendered to other carers, to peers, to employing authorities and eventually to society at large. Self-accountability is also important. Nevertheless, whilst practitioners may pledge themselves to provide safe, efficient care for seniors, it must be appreciated that this must also be seen to be done. Unlike hospital settings however, where work is mainly publicly observed, the interactions between older clients and health visitors are often conducted in the privacy of homes, and thus are mostly unobserved. Under such circumstances, therefore, accountability can only be indirectly demonstrated, and this is done mainly through the record of the visit. This raises many issues, including the authenticity of records; practitioner integrity, objectivity and perceptual ability; standards of confidentiality; and comparability of records. Consequently the comprehensiveness and the availability of health visiting records are central to accountability. For this reason records should contain a written declaration of the purpose of each visit, and the views of both client and worker should be recorded, concerning aims, objectives, plans and outcomes of care. If this is to be achieved it follows that the written record should be shared with the client and, where appropriate, client-carers as well. Only in this way will misconceptions about care be reduced. For this reason many health visitors find the application of the health visiting process provides a systematic way of ensuring that problems, goals, action and evaluation are shared activities (see Ch. 5). For some others, however, the idea of sharing records with clients is still innovative. Some practitioners are uncertain about implementing such an idea, possibly because they fear the negative aspects of accountability, and the risk of managerial censure, sanctions or control.

At present most health visiting records for the elderly contain biographic data; medical and social history; brief details of personal and situational progress; and a practitioner assessment. Process recordings of action taken, and details of interactions, subjective perceptions and evaluations, are less common. This could prove a serious drawback to health visitors, if the system of professional peer review were to be implemented. If a small group of independent professional peers, checking retrospectively for evidence of quality of care, had insufficient data on which to base their evaluations, inadequate or false judgments might be made. For these reasons an urgent review of record format, storage and retrieval facilities, and the time required for correct documentation, is needed, in order to protect both practitioners and elderly clients. Meanwhile health visitors need to give careful attention to the way they explain, disclose and report their actions and outcomes of care, as such safeguards may be even more important when dealing with older people, who are so often over-tolerant and may be uncritical of their care, or who may at times experience distortion of reality.

THE NATURE OF THE PROFESSIONAL RELATIONSHIP

Closely linked to the professional commitment is the quality of the professional relationship. This is one of the most sensitive aspects of the care of the elderly. Through such a relationship clients present their needs and expectations, and practitioners demonstrate their knowledge, skills and attitudes. By exchanging information, ideas and feelings both parties can learn and develop. Such a relationship, however, depends on the extent to which both persons feel comfortable within it, can trust each other, act freely and show respect for each other. In order to achieve this, honesty, integrity and reliability must prevail.

Older people come to these relationships with a different, and sometimes much wider, frame of reference than practitioners. By virtue of their age they have long histories, clear identities, and much life experience. They will have filled many different roles, encountered various status transitions and developed different coping strategies which they can bring to bear on current situations. Some of their attitudes towards old age will have derived from their perceptions of it in others. However, their experiential learning will depend on their circumstances, their personality attributes, cognitive abilities, physical and mental health and the rate and form of their ageing. Sometimes, therefore, seniors may be interested, tolerant, upset or puzzled about their state; they may also possibly show marked differences in their reactions between the 'young elderly' and 'the very old'.

Not all seniors grow old gracefully. Some become cantankerous, hostile or aggressive; others may be dejected, apathetic or confused. Some may project their feelings on to practitioners. Whilst most are likely to show indomitable spirit, and having spent many years developing independence, will be reluctant to lose it, a few may become over-dependent. Many will have developed a philosophical manner and often marked humour. They may frequently indulge in gentle teasing or use jokes to ease their tension, increase rapport, test out practitioners, or demarcate the boundaries of the relationship. Recognising the value of humour and using it to motivate clients is, therefore, an important health visiting technique.

Ethnic and cultural influences also affect seniors' behaviour and can explain the sometimes strong reactions they show to others' dress, speech or manner. Recognising and allowing for these differences, and addressing older people in terms which afford them dignity and take account of their value-system, are, therefore, essential courtesies.

At times in the professional-client relationship, older persons· may associate workers with authority-figures from their past, and this may sometimes evoke reactions which appear incongruent in present circumstances. Conversely they may sometimes identify with the parental or grandparental role, regarding practitioners as 'children' and becoming over-solicitous, over-protective, or even dominating in their manner towards them. Being aware of this phenomenon of transference can help health visitors to deal with any emotional reactions from clients which seem inappropriate, or to use the mechanism to help propel older clients towards mutually desired goals.

Another point is that sometimes older people feel they 'should have all the answers' because they have lived so long. In such circumstances they may feel ashamed to reveal their needs, admit weaknesses or ask for help. They may then display bravado, or adopt such stances as 'what can you teach me?' Such a response can prove disconcerting, especially to inexperienced health visitors. Under such circumstances it is helpful to realise that it is the professional knowledge, derived from education and experience, which enables workers to contribute effectively. Occasionally older clients react by listening politely and concurring with all suggestions, only to ignore them afterwards! When this happens health visitors need to search for relevance in what they are recommending, since this is the key to motivation. However, most older people are outgoing and co-operative, eager to relate and appreciative of help given; they, therefore, bring very positive contributions to the relationship and can teach practitioners much.

Nevertheless, the relationship is not one-sided. Like clients, practitioners are also constrained by personality attributes, life experiences and attitudes. Their frames of reference, drawn from personal and professional life, may clash with those of clients, thus creating potential misunderstanding. Sometimes health visitors unconsciously react to older clients to the basis of former relationships with their own parents or grandparents. They then demonstrate counter-transference. One student found that she was virtually unable to implement professional-type care, because she cast herself into the role of a 'daughter' to an elderly client. Prior awareness of these risks can help practitioners guard against them, but if such situations do arise they should be discussed with a senior professional in order to allow effective work to continue with the client.

Occasionally anger or fear may enter into the relationship because workers have not resolved their own reactions to ageing, or they may have difficulty handling the dependency-independency conflicts which clients sometimes demonstrate. If practitioners have hitherto regarded all seniors as 'near-omnipotent beings', they may sometimes experience revulsion at the helplessness of frail old people. Additionally there may sometimes be over-attachment to, or over-possessiveness of, older clients, especially if they have appealing attributes. Recognising the gamut of possible reactions evoked in work with the elderly can enable health visitors to develop the disciplined and objective approach needed to care effectively, and to maintain professional rather than social relationships. It is noteworthy that most practitioners experience great pleasure when working with seniors and gain much from them.

The basic ingredients of professional relationships between clients and practitioners include acceptance, empathy and purposeful communication. These apply equally to contact with all age groups.

Acceptance

Although sometimes used rather glibly, conveying an impression of resignation or weakness, acceptance is in fact a very active concept, meaning a ready acknowledgement of client uniqueness and worth. It does *not* mean agreeing with inappropriate behaviour, but it does include the belief that elderly clients have the right to continuing professional attention, regardless of their behaviour. It includes responding to older persons in a positive and non-judgmental manner, without either altering one's own standards, or imposing these on others. Not everyone is easy to accept. Nevertheless, reaching out to older clients, even when they show negative reactions, can enable practitioners to gain insight into the reasons for their behaviour. Caring for clients is thus displayed through the sustaining of helping contact with the less attractive, as well as with gracious and responsive seniors.

Case study

One of the many interesting examples of acceptance was demonstrated by a student assigned to study the care of Miss E., aged 79 years and a former nursing sister, now partially disabled after a cerebrovascular accident. The client lived alone in a ground-floor flat, and her querulous and demanding manner had alienated many of her neighbours and most of her relatives, so that she became isolated and depressed. The health visitor student initiated and maintained an openness of contact, refusing to be daunted by the client's carping comments. Focusing on their shared experiences, the student elicited accounts about the client's rigorous nursing training, which helped her to understand Miss E.'s high expectations, and explained some of her exacting behaviour. Over several weeks the student led the client on to express and explore some of her fears about total dependency, and to discuss the hurt she had experienced, when her image of herself as 'one in command' had been forced to change to 'one needing help from others'. Frequently Miss E., reverted to acid comment; often she compared her own treatment unfavourably with the care she felt she had given to others. At times she abruptly terminated visits, or scorned suggested interventions. Each time the student pointed out the inappropriateness of such behaviour, but maintained the open relationship, until the client, somewhat grudgingly at first, allowed her to mobilise much needed services. Eventually a small cadre of caring workers were able to assist Miss E. to maintain optimal functioning, within her own home and within the limitations of her own lifestyle.

Empathy

Empathy is the ability to see the problems and needs of others, as it were through their eyes, in order to appreciate their attitudes and reactions. It differs from sympathy, in that objectivity is retained, in order to offer non-emotive help. Because older people are often the victims of pity or sympathy, they look to professional practitioners to offer them deeper understanding and more practical help. Practitioners display their empathy through the medium of verbal and/or non-verbal communication, and in the marshalling of resources to meet need.

Empathy can be developed, provided that workers have warm, flexible personalities; the capacity for imaginative thought; perceptual and social skills; and a readiness to listen. Interpretation and insight can also be fostered, especially if practitioners maintain sound physical, mental and emotional health and can control their personal stresses and free themselves from undue anxiety and negative emotions, which distort perception.

Communication

Communication forms an essential part of all health visiting. It requires special skills and has been studied and discussed by many researchers and several practitioners, including (Raymond 1983). In the care of the elderly, however, communication is not only particularly important, it is also extremely complex. It is important because it is a vital ingredient in maintaining relationships, thus enabling mutual understanding to be developed between elderly clients, practitioners and others, and also because it serves to prevent the client's social isolation and affords scope for client participation. It is through communication that assessment can be made, goals be mutually determined and plans developed.

Nevertheless it is complex because communication in the elderly is often hampered by sensory or neural deficits which result from the ageing process. For example, there is generally slower word-association and word-retrieval with age; greater dysfluencies, more frequent interjections, word repetitions and dysrhythmic phonations. In addition, presbycussis (auditory deterioration associated with ageing) leads to some loss of acuity, especially for higher-pitched tones; consequently older people have more difficulty in hearing women's and children's voices, and may miss certain consonants. Furthermore some 60% or more of older persons have specific hearing impairments, whilst the majority of those with visual disabilities are also elderly. Thus, whilst all the rules for successful communication on verbal and non-verbal levels apply equally to the elderly client, special attention must be given to those seniors who experience sensory deprivation, speech impairments (whether arising from 'stroke' or other neurological disorders), perceptual difficulties, or disturbances of affect, such as depression or emotional illness. Suspicious elderly clients, or those who are non-English speaking, also need particular care. Deliberate techniques may have to be selected to meet specific problems, and liaison with speech therapists is then strongly advised.

When dealing with elderly clients from ethnic minorities, or differing cultural groups, it is helpful to try to gain some understanding of the more common languages met with in practice, if only to greet seniors correctly. Appreciation of dialect and vocabulary is also important, as the latter, whether expansive or restricted, is always rich in meaning.

Because of these various factors which affect communication, some modifications in technique are necessary with the elderly. Whenever possible contact should be made in a quiet environment, with few auditory or visual distractions. Health visitors should sit reasonably near to, and facing, clients, in a good light to facilitate lip-reading if necessary. Sometimes it may be helpful to kneel beside less mobile or handicapped older people. Enunciation should be distinct, with rate slightly slower, pitch rather lower and volume rather stronger than for younger people, although shouting and elaborate speech mechanisms should be avoided.

Whilst 'leading' is a technique frequently adopted by health visitors, it must be used selectively with the elderly. Closed-ended questions, which are used to elicit specific data, usually of a factual nature, can often give old people an impression of catechisation, so should be introduced with care. Whilst open-ended questions are usually preferable, since they promote understanding and help communication flow, they can lead to irrelevancies, clouding of original issues, or confusion.

A useful tabulated list of techniques, modified for use with elderly clients, is given by Leitch & Tinker (1978). A summary of important helping functions for communication-disordered elderly people is given by Ebersole & Hess (1981). Perhaps closing conversations may be the most difficult part of communicating with the elderly, especially if clients are lonely and seek attention. When time is limited it may be helpful to indicate in an unhurried way at the outset of the conversation, just how much time can be given. Time must of course be allowed for the establishment of rapport, and scope for clients to present their needs and to feel they have practitioners' full attention. When interaction is drawing to a close, this should be indicated by a re-capping of salient points, with an accompanying written account of decisions made, goals set and plans agreed being left to facilitate comprehension and explain actions. One helpful maxim often quoted concerning communication is that professional workers should be noted for their large ears, wide eyes and small mouths! (Schulman 1974, Beaver 1983).

SUMMARY

This chapter began with two questions, one concerning what health visiting could offer the elderly, the other regarding what differences, if any, such care might involve. By exploring the nature of the professional activity, and examining the early and later characteristics of health visiting, together with its principles, values and goals, some inferences have been drawn about the forms and the directions of care. There are, however, many issues about the nature of the service which demand further discussion. The professional commitment was examined, because the service which health visitors can render elderly persons rests on practitioner ability, responsibility, accountability and sense of vocation. The professional relationship has been discussed in some depth because it constitutes the medium through which care is given, although principles rather than great detail have been emphasised.

That there are differences sometimes in the way health visitors offer care to older clients, compared with other age groups, has been indicated, but these have been seen to be related to individual differences, specific developmental needs, levels of functional ability and client uniqueness. Throughout the discussion the thrust has been towards stimulating thought about what underlies health visiting care for any age group, but chiefly, in this context, for older people. Whilst existing work with the elderly appears considerably under-rehearsed, it is our contention that health visiting has much to offer the elderly client, providing practitioners resolve some of their equivocalness and given that essential resources are forthcoming to allow professional claims to be demonstrated.

REFERENCES

Batey M V, Lewis F M 1982a Clarifying autonomy and accountability in Nursing Service. Part I. The Journal of Nursing Administration Sept: 13–18
Batey M V, Lewis F M 1982b Clarifying autonomy and accountability in Nursing Service. Part II. The Journal of Nursing Administration, Sept: 10–15

Beaver M L 1983 Human Service practice with the elderly. Prentice Hall, Englewood Cliffs, New Jersey, p 175

Bergman R 1981 Accountability: definition and dimensions. International Nursing Review 28(2): 53–59

Chapman C M 1980 The rights and responsibilities of nurses and patients. Journal of Advanced Nursing 5: 127–136

Council for the Education and Training of Health Visitors 1969 Fourth Report. CETHV, London

Council for the Education and Training of health Visitors 1977 An investigation into the principles of health visiting. CETHV, London

Ebersole P, Hess P 1981 Towards healthy ageing. Mosby, St Louis, p 199–226

Freeman R B, Heinrich J C 1981 Community health nursing practice, 2nd edn. W B Saunders, Philadelphia, p 36

Health Visitor Association 1970 Health visiting manifesto. HVA, London

Health Visitor Association 1980 Health visiting in the 80s. HVA London

Leitch C, Tinker R 1978 Primary care. F A Davis, Philadelphia, p 475–480

Luker K 1982 Evaluating health visiting. RCN, London

Murray R B, Zentner J 1975 Nursing concepts for health promotion. Prentice Hall, Englewood Cliffs, p 123

Raymond E 1983 The skills of health visiting. In: Owen G (ed) Health visiting, 2nd edn. Bailliere Tindall, London, p 221–231

Robinson J 1982 An evaluation of health visiting. CETHV, London

Royal College of Nursing 1972 The role of the health visitor. RCN, London

Royal College of Nursing, Health Visitor Advisory Group, The Society of Primary Health Care Nursing 1983 Thinking about health visiting. RCN, London, p 11–29

Royal College of Nursing, Health Visitor Advisory Group, Society of Primary Health Care Nursing 1984 Further thinking about health visiting; accountability in health visiting. RCN, London

Schulman E D 1974 Intervention in human services. Mosby, St Louis

FURTHER READING

Helvie C O 1981 Community health nursing. Harper & Row, Philadelphia

Spradley B W 1982 Readings in community health nursing, 2nd edn. Little Brown, Boston, p 71–79

5

Frameworks, models and processes of health visiting care

Chapter 4 took as its theme what health visiting *is* and, therefore, what it can offer the elderly client. This chapter is about *how* health visiting the elderly may be carried out. It uses a conceptual approach, rather than a firm recipe for practice, on two main counts. Firstly, there are as many differing health visiting situations as there are clients; hence practitioners need to be flexible in their response. Understanding the ideas and principles which underlie practice helps health visitors to adapt and apply these to differing circumstances. Secondly, although health visiting is essentially a practical activity, its practitioners require a body of knowledge which is constantly reviewed and updated, as well as a range of skills and techniques, and appropriate attitudes, traits and values. Examining these components can help us to draw inferences about how this particular professional activity might be best demonstrated. If some points are considered unusual or controversial, they are offered in the hope that students and practising health visitors will be stimulated to explore them further.

KNOWLEDGE

Knowledge is acquired in two ways. The first way is to seek

out theories which are held by others, and then examine and apply these to one's own practice. A plumber, for example, does this when he uses the science of physics and the laws of hydrodynamics to enable him to repair a leaking pipe. This deductive technique was advocated in Chapters 2 and 3 on the ageing process, and is also the method used in much of health visitor education, where the syllabus is based on theories from many disciplines (see Appendix 2). This is a helpful approach, especially if such theories are constantly challenged, and if the deductions drawn for health visiting practice are regularly re-appraised and tested.

The second way of acquiring relevant knowledge is the method of inductive theory development. Events met with in practice are carefully observed, then defined, described and classified, before being used to generate hypotheses which can then be tested. Evaluating theories in this way means they are then firmly grounded in practice. Health visitors are increasingly employing this method, either by carrying out investigations themselves, or by studying other practitioners' work, and then testing out their ideas in practice (Clark 1983). Such action is a necessary process, because if health visiting is to establish itself as a scientifically credible and socially useful discipline, it must collectively identify and refine its concepts and test its theories and principles (CETHV 1977, 1979).

Concepts: the first stage in theory building

Some readers may wonder why a chapter about *how* the elderly may be cared for within health visiting practice should begin so theoretically. The answer is that the concepts, or global ideas or constructs, which workers hold largely determine how they operate. Therefore, concepts may be regarded as the first stage in theory building and such knowledge will eventually underpin practice.

Health visiting employs many complex concepts, but all too often they are taken for granted, being held and used implicitly, in the mistaken belief that everyone else understands and acknowledges them. Unfortunately, this belief can sometimes lead practitioners into conflict, because different meanings are attributed to words and ideas; therefore differing frameworks underlie care, causing variation in practice. Since practice rests on knowledge, theory development depends largely on making concepts explicit, and then analysing them. This is an issue stressed by many writers, including Dickoff & James (1968), McFarlane (1977), and Riehl & Roy (1983).

The concept of holistic care

Fundamental to the way health visitors relate to and care for elderly clients are the ideas and beliefs they hold about people. Believing that they are biological, psychological, social and spiritual beings, who live in matching environments, health visitors claim to adopt an integrated approach based on an assessment of the whole person. This has given rise to the concept of 'holistic care'. Of course this does not mean that health visitors regard themselves as responsible for the entire and sole care of clients, but rather that they see the client as the prime determiner of his, or her, needs, and workers as seeking to provide complementary help in order to meet these in each of these dimensions. Although the idea is sound, its implementation fully may sometimes be very difficult. Nevertheless practitioners strive towards this as part of their role as one of the major caring professions.

The concept of health

Another concept basic to health visiting care is the concept of health, since the aim of all practice is to promote optimum well-being. However, although most practitioners have strong ideas about what health means, a precise definition is difficult and concensus is lacking. Nevertheless the way health is perceived, and the way in which health visitors consider elderly persons to be healthy or not healthy, will affect the ways they deliver care. Thus the frameworks and models used for health visiting action rest upon fundamental beliefs.

Five different conceptions of health are now considered, each of them giving rise to particular models of care, which are relevant to health visiting practice with the elderly. These five conceptual ideas are:

health as the absence of disease
health as a positive state
health as a fluctuant experience
health as independence in living
health as adaptation.

Health as the absence of disease

Traditionally health was perceived as freedom from disease. Logically, therefore, the model of care which followed was the medical one. Using this framework, disease must first be identified and differentiated so that a diagnosis can be made. However, diagnosis rests upon knowing and recognising the unique course which each disease follows, and the specific signs and symptoms which are exhibited. For this reason a knowledge of aetio-pathology and the natural history of disease are important contributory factors. Once diagnosis has been correctly established, specific remedies can be applied, which hopefully will lead to cure or control. Thus treatment and follow-up, in order to determine outcome, are other neccessary components. Of course, where natural resistance or specific therapy are ineffective, deterioration and/or death may follow.

Like all nurses, health visitors are very familiar with this framework, since their basic nursing education currently rests largely on it, and the prescribed elements of their role frequently stem from it. Practitioners using this model can, therefore, engage in secondary prevention, acting on the assumption that if disease can be detected early, preferably at the pre-symptomatic stage, it may be more amenable to treatment. It is for this reason that screening and surveillance form part of health visiting functions with the elderly (see Ch. 6). Similarly, tertiary prevention can be justified, since by accepting referrals and carrying out follow-up to elderly people who are more prone to disease and disability, health visitors can help to ameliorate their effects. Applied to the community, this concept allows for an epidemiological approach to be adopted, aimed at identifying health and disease states in aggregates of elderly people, and the causal environmental influences and stressor agents which act upon older hosts. In this way health visitors can play a part in the control of community disease.

However, the limitation of the concept of health as an absence of disease is that it focuses on the pathological process, rather than on the person, and it is therefore, negative in approach. If health visitors were confined to this model of care only for their elderly clients, they would not undertake health promotion activities nor engage in primary prevention to any large extent, which would of course negate their professional values. Also they might feel less job satisfaction, since fewer older clients may achieve complete freedom from disease. For these reasons most health visitors adopt alternative frameworks on which to base their care, although they use this concept as an adjunct.

Health as a positive state

This framework, established by the World Health Organization, defines health as 'a state of physical, mental and social well-being not merely the absence of disease or infirmity'. This positive concept, therefore, lays emphasis on *potential* setting out total well-being as a goal to be aimed at. Thus health visitors using this developmental model direct their efforts not to finding out what is wrong, but rather to improving optimum performance in all three realms. Major activities are therefore, concerned with personal and community health education and development.

Maslow's hierarchy of needs model adopts a similar approach (Maslow 1962 — see Fig. 5.1) and Ebersole & Hess (1981) have usefully applied this model to the older client. Using this framework at the level of individual client care, efforts are first directed towards discovering and meeting basic biological and safety needs, so that attention can next be directed towards increasing client self-esteem, and thence self-realisation. Whilst such an approach has much to commend it, and many health visitors make use of the model (albeit implicitly), practitioners are often aware that it is much easier to identify and meet the clients' lower-order survival and safety needs, than it is to help older people feel loved, recognised, protected and fulfilled. Nevertheless it is in

Application of model to the needs of the older person

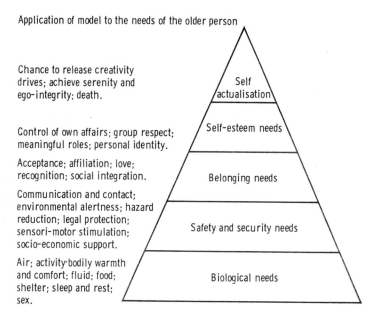

Chance to release creativity drives; achieve serenity and ego-integrity; death.

Self actualisation

Control of own affairs; group respect; meaningful roles; personal identity.

Self-esteem needs

Acceptance; affiliation; love; recognition; social integration.

Belonging needs

Communication and contact; environmental alertness; hazard reduction; legal protection; sensori-motor stimulation; socio-economic support.

Safety and security needs

Air; activity·bodily warmth and comfort; fluid; food; shelter; sleep and rest; sex.

Biological needs

Fig. 5.1 Maslow's pyramidal model of human needs (Maslow 1954, Ebersole & Hess 1981)

endeavouring to achieve these higher-order levels of well-being that the main challenge to high-quality health visiting care lies.

Health as a fluctuant experience

The positive state described above has been criticised by some as being somewhat unrealistic as it is hard to achieve and almost impossible to measure. One such critic, Dubos (1959), regards health as a mirage: not a state but rather a dynamic process, with the organism striving constantly against a changing environment, in an endeavour to achieve homeostasis. Dunn (1959) also took a somewhat similar approach, perceiving health as a fluctuant experience, rather than a constant state. As a result he depicted health as a continuum, ranging from high level wellness at one end, to imminent death at the other (Fig. 5.2). Individuals were then seen as occupying positions at different points between these two poles, depending on the degree of environmental threat they faced and their levels of personal resistance. This notion

The health-illness continuum

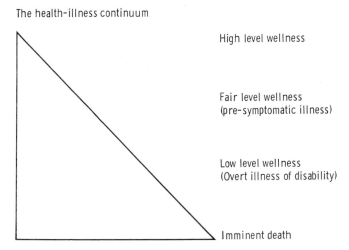

High level wellness

Fair level wellness
(pre-symptomatic illness)

Low level wellness
(Overt illness of disability)

Imminent death

Fig. 5.2 Health conceptualised as a fluctuant experience

of health status as differing from day to day is one which seems highly pertinent to the elderly, who so often have a tenuous grasp on well-being and may shift their hold very readily.

Health visitors who adopt this perspective would require to obtain data to enable them to estimate and plot the position of their elderly clients along such a health continuum. They could then determine the amount and direction of care needed to bring these older people as near as possible to high-level wellness. Hobson & Pemberton (1956) used a version of this model, when they coined the phrase 'effective health levels', to help them study functional ability in their sample of elderly people. 'Good effective health' they applied to those functionally independent elderly people who were maintaining reasonably high levels of well-being. 'Fair effective health' denoted those who were house-bound and somewhat functionally restricted, but were coping, in spite of medium-to-low levels of well-being. 'Poor effective health' was the term they used to describe those who were physically and mentally unwell and dependent.

Another example of the use of this concept of health, is shown by one general practitioner (Williams 1979). He used this modified version to help him categorise the elderly people in his practice. In this way he was able to identify some 4% as being at the lowest point on the health continuum, i.e. 'in poor effective health'. This enabled him to focus scarce medical resources more effectively. He then was able to identify the 36% whom he considered were in 'fair effective health'. Although they were coping they were in danger of being overwhelmed and thus slipping further down the health scale. Thus he considered they required more medical surveillance than the 60% whom he graded as being in 'good effective health'. Health visitors can learn much from these examples which use this notion of health as a continuum, with individuals fluctuating in their position on it. For instance it can cause them to think about devising criteria for recognising levels of well-being amongst their elderly clients, as a prelude to priority-setting. It can also remind them of the precarious balance some older people experience and therefore the need for constant vigilance. It is particularly useful for practitioners working in a team setting, where doctors and district nurses can direct their main efforts towards secondary and tertiary prevention and health visitors can concentrate on promoting and maintaining the health of the apparently well elderly.

Health as independence in living

Closely allied to the concept of health as a fluctuating experience is that of health as independence in living. The strength of this idea is that it focuses not so much on an individual's limitations, as on how well he can manage within these. Thus even those who are experiencing illness or disability are regarded as achieving some degree of health, commensurate with their levels of independence.

Roper, Logan & Tierney (1980, 1983) utilised this concept when they formulated their 'Activities of Living' model, which they designed specifically for nursing. They regard individuals as holistic beings who are constantly, actively and uniquely striving towards independence and self-fulfilment from conception to death. This independence is demonstrated through 12 common activities of living, which are shown in Figure 5.3. Thus under this model individuals are visualised as moving uni-directionally and inevitably along the life-span, whilst at the same time occupying fluctuating positions on a

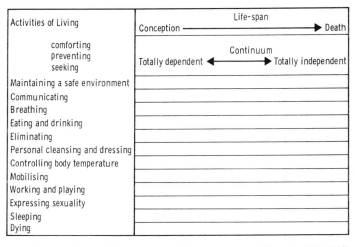

Fig. 5.3 The Activities of Living model (Roper, Logan & Tierney 1980, 1983)

parallel independence-dependence continuum (Fig. 5.3). At certain times, such as when people undergo developmental transitions like adolescence or retirement, or when illness or accidents occur, their independence is threatened and the level achieved may be altered.

Practitioners are, therefore, regarded as adopting an interventionist role. They may either assist people to retain their independence, by preventing or alleviating threats to their functioning, or they may help them to regain such independence if it is lost. Although this was primarily designed as a general nursing model one health visitor/researcher considers it well suited to the care of the elderly.

> It would provide a frame of reference which would make assessments or surveillance by health visitors meaningful, in giving quality of life for the elderly its due recognition.
>
> Luker, 1982a

An example of one way in which this model might be applied to the care of a very old client is given at the end of this chapter in Tables 5.1–5.3.

Health as adaptation to stress

This last concept perceives health as synonymous with adaptation. The theory, which is based on ideas propounded by

Selye (1956), postulates that throughout life individuals are constantly bombarded with stimuli from changing internal and external environments. They respond to these stress-stimuli by a series of inherent and learned behaviour patterns, which are designed to maintain or restore equilibrium, comfort and stability. Sometimes, however, stimuli are overwhelming and then balance is lost. In such circumstances individuals need help to regain homeostasis.

This concept, therefore, sees health visiting intervention as being logically directed in two ways: one towards manipulating the stimuli, so as to minimise their harmful effects, and the other towards strengthening the coping abilities of individuals, groups or communities, so that they can adapt and achieve balance. This idea appears relevant to the care of the elderly, who have had long experience in adapting to different types of stress situations, and who have developed coping abilities in consequence. Furthermore, older people are often susceptible to upsets in their circumstances, because their adaptive processes become more delicately poised. Therefore, a simple infection, which a younger person might easily shrug off, may constitute an acute event for a frail senior. Changing house; modifying lifestyle, as in retirement; losing supportive networks such as a helpful neighbour leaving the district; coping with a chronic disorder; or the loss of a loved person or pet may prove devastating to an older person.

Health visitors make use of this concept of health as adaptation, when they use anticipatory guidance techniques; advocate prophylaxis; develop systems to predict potential crisis-events and then institute 'early warning measures'; or mobilise resources to meet needs and so strengthen and support the vulnerable elderly. Four main nursing models currently make explicit use of this theory:

Neuman Health Care Systems Model (Neuman & Young 1972, Neuman 1980)
Crisis intervention model (Caplan 1964, 1974)
Roy's adaptation model (Roy 1970, Riehl & Roy 1983)
Stress adaptation model (Saxton & Hyland 1979).

Within the constraints of this chapter only the first model is discussed here, but a summary of the other three, together with some additional models which are used in nursing generally, and which may have some application to health visiting, is given in Appendix 3.

The Neuman Health Care Systems model depicts individuals as unique beings, who constantly face stresses, to counter which they have certain lines of defence. These are conceptualised as:

an outer or 'flexible line of defence,' which is constantly utilised to maintain equilibrium

a second or 'normal line of defence,' which is brought into action when stressors breach the flexible line and disturb equilibrium'

still deeper 'lines of resistance' which help to stabilise people and return them to equilibrium when stresses are overwhelming and have overcome normal and flexible lines of resistance.

One health visiting practitioner considers that the Neuman model fits well into the nature and purpose of health visiting, because it sees the individual as being mostly in balance, and the practitioner's job as being to maintain that steady state (Clark 1982a, 1982b). When this model is used in practice it fits well into the framework of primary, secondary and tertiary prevention which characterises health visiting care. For example primary preventive care is directed both towards reducing the possibility of individuals encountering stresses, and strengthening their 'flexible lines of defence' through raising their general and specific resistance and improving their coping abilities. Secondary preventive care, recognising that deviation has occurred, seeks to repair the breach quickly through early detection and prompt treatment. In this way the 'normal line of defence' is strengthened, so that balance can be maintained or restored. Tertiary preventive care is employed when balance has been lost in physical, mental, emotional social or spiritual realms and the client needs help to enable him or her to readapt, and thereafter to maintain stability. Thus the 'deeper lines of resistance' are restored and the client re-educated to help prevent future stress-reactions.

By now readers will probably have perceived some linking of ideas between these various concepts of health, noted some similarities as well as differences in the models derived from them, and seen some overlap in the inferences drawn for practice. However, it is not only workers who formulate conceptual frameworks to help them think about health and so plan and organise their care; clients too have their ideas about what constitutes health. Dunnell & Cartwright (1972) showed how entrenched the health perceptions, and hence the health behaviours, of older people are, and how strongly they are influenced by cultural and social class factors in deciding what makes for well-being. Such differences in conceptualisation between clients and health visitors, and between various workers, can mean that they may pursue very different approaches and may therefore set different goals in care. This is one reason why it is so important to make ideas explicit and to seek to find congruence in perceptions.

Another way to reduce the possibility of 'clashes' of ideas in teamwork is to adopt one particular model for all to follow. This is a current fashion in some hospitals or educational establishments; but is less common within the community setting. It has certain merits since it means all involved are aware of the shared theory base, and are likely therefore to look at problems from similar viewpoints. However, there are times when a specific model may be a more appropriate framework for a particular client; so retaining an eclectic stance may be wise. Those who wish to explore further the issues of models, frameworks, concepts and theories as they mould and shape practice, are referred to Clark (1982a) and Binnie et al (1984).

SKILLS IN HEALTH VISITING PRACTICE

Argyris & Schon (1974) state that 'learning a theory of action, so as to become competent in professional practice, does not consist of learning to recite the theory: the theory of action has not been learned, in the most important sense, unless it can be put into practice.' For this reason the concepts described above, which form an important part of the health visitor's knowledge base, must be accompanied by commensurate skills and appropriate attitudes, values and traits. These various components are welded together in the processes of delivering care. This is why health visiting may be regarded both as a science and an art. Possibly no other client group needs this blend more than older people.

The dictionary defines skill as 'adroitness, dexterity, expertness, ingenuity, or practised ability'. Thus an idea is conveyed of smoothness in the execution of a task, procedure or technique. Skills may be practical or intellectual, and those used in health visiting are as diverse as the clients and their settings. The CETHV (1967) and Raymond (1983) have discussed these skills in some detail, relating them to the overall health visiting role. However, in the care of the elderly client, certain skills assume even greater importance and are briefly considered below under the following headings, even though in practice it is difficult to separate them:

- perceptual skills
- interrelational skills
- teaching and counselling skills
- skills in organisation, planning and decision-making.

Perceptual skills

Because old people are often reticent about their state, are sometimes unaware of the significance of events, and frequently display non-specificity in illness, with atypical symptoms, the observational and interpretive skills of the practitioner must be highly developed (see Chs. 2, 3, 8 and 9). Astute observation includes learning to read body language, displayed through posture, facial expression, gesture and dress. Often the relaxed attentive position, or the blank uncomprehending stare, the covert twinkle in the eye, or the nervous movements of the fingers, tell their own story. Similarly so do gross or subtle changes in personal appearance, or surroundings. Study of the environment helps practitioners to note the presence or absence of artefacts, such as books, photographs, pictures, ornaments, or of pets, all of which may give clues to personality and lifestyle, mood or status. Particular resources, or specific problems, may be discovered through an unobtrusive examination of the environmental lay-out.

Of course, nursing education will have helped to develop

skills in observation, listening and interpretation, whilst health visitor preparation should enhance awareness and insight, but each practitioner has the ongoing responsibility to sharpen and refine these abilities. The perceptual skills of the health visitor will also be extended to any family or group members with whom the senior may have contact, as well as the community of which they form part. Identifying community needs and perceiving levels of community support for the elderly are important adjuncts to personal client care.

Interrelational skills

Closely allied to perceptual skills are those in developing interpersonal relationships. These include the techniques of verbal and non-verbal communication, already touched on in Chapter 4. Interviewing skills are particularly relevant to the elderly, since it is within the context of purposeful conversation that rapport and confidence are developed and information is elicited which is pertinent to care.

Modification of these skills for older clients is related to the slower reaction time which may be present; the constraints of sensory ageing; sometimes the narrowing of the clients social networks, so that suspicion and hesitancy initially characterise contact; or the limitations of physical illness and/or disability.

Teaching and counselling skills

Mention has been made in several places of the teaching skills of the health visitor. For the elderly these skills are frequently employed on a one-to-one basis, or in small groups. Contact may be in the home, or in clubs, day centres, clinics, residential homes, or similar settings. Teaching may also involve work with larger groups, not always the elderly themselves, but those seeking to understand the needs of older people. Teaching skills include information-giving, demonstrations, conducting discussion groups, lecturing, participation in exhibitions, the mounting of displays and participation in special programmes including radio. Socio-drama is a technique much enjoyed by some older people, so health visitors may make use of this during health education, as well as such sophisticated equipment as video recordings or closed circuit television. Each of these activities requires different skills, as well as a wide knowledge about educational processes. When applied to the elderly, practitioners must take account of relevance, motivation, the constraints of ageing, differences in learning styles and the need for spaced repetition and time to consolidate learning.

Counselling differs from teaching in that it encourages clients to become more aware of alternative courses of action and invites them to take the lead in the problem-solving and decision-making processes. In work with older people such counselling may often relate to decisions about the type and settings of care. Counselling is also a skill much used with carers of the elderly. Some practitioners say they have found it helpful to take additional study in the techniques of counselling, after they have gained initial health visiting experience.

Skills in organisation, planning and decision-making

Closely linked to, and utilising, the previous skills are those affecting the organisation and management of a case-load. The ability to identify need and determine priorities, especially from among a welter of competing demands, is clearly of relevance to elderly clients, who do not always recognise their own needs and may play down, or ignore, the severity of some difficulties. Skill in exercising judgment, in weighing up the relative merits of alternative strategies, as well as the timing and execution of tasks, also fall under this heading. Similarly health visitors may head up a team of other workers, so they need to be able to exercise skills in appraisal, delegation, supervision and control. Planning must also take place at the community level. Strategies frequently have to be forged with different groups who are involved with the elderly, so that collaborative programmes can be developed. Sometimes such plans may be longer-term, and practitioners may then have to motivate and encourage people, so that they do not grow weary in their well-doing.

ATTITUDES, TRAITS AND VALUES

> What nurses and health visitors do depends not only on their educational and professional ability, but also on the type of people they are — the attitudes and expectations they bring to their work and the organisational frameworks within which they operate.
>
> Hockey, 1979

The frameworks are discussed in Chapter 6, whilst some of the attitudes which practitioners need to display were mentioned in Chapter 4. These included positive attitudes towards accountability, commitment, acceptance and empathy. However, with the elderly, approachability is a much-needed trait, since little can be achieved if older people feel practitioners are remote from them. Flexibility, tolerance, a high degree of self-knowledge and awareness, adaptive capacity and resourcefulness are also required. Other necessary traits include humour, practicality, a spirit of co-operation and an appreciation of professional values. Perhaps tenacity in the face of difficulties is one of the most valuable assets, since frustration is common in all health visiting work. It is easy to depict an 'ideal type' of practitioner, who rarely exists; but warm and insightful workers with a variety of different traits can learn to develop attitudes appropriate to the care of elderly clients, provided they are patient and willing to do so. Most of all, practitioners will find how much they can learn from their older clients, so that they can benefit from the contact as well. This is most likely to happen when practitioners are prepared to make the effort to work within the clients' value systems and develop respect for their culture.

PROCESSES OF CARE

Processes of care involve not only the knowledge, skills, attitudes and values held by practitioners, but also the service received by the client. Health visitors use several different processes in the course of their work, including those involving research, communication and team-building. Sometimes these may be used concurrently, although their foci and goals may vary. Only the health visiting process is discussed here.

The health visiting process

More recently there has been an effort to make explicit the process by which practitioners systematically identify, describe, define and classify initial events, situations or problems, and the way they collect, record, analyse and interpret data, as a prelude to clarifying issues, and planning and implementing care. This sequence has become known as the health visiting process, and has similar elements to the nursing process, with which practitioners may be familiar. A number of health visitor students and practitioners find this systematic approach helpful as a means of co-ordinating their knowledge and skills and enabling them to structure their practice, so that they can see clearly what they are doing and where they aim to go. Furthermore, when such data is adequately recorded, other persons, including clients, can see how decisions have been made and thus are informed about the rationale of care. Such records need not have complicated formats, although their initial completion is likely to be rather more time-consuming. They should eventually save time, when practitioners can see at a glance exactly what is intended for a particular client, and can quickly pick up the threads from a previous visit or take over from a colleague. Of course the recording system should never be allowed to become a ritualistic performance, but kept flexible enough to follow, rather than dictate, care.

Some practitioners find the mnemonic **SOAPIER** helps them to check out the sequences of the process, which are ordered as follows:

S subjective data gathering — or what the client *says*
O objective data gathering — or what the health visitor *sees*
A analysis and interpretation of data — in order to *assess* and set *aims*
P planning — immediate, intermediate and longer-term
I implementation — the actual action taken to put plan into operation
E evaluation — judging results against goals set and relevant criteria
R review and reorganisation — re-assessing and revising plans as needed.

Subjective data gathering

Subjective data gathering is of paramount importance when working with older people, because practitioners are often unaware of their clients' perceptions of problems or their expectations of care. This is demonstrated at the individual level of activity, by the following study.

Case study

One elderly lady, who was receiving visits from a health visitor with the intention of encouraging greater independence and a restorative perspective, was concerned because she had severe varicose veins and general circulatory problems. She complained that she could not comply with the practitioner's advice and increase the amount of walking she did, because she could not apply her supportive stockings. Further investigation showed that she had tried stocking appliers but did not have the strength to manipulate them because of arthritic hands and general muscle weakness. Asked what *she* thought she needed, she said, 'Someone from the health or social services should visit me daily to help me put on these stockings, or how else am I to prevent worsening of my condition?' Because such help was not forthcoming, nor had any other measures been proposed, this client was frustrated and critical of services.

Whilst such subjective data is of great importance at the individual level, giving scope for estimating congruence between health visitor and client perspectives, and thus enabling more appropriate action to be taken, it is equally so at the group and community levels of care. It is not possible effectively to stimulate an awareness of health needs, nor to facilitate self-help and encourage people to take positive steps to control their own ageing, unless one has a clear grasp of *their* views and goals.

Objective data gathering

Practitioners will realise this must be as comprehensive as possible; so observation and measurement must be widely employed. Sight can point out incongruities in the elderly client's view of his or her domestic state, food supplies, general amenities or coping ability. Smell reveals the presence of soiled linen, stale food, damp housing, inadequate personal or domestic hygiene, the presence of animals or the characteristic odour of specific diseases. Touch indicates temperature, skin texture, muscle tone and may reveal problems. Cognitive assessment can be made through listening to the client's answers to questions which involve thinking, memory, judgment, problem-solving or the carrying out of simple instructions. However, whenever possible these observations and interpretations should be supplemented by the use of valid measuring devices. These include not only the recordings of vital signs such as temperature, pulse, respiration, blood pressure, urine analysis and checks of height, weight and skin-folds, but also screening tests for vision and hearing; the measurement of pain levels; and the use of health questionnaires and life satisfaction indexes such as those used by Neugarten, Havighurst & Tobin (1961) and Luker (1982a). These forms of measurement are relevant to health visiting practice, even though the practitioner may not necessarily obtain them all herself, and is not engaged in clinical nursing duties.

Assessment

Perhaps one of the major difficulties which some practitioners have raised about adopting the health visiting process lies in finding an appropriate model to use as a framework for care, and then developing an operational tool based on it. Such a tool needs to be sharp enough to cover all types of client needs, yet capable of being used by a variety of practitioners as well as incorporating the demands of differing employing authorities. Although students receive education in the natural and behavioural sciences, and training in the use of many skills and techniques, one weakness of their preparation seems to be that they are often expected to conceptualise care in their own way, synthesising knowledge and skills for themselves. They may, however, sometimes need guidance in bringing together the conglomeration of ideas, skills and values, in order to produce commensurate operational tools.

In the constraints of this chapter it is not possible to give examples of operational assessment/intervention tools for each model which has been discussed. This would, however, be a useful exercise for students as well as practitioners to undertake and one that field work teachers might find helpful. Instead mention is made below of some operational frameworks, with more detailed examples being given for two of the models at the end of the chapter. These are 'the Activities of Living model' and 'Neuman's health care systems model'.

In presenting these illustrations it should be noted that they have had to be restricted to work at the individual client level. The use of these two models does not imply superior merit, and the examples are intended to provoke thought and discussion rather than to serve as a firm guideline for practice. Each example deals with very old clients, and both are set within the context of tertiary prevention, although primary prevention is involved in the outworking of care. The selection of clients with established medical states, even though temporary, should in no way be considered to negate the contention that the major role of the health visitor is, and remains, in primary prevention.

Some operational tools for assessment

Those who advocate the medical model and conceptualise health as the absence of disease are thus most likely to use the body-systems approach, using such headings as sensori-motor state, mental-emotional state; nutritional state; circulatory, respiratory, elimination and skin state; comfort and sleep state, and environmental and economic state (Mitchell 1977). Price (1981) uses a similar approach, assessing from 'head to toe'. Smith (1983) discusses the advantages and disadvantages of this model and its associated framework for assessment.

Those who conceptualise health as a positive state, and adopt a developmental approach, are likely to use a framework of human needs (see Fig. 5.1) as an assessment tool. Thus they may follow Maslow's example and use headings such as physiological needs; safety needs; belonging needs; self-esteem needs; and self-actualisation needs, to help them assess clients. Others may use Bradshaw's taxonomy (1972);

normative needs; felt needs; expressed needs; and comparative needs. A framework more commonly adopted by health visitors using this concept employs the headings physical needs; mental and emotional needs; social needs; financial and environmental needs. This is described by Yura & Walsh (1978).

When health is viewed as a fluctuant experience, the assessment tool used is likely to include headings which reflect functional ability, and levels of wellness, in order to allow practitioners to plot the client's position on a health scale. Lawton (1971) recommended this approach, using headings such as physical health; capacity for self-maintenance; role performance; intellectual, emotional and social capacity; and attitudes towards self and others.

The idea that health is synonymous with independence in living is a combination of the developmental approach, a systems approach and the functional ability framework. Thus the assessment tool determines client ability in a number of common activities. The Activities of Living model, already described, and shown in Figure 5.3, is one such framework. It is used as an example at the end of this chapter, and deals with Mrs M. Davison, an elderly woman living alone. Table 5.1 sets out her health visiting history and Table 5.2 shows her initial health visiting assessment. Figure 5.4 gives an estimate of the client's position on both the life-span and the independence continuum. Table 5.3 outlines the health visiting care plan. It will be noted that this illustration deals mainly with care at the tertiary level, although primary and secondary prevention are indicated.

Lastly, when health is regarded as an adaptive process, the assessment tool logically takes account of the stresses which the client encounters. Thus headings might include stress agents; client perceptions of stress stimuli; adaptive/maladaptive behaviour patterns; client coping mechanisms; and client expectations. The second case study involves the assessment of an elderly woman client, Mrs Black, and uses the Neuman model. For illustrative purposes these details have been elaborated rather more than might be possible to record in practice. They have also been separately tabulated, although in practice they would form one continuous record. Table 5.4 gives the general content of the model. Table 5.5 gives Mrs Black's (subjective) view of her stresses, problems, coping patterns, anticipations and expectations. Table 5.6 provides the practitioner's (objective) account of the client's problems, stresses and coping patterns and seeks to identify the extent of client-practitioner congruence. Table 5.7 gives the practitioner's summary of impressions, and formulates the major problems requiring health visiting action. These are then rank-ordered. A detailed care plan is *not* given. Readers will appreciate that this example of the possible use of such an assessment tool is open to debate.

Nevertheless, students and practitioners will appreciate that whichever, framework and headings are used for assessment, the approach must always be systematic, and the data collected should relate whenever possible to each dimension of client need. Furthermore the ageing process may modify the techniques which can be used to gather data. For this reason and in order to ensure comprehensive care whenever possible, health visitors should try to obtain as much family and community data as they can. This not only acts as back-up material, reducing the risk of inaccuracies in data collection, and consequent skewing of care, but helps to set the clients into context and enables the health visitor to help families as units, and communities as well (see Ch. 4). An illustration of the form such family and community assessment might take is given in Appendices 4 and 5.

Planning care

Once subjective and objective data have been obtained and analysed and assessment has been made, the major needs and/or problems can be identified and the problem-solving process begun. Some practitioners call this stage, 'making a health visiting diagnosis', by which they mean 'a professional decision or opinion, formed after careful consideration of all relevant material'. This may not be a familiar term, and it should be realised that this formulation will probably not correlate with any medical diagnosis, although of course it will take this into account. This is because the nature of the problems investigated differ, and the assessment refers to those needs which can best be helped by health visiting intervention. For this reason the goals of care, which by this process will have been mutually determined, will reflect the client and family behaviour patterns and their culture. However it should allow for inputs from other team members as necessary. Immediate goals will shape short-term plans. Likewise longer term goals will cover broader activities, including the overall aim of health visiting intervention. Whenever possible the goal statements should be given in behavioural terms, but this may sometimes prove rather difficult. Goals should always be concise, feasible, relevant and realistic. Plans derived from them should be personalised, comprehensive, yet succinct, so that others can quickly detect purposes and proposed action. Where possible the time-scale expected for the accomplishment of specific activities should be given, but this is sometimes more problematic when visiting the elderly, whose reactions may be less predictable. Every participant in the planning process must be clear about their own and others responsibilities.

Implementation

This is the active phase of the process and is a record of all the activities involved in trying to reach the set goals. It therefore includes all that clients, carers and significant others, as well as practitioners, do to accomplish the aims. Active participation is the key-note of this phase, and each step should be monitored to check that it fulfils part of the overall plan.

Evaluation

Health visiting practice should be evaluated with respect to both client outcomes and the process of care. Without measuring outcomes against desired goals it is not possible to identify or compare client progress; without measuring the care process it is not possible to demonstrate how far the health visiting practitioner has contributed to care (Luker 1982b). The secret of effective evaluation lies in determining relevant criteria. Client outcomes can usually be determined through criteria arising from the goals set, but the criteria for determining process and health visitor contribution must relate to effort, efficiency and effectiveness. Negative as well as positive evaluation should be encouraged, since setbacks as well as successes can indicate which courses of action should continue, and which must be changed.

Review and reorganisation

As a result of the evaluation against set goals, plans should be reviewed and reorganised. Re-assessment may well be needed; new goals may have to be set; new actions considered. The whole activity is thus seen as a dynamic, interactive and continuing process, which operates throughout a client's life. For further reading on the application of the health visiting process readers are referred to Clark (1982b) and to Burgess & Ragland (1983). Ebersole & Hess (1981) have covered the application of care to elderly clients quite extensively.

SUMMARY

This chapter has examined the practice of health visiting the elderly, within the context of knowledge, skills, attitudes traits and values. It has looked at *how* health visiting may be undertaken with elderly clients, using a conceptual approach rather than a detailed account of procedures. It has particularly explored ideas of holistic care and health, seeing these as basic to health visiting practice. Attention has been directed towards the various models which may be used as frameworks for care, on the assumption that an explicit model is likely to assist the practitioner to structure her diverse observations, and to reach a knowledge-based assessment, which can be explained in a written record for others to follow. The need for a systematic approach to the delivery of client care has been stressed, at a time when the unstructured nature of some health visiting has been a controversial issue. Two case studies have been given to illustrate possible ways of applying these to the assessment and care of older people. However, it has not been possible to discuss the application of appropriate models to group and community level care. Underlying the chapter has been the belief that a major part of the health visiting role with the elderly is to encourage older people to take a lively interest in the preservation and enhancement of their own well-being as a means a controlling some of the problems associated with ageing. Emphasis has also been laid on the priority to be given to improving the quality of life for older clients, through a consideration of their views and expectations.

If some readers are disappointed that they have not been given more detail about specific procedures relating to practice, we can only point out that the strength of a professional preparation is that it provides its members with principles, concepts and theories in order that professional judgment may be exercised in their applications. If the reality of practice is thought to fall short of the intent and potential of the service as discussed here, it may be that this indicates a need for collective professional re-examination of role-performances and service priorities in the light of post-basic and continuing health visitor education. If **one** reason for any incongruence between professional intent and professional performance is gross underresourcing and underdevelopment of the health visiting service, could it be that the time has come for a corporate posing of the question 'Can society afford to ignore the preventive care and health education role which health visitors, given the resources, could offer its middle-aged and elderly members?'

Case study
Mrs M. L. Davison, an elderly woman, living alone
Mrs Margaret Davison, aged 88 years, normally lives alone, and copes well. She sustained a fall whilst gardening, twisting her left ankle and causing extensive bruising to her left leg and both arms. She was relatively shocked. Medical aid was summoned by a neighbour and after initial examination and diagnosis, Mrs Davison was prescribed Ponstan 100 mg tds and advised to rest with her left leg slightly elevated. Cold compresses were advised tds and a supportive Tubigrip bandage was applied to her left foot and ankle. Because she had difficulty weight-bearing and could not easily manage personal dressing or washing, nor cope with domestic duties, she was invited to stay with her daughter, Mrs Penelope Charger.

Mrs Charger is a retired teacher, married and living with

her husband in another district of the same town as her mother. Mrs Davison and her daughter and son-in-law do not get on well. However, Mrs Charger signified her willingness to care temporarily for her mother during the post-trauma period. At a short meeting of members of the primary health care team, decisions were made that clinical nursing care was not required, but that Miss Brand, the health visitor who has been paying surveillance visits to this client at 4-monthly intervals, should visit Mrs Davison at Mrs Charger's address, to maintain continuity. Miss Brand arranged to pay an assessment visit and subsequently maintained a supportive and teaching role to the client and her family.

Table 5.1 Example of a health visiting history

Surname	*Forenames*	*Marital status*	*Date of birth*
Davison	Margaret Louisa	Widowed 1974	21.2.1896

Address	*Tel. No.*	*Former occupation*	*Retirement date*
1, Lower Street Old Town Boldsworth	223344	Biology Teacher	1959

Next of kin

Name	*Address*	*Relationship*
Mrs Penelope Charger	6, Brook St New Town, Boldsworth	Daughter

Present residence and composition of household
Staying with daughter at 6 Brook St, New Town, Boldsworth

Self (Client)		
Mrs P. Charger	daughter	Retired Teacher (62 yrs)
Mr F. Charger	son-in-law	Engineer (64 yrs)

Significant others

Name	*Address*	*Relationship*
Mrs Barbara Thomas	6 West St Taunton	Granddaughter
Mr David Thomas	S/A	Grandson-in-law
Paul Thomas	S/A	Great grandson (8 yrs)

Health care team

Mrs V. Jones	District Nursing Sister
Miss J. Brand	Health Visitor
Dr B. Quick	General Practitioner

Address	*Tel. No.*
Health Centre, Old Town, Boldsworth	556677

Table 5.1 Contd.

Client's health history
Prolapsed uterus, treated by pessary insertion, 1974. Cataract operation, lens extraction Rt eye 1972: Lt eye 1974 Fractured Lt. wrist 1977. Has osteo-arthritis: occasional vertigo. 2-yearly medical appraisal carried out by General Practitioner. 4-monthly health surveillance carried out by Health Visitor.

Significant social history
Husband died Jan 1974 (former solicitor).
Son killed 1975: road traffic accident.

Details of present event
Twisted/sprained left ankle, due to fall whilst gardening. Unable now to weight-bear: has extensive bruising of left leg and both arms. Complains of pain: was initially shocked. Neighbour called GP who prescribed Ponstan 100 mg tds for pain relief; elevation of left leg, with application of cold compresses tds. Tubigrip support applied. District nursing help not sought as client temporarily transferred to care of her daughter who 'feels she can manage for a time'. Referral from Dr Quick to health visitor requesting visit and maintenance of continuity of care.

Impact of precipitating event on client

Subjective account (client)	*Objective account (HV)*
'I'm in pain and feel shaky. Because I cannot stand or walk at present nor manage to look after myself, I have to go and stay with my daughter. I fear she and her husband will not really like this.'	Client quite distressed. Has obvious pain which is eased by medication. Left ankle swollen, cannot weight-bear. Daughter offering help but relationships are strained.
Perception of significance of event 'This fall indicates I am at risk. It means I must re-plan my future. I don't want to go into care and fear my daughter may make me do so. I need help to sort things out quietly.'	Temporary incapacity, but indicative of increasing vulnerability. Needs immediate care and rehabilitation. Will need to consider future, but no haste. Family pressures may well need countering.

Available resources
Self (client)
Physically: has limited capacity: increasing frailty.
Mentally: has good reserves. Emotionally: strong will and an independent spirit. Well-motivated towards self-help.
Socially: good rapport with neighbours; moderate supportive network from friends and church members: attends OAP Club regularly.
Spiritually: is a member of St John's Church, Old Town. In contact with Minister; participates in church activities.
Economically: has both retirement pension and a teacher's pension; has savings: owns own home.
Socio-culturally: generally exhibits middle class values. Traditional lifestyle.
Environmentally: home in good repair. Close to shops and other amenities. House rather large for present needs. Some difficulty in doing housework, but does not currently have any domestic help.

Table 5.1 Contd.

Usual coping strategies Client's view	
'I usually size up situations and then do my best to soldier on.'	Health Visitor's view Practical client. Usually seeks help early, follows advice. Rather stoic manner.

Family resources
Daughter: retired teacher, very capable person. Homeowner, with good facilities. Has never been close to mother.
Son-in-law: presently in full-time work, but planning to retire at 65. Does not get on with client. Couple are not willing to have client live with them permanently, but are 'prepared to do their duty by her, as far as possible, without this.'

Client's use of health services
Infrequent to date. 2-yearly medical check, 4-monthly health visiting surveillance. Chiropody at six-week intervals. Ophthalmic examination 2-yrly, bi-focal glasses worn (cataract lens).

Use of social services
No contact so far. May need aids and adaptations later.

Client's capacity to meet present basic needs
Unable to move freely, cannot prepare own food, manage housework, personal washing or laundry. Has some difficulty getting to toilet, will require use of commode. Must have temporary care from daugther.

Ability to identify and deal with problems
Has knowledge of biology, simple home nursing, and much life experience. Perceives threat to independence from increasing physical frailty. Anxious about dependence on her daughter. Heeds teaching and tries to adapt to changing circumstances.

Desired direction of care
Seek pain relief, restoration of function and independence. Maintenance of future independence for as long as possible. Requires help to examine alternatives for future care. Hopes to effect improvement in relationship with daughter and son-in-law; welcomes help in effecting greater communication with them.

Table 5.2 Health Visitor's initial assessment of independence in Activities of Living for Mrs Davison

Activities of Living	Usual routines What client can/cannot do independently	Client needs and problems (a = actual) (p = potential)
Maintaining a safe environment	Reasonably independent until now. Requires help to assess hazards/guard against future accident.	Some instability: sight diminishing (a) unstable balance (a) takes some risks (p) Needs help to balance drives and risks

Table 5.2 Contd.

Activities of Living	Usual routines What client can/cannot do independently	Client needs and problems (a = actual) (p = potential)
Communicating	Cognitively clear: speech good. Feeling some pain: distressed at present dependency. Some relationship problems with her daughter and son-in-law.	Fears deterioration of emotional climate if stays with daughter (p) Depressed about rapport. Wants to improve future relationships (a)
Breathing	Normal	Risk of respiratory infection if immobile (p)
Eating and drinking	Small appetite. Cooks and shops for self usually. Temporarily unable to do so.	Nutritional impairment if not fed well after injury (p)
Eliminating	Normally independent. Occl: stress incontinence. Occl: constipation: Temporarily unable to get to WC	Requires commode (a) Help to combat risk of incontinence: Immobility increases constipation risk (a)
Personal washing and dressing	Usually well groomed Temporary difficulties	Needs help from family to obtain wash/get clothes: avoid skin soreness (p)
Controlling body temperature	Normal	Sl. risk infection (p)
Mobilising	Normally very active. Injured ankle: temporarily cannot weight-bear	Stiffness (a) pain (a) Thrombosis (p) Needs help short-term
Working/playing	Normally very active, cannot manage housework at present.	Requires temporary care (a) Risk of boredom (p) and strained family relationships
Sleeping	Usually fair, may be fitful due to change in environment.	Insomnia (p) Fatigue (p) Reduced resistance (p) Need to ensure pain relief: simple means for meeting body comfort promote relaxation, (a).

Table 5.2 Contd.

Activities of Living	Usual routines What client can/cannot do independently	Client needs and problems (a = actual) (p = potential)
Expressing sexuality	Widowed. Good social relationships with both sexes.	Strained relationship with son-in-law (a) Likely to miss friends during temporary stay with daughter (p)
Dying	Not imminent but is likely in next 20 yrs.	Awareness of risk now heightened (a) Needs to prepare self for event (p)

Summary
Presenting problem is post-traumatic immobility/dependence. Family capable of giving adequate care provided they have appropriate information and guidance: understand needs and can meet same, especially for pain relief and gradual return to mobility and independence.
   More significant and underlying problems: increasing frailty; increased accident risk; need to seek longer-term solutions for care yet maintain optimum independence. Major difficulty strained family relationships: need to explore source of tensions, reduce same if possible. Encourage improved rapport and build up more stable and caring relationship for future. Help client and family to relax with and enjoy each other — discover practitioner role and feel free to call on help in future as needed.

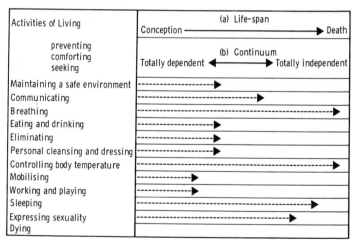

Fig. 5.4 The assessment of Mrs Davison, using the Activities of Living model

Table 5.3 Health Visitor's plan for Mrs Davison (based on Activities of Living model)

Activities of Living	Need or problem (a) = actual (p) = potential	Goal of care (s) = short-term (l) = longer-term	Health visiting intervention (s) = short-term (l) = longer-term	Evaluation criteria (s) = short-term (l) = longer-term
Maintaining a safe environment	Need to remain accident free	Maintain safety (s) (l) Identify risks compatible with quality of life	Check safety of client in own and daughter's home Alert family to hazards: invite improvement	Client and family regard safety needs remove risks: maintain vigilance (s) (l)
	Problem 1. Instability (a)	Discover cause: remove/reduce if possible	Arrange medical check: explain any subsequent treatment	Full medical check/needed treatment prescribed before return home
	2. Failing vision (a)	Maintenance of optimum sight	Visual check encouraged: advise on low vision aids if needed (s) (l)	Check carried out (s). Aids used correctly (s) (l)
	3. Risk of further falls (p)	Restore client confidence	Encourage client to move freely as improves: to act confidently (s) (l)	Client regains confidence (s) Balances care with confidence on return home (l)
	4. Risk of incorrect handling of medication (p)	Safe administration of drugs	Check client and family understand use of medication and can handle same safely	Medication is taken correctly. Medicines are stored safely. Client has no adverse reactions. Maintains respect for care of drugs
Communicating	Client needs 1. To release feelings about accident (a)	Appropriate release of emotions: positive adaptation towards restoration (s) (l)	Encourage verbalisation Interpret behavioural needs to family. Help family adapt to situation and behave restoratively (s) (l)	Client talks out feelings (s) Family are aware of of effects of shock and meet care needs in a helpful manner. Client acts positively and discusses ways of restoring normal function (l)

Table 5.3 Contd.

Activities of Living	Need or problem (a) = actual (p) = potential	Goal of care (s) = short-term (l) = longer-term	Health visiting intervention (s) = short-term (l) = longer-term	Evaluation criteria (s) = short-term (l) = longer-term
	2. Client needs to understand/explain reaction to dependency state	Reduction of adverse dependency reactions (s) (l)	Carefully explain dependency reactions to family: explore appropriate family actions with them Encourage caring within a rehabilitative approach	Client and family learn to understand dependency reactions Family accept client reactions but move towards restoration of full independence, compatible with physical potential
	3. Client needs to obtain relief from pain	Pain relief and restoration of normal function (s)	Check family understand simple pain relief measures and can/will use them to help client obtain comfort/restoration (s)	Family act appropriately to relieve pain, e.g. apply cold compresses as needed Client is relieved of pain within 1 week/function is gradually restored
	4. To recognise source of family tensions and modify own behaviour which helps to create same	Tension reduction	Elicit behaviour which creates tension. Identify family flash points Explore with family more appropriate alternatives	Client relaxes: both parties try to modify their behaviour (s) (l) Family learn HV role in care Family use contact to discuss their own health needs
	5. Improve rapport	Build warmer relationships	Encourage interaction: study needs of each member: monitor progress Promote care actions	Family do discuss more freely with one another. Rapport improved

	Maintain normality. Risk of infection (p)	Respiratory health Freedom from infection	Demonstrate/encourage breathing exercises Advise on measures for preventing infection following trauma	Client carries out exercises (s) Breathing remains normal Client is infection free (s) (l)
Breathing	Maintain normality. Risk of infection (p)	Respiratory health Freedom from infection	Demonstrate/encourage breathing exercises Advise on measures for preventing infection following trauma	Client carries out exercises (s) Breathing remains normal Client is infection free (s) (l)
Eating and drinking	Small appetite (a) Temporarily unable to obtain/prepare own food (a)	Maintain adequate nutrition and promote healing	Review diet with client/and carers: advise on content: ensure vitamin intake. Restore independence but monitor future plans	Diet maintains weight within desirable limits. Daughter/son-in-law give suitable diet. Family arrange for future eating patterns after client returns home
Personal washing and dressing	Requires help from family to wash and dress. (a)	Facilitate personal grooming Restore independence	Encourage carers to help Suggest measures Early return to self-care	Family assist client (s) Full independence restored 1 month.
Mobilising	Temporarily unable bear-weight (a) Ankle swollen (a)	Maintain flexibility Avoid stiffness Restore independence	Advise/teach leg exercises. Check client and family can understand use of walking frame (s) Encourage gradual mobility	Family monitor exercises. Client gradually assumes weight bearing. Client improves within 3 weeks.
Eliminating	Temporarily unable to get to WC (a) Has sl. stress incontinence (a) Fears lapses: (p) falls: daughter's displeasure (p)	Interpret needs to family Use alternative methods safely Maintain continence Improve pelvic tone: increase confidence	Explain problems to family Help them obtain commode Advise on use (2-hourly by day) Teach pelvic exercises.	Client-carers appreciate needs Obtain commode: site safely Client manages commode safely (s) Toilet needs are monitored and pattern of continence established

Table 5.3 Contd.

Activities of Living	Need or problem (a) = actual (p) = potential	Goal of care (s) = short-term (l) = longer-term	Health visiting intervention (s) = short-term (l) longer-term	Evaluation criteria (s) = short-term (l) = longer-term
	Constipated: (a) anxious (a)	Avoid constipation Restore independence	Explore fears and reduce risks of falls Review diet: increase fibre/fluid content Encourage early return to full independence	Client continues pelvic exercises (l) Source of family tension reduced Client eats a higher fibre diet Avoids constipation Client returns to full independence in elimination with 1 month
Sleeping	Usually sleeps well Currently fitful (a) Fatigue (p)	Restore normal sleeping pattern (s) (l)	Teach natural sleep measures. Monitor	Client's sleep improves. No undue fatigue present (s)
Working and playing	Cannot manage own housework at present. (a) May need domestic help on return home	Daughter cares without undue stress. Client considers her future needs (s) Plans for the longer term (l)	Discuss domestic help Maintain client self-help in future Outline alternative courses of action, including need to plan for longer-term	Client accepts help from daughter with good grace (s) Examines future needs reaches own decision (s) (l)

	Unable to socialise (a)	Client resumes contact with friends 2 weeks returns to clubs in 1 month	Discuss need to keep up interests. Encourage contact with friends. Check client has notified club leader. Encourage return	Client takes up diversionary interest (s). Contacts friends (s) (l). Plans to return to club activities (s). Maintains positive attitude (s) (l)
Expressing sexuality	Maintain contact with both sexes (a)	As above	As above	As above
Dying	Need to consider eventual death	Approach future death with equanimity	Encourage client to meet spiritual needs as indicated by client	Client adopts healthy attitude to future death: seeks own form of spiritual support

Case study

Mrs R. Black, an elderly woman, living in warden-supervised sheltered housing

Mrs Rose Black, aged 83 years, was referred by the Warden to the Health Visitor, Mrs East, during the latter's regular weekly liaison visit. The client moved to her new home 3 weeks ago, but now appears very anxious and unsettled. Previously she had lived in another area of the town, for 20 years. She was widowed 2 years ago.

6 months ago Mrs Black was an inpatient for 4 weeks at North Town District General Hospital suffering from 'jaundice '. Was treated successfully by medical means but incorrectly assumed surgery was contemplated. Refused same. Since discharge she has been rather apathetic, reluctant to resume earlier activities, and functionally less able. Transfer to sheltered accommodation expedited because of lessened coping ability.

Client has history of mild maturity-onset diabetes first noted in 1981. Now attends Diabetic Clinic North Town District General Hospital 6-monthly, under supervision of Dr Stewart (Consultant). A 2000 Kcal diet is prescribed, and client's condition is stable. Cataract operation (lens extraction) performed in 1978: spectacles prescribed and worn.

Client lives alone but is visited weekly by her only daughter, who lives in a neighbouring town, is married and has 4 young children. There are 2 sons: 1 living in Canada and 1 in Norwich (England). The client was very attached to one helpful neighbour in former location. Is a member of several Elderly People's Clubs.

Has recently registered with Dr Green; medical records currently being transferred.

Table 5.4 An assessment/intervention tool adapted from the Neuman Health Care Systems model — content of model

---

1. Client details
2. Stressors and responses to same

Subjective data
a. Client's view of his/her major difficulties/stresses
b. Client's perception of present circumstances and whether these differ from usual pattern of living
c. Client view of whether he/she has experienced similar problems, needs, concerns, before. If so, how dealt with.

Table 5.4 Contd.

d. Client anticipations for the future as a consequence of present situation (whether these anticipations are feasible and reality-based)
e. Client views on what he/she is doing to help self
f. Client expectations from friends/family, practitioner and others.

3. Stressors encountered and responses to same

Objective data practitioner-derived, supplemented by information from records, colleagues, other carers
a. Major needs, problems, stress areas or concerns (degree of congruence with client perceptions)
b. Client's present circumstances compared with usual lifestyle
c. Client experience of similar situation
   (objective evaluation of client response in similar situations: outcomes on previous similar occasions)
d. Practitioner anticipations for the future, re: the consequences of present situation
e. Practitioner view on client levels of self-help
f. Practitioner view of client expectations
   (degree of congruence between client and practitioner views).

Summary of impressions
 (i) Intra-personal aspects
 (ii) Inter-personal
 (iii) Extra-personal
Formulation of problems, needs, concerns, ranking same in priority order.

Table 5.5 Assessment of Mrs Black using the Neuman Health Care Systems model — subjective data

1. Client details

Name	Date of birth	Marital status
Mrs Rose Black	19th April 1901	Widow
2 Gayler Terrace		
North Town		

Socio-economic status Social Class 5 (by Registrar General's classification of former occupation of husband)

Newly transferred to	Dr Green	General Practitioner
General Practice Team	Mrs Fox	District Nursing Sister
based at North Town	Mrs East	Health Visitor
Health Centre.		
Formerly cared for by		
General Practice Team		
at Merryfield Surgery,		
North Town.		

Referred by: Mrs Ann Jones, Warden, Gayler Housing Assocn.
Concerned at client's anxiety level and general lack of coping ability, since transfer to sheltered accommodation.

Table 5.5 Contd.

2. Stressors and responses to same

A. *Client's view of her major difficulties/stresses/concerns*
'My worst problem is diabetes, but it's not very bad. If I keep to my diet I'll be all right. I want to do this because I lost a sister from gangrene of her feet. 6 months ago I spent a month in hospital and still feel weak. I went in because my legs were like jelly and I was yellow all over and felt bad. I think they wanted to operate but I refused, as it's my flesh and I wish to keep it.

I've been waiting to move here for 2 years, but I don't know if I'll like it here; the move has been a nightmare. I miss my old home and neighbour.

I've not been out much since I came here. It worries me to do my washing in this communal machine.

My legs will not go like they used to; but I manage.

This move has cost me a lot of money and I'm very worried about this.'

B. *Client's perception of how her present circumstances differ from her usual pattern of living*

Usual lifestyle	Present lifestyle
I used to do everything for myself. I looked after my husband before he died. You have to get on with it.	'I don't seem to have the same interest here. I can't be bothered. I feel too weak and wobbly.'
I usually get up at 7 a.m. and go to bed about 11.30 p.m.	I don't want to get up before 9 a.m/go to bed any time after 7 p.m.
I used to sleep well. I try to follow my diet — meat and 2 veg every day. I visited my daughter and her family on Sundays.	I wake a lot now. I don't feel hungry now but I force something down. I don't go out now. My daughter cooks for me for Sundays.
I used to do my own laundry.	I worry about washing. I don't like this machine.
I went to my club on Mondays and collected my pension after. I also went to clubs on Tuesday and Friday.	I think it's too far to get to my Clubs now. The Warden gets my pension.
I get the Supplementary (SB) and they pay my rent. It's not much but I managed with care.'	I don't know how I will afford this central heating. It worries me so.'

C. *Client's view of whether she has experienced similar needs or problems before*

'I've never been "yellow" before, but I have felt weak. I worked it off: you see I knew everybody round me and it helped.'

'I worry if the yellow will come back. I have no strength to work it off: they are all strangers here.'

D. *Client's anticipations for the future as a consequence of her present situation*
'I can't see things will ever be right for me again. I can't seem to tackle this place like I did.

Table 5.5 Contd.

E. Client's perceptions of what she is doing to help herself
I'm very busy getting myself straight. I've no time to go shopping even if I
wanted to, because I've all this housework and washing which I do.
I do as I'm told from the diabetic clinic.
I'm quite independent now.
I manage although I feel so tired and miserable.'

F. Client's expectations of family, friends, practitioner and others
'My family will do all I need, my daughter will come and help and my eldest
grandchild especially. The diabetic clinic will stop me getting gangrene. I
don't suppose I will need to bother this new Dr Green very much, because
the yellow has gone away, but I expect he'll help me if I need him. He will
come and see me here.
I don't expect to need the hospital again.
The Warden is very good and will do anything I ask her.
I know you will come and see me, but I shan't need much.
I do wish the Supplementary would give me a bit more for the heating.
Perhaps some of my friends in my old area will move here when they close
those old houses. I know they will visit me a lot here.'

Table 5.6 Assessment of Mrs Black, using the Neuman Health Care Systems
model — objective data

---

a. Major needs, problems, stress areas or concerns
Octogenarian with history of increasing frailty, some instability and vague
abdominal discomfort, increasing over past year. Familial history of diabetes/
1 sister died from it. Diagnosed maturity-onset diabetes 3 years ago, well
controlled by diet alone. Widowed 2 years ago after a 4 year period of caring
for sick husband in very poor environmental circumstances.
   Health visiting support given by colleague intermittently following
bereavement. Planned move to sheltered accommodation expedited as a
result of hospital admission for jaundice 6 months ago. Diagnosis not fully
established: treated medically although client incorrectly assumed surgery
was contemplated, and refused this. Became very distressed. Otherwise
independent. Moved here by Local Housing Authority 3 weeks ago. Has
found experience threatening and seems overwhelmed ? slightly
disorientated. Has registered with Dr Green but not yet consulted: will
need immediate referral and full check-up. Is mobile but rather unsteady,
has a walking frame for use in home.
   History of strict personal and domestic cleanliness but is now untidy in
home and rather dishevelled in appearance. Sleeping and eating routines
disturbed, stability of diabetic state potentially threatened.
   Clearly grieving for loss of old home and security of known
neighbourhood. Highly anxious, tension habits present, emotionally labile.
Flattened responses, depressive manner. Previous account of resilience
now incongruent. Own perceptions of coping ability are rather unrealistic.

b. Client's present circumstances compared with usual lifestyle

Usual lifestyle	Present lifestyle
Independent:	Becoming dependent
coping with diabetic diet.	Functionally restricted

Table 5.6 Assessment of Mrs Black, using the Neuman Health Care Systems

Managing full domestic duties.	Dietary intake uncertain.
	Domestic care poor.
	Unable to establish routine
Budgeted well.	Anxious about finances.
Socialised well.	Withdrawing.

c. *Practitioner view of client experience of similar situation*
Has not moved for many years. Clearly uncertain of how to adapt. Limited experience of illness and hospitalization, very disturbed by recent experiences, fearful of repetition and eventual outcome.

Health visitor colleague reports 'Colourful character: usually very resilient, adamant manner and decided views.' Clearly present reaction is out of character.

d. *Practitioner anticipation for future as a consequence of present state*
Client deterioration likely unless prompt action taken. Will likely need intensive rehabilitative measures, possibly short-term, but depends on establishing diagnosis/prognosis of medical condition.

Will require greater involvement of family.

Anticipate programme of social support/restoration, mobilising home help: (at least short-term).

Increased input from health visiting service.

Possible use of luncheon club/voluntary visiting service.

Increased liaison with social services department, hospital staff, and general practice team.

Likely treatment for ? depressive state.

e. *Practitioner view on client levels of self-help*
Potentially sound in short-term given intensive help now. Likely need for increasing involvement of caring services in longer-term.

f. *Practitioner's view of client's expectations of care-givers*
'Low level of fit.' Client generally rather unrealistic. Daughter burdened with family responsibilities and some transport difficulties. Relationships caring.
Old friends interested but circumscribed by age from giving much practical help. Diabetic clinic will supervise but cannot guarantee her condition. Will likely need more help from social services than she envisages.

Table 5.7 Summary of impressions formed by practitioner assessing Mrs Black, using the Neuman Health Care Systems Model

(i) *Intra personal factors*
Biological. Client's functional ability and nutritional status fair, but under threat. Sleep and appetite disturbed: skin in good condition. Other systems functioning, apart from instability and limited mobility. Some self-neglect from emotional upset.

Psycho-social. Agitated, emotionally labile and depressed. Limited insight Low motivation at present. Still communicating but tending to withdraw. Open to family and friends. No request for spiritual help.

(ii) *Inter-personal factors*
Loving family relationships. Some loss of contact with friends and acquaintances in clubs.
Normally outgoing — currently flattened responses.

Table 5.7 Contd.

(iii) *Extra-personal factors*
Others in housing complex able to visit and support.
Community is an inner city area: heavy demand on health and social services. Limited places in day centres/luncheon clubs/community nursing services and social services below establishment.

(iv) *Problem formulation — priority rated*
(a) Maintain safety and comfort
Immediate referral for medical investigation: liaise with hospital staff for full data: contact social services: arrange for home help if possible. Later luncheon club placement: Transport for attendance at resumed club activities.

(b) Raise and maintain morale
Treat underlying depression. Encourage friends and family to visit. Improve mobility: continue intensive short-term support.

(c) Maintain nutrition and dietary stability of diabetic state
Determine accurate dietary intake, liaise with diabetic clinic and ensure correct balance. Discuss shopping and cooking arrangements with daughter and Warden, ? home help. Later possible use of luncheon club.

(d) Maintain integrity of skin
Encourage attention to personal hygiene and reduce risk of skin infection.

(e) Review socio-economic state
Relieve source of immediate anxiety by discussing needs with client and encouraging contact with local officer from DHSS Supplementary Benefits Office.
With client permission, discuss position with Local Authority Social Worker. Advise on local voluntary services who may be able to meet needs for any pressing deficiency in requirements following removal from previous home.

(f) Once agitation has subsided assist client to gain insight into circumstances and re-establish independence in living
Encourage client to talk out difficulties and consider problem-solving measures.
Encourage client to take interest in new environment and to participate in activities held within the housing complex.
Inform about local-based group activities which she may wish to join, as substitute for some previous activities.
Assist client to regain full equilibrium and maintain stable state as long as possible: gradual withdrawal of intensive support.

Summary
Normally resilient individual.
Flexible line of defence breached by stressor — loss of husband
Normal line of defence breached by stressor — loss of health
Inner line of defence breached by stressor — loss of old home.
Requires help to recover equilibrium.

REFERENCES

Argyris S, Schon D A 1974 Theory in practice: increasing professional effectiveness. Jossey-Bass, San Francisco.
Binnie A, Bond S, Law G, Lowe K, Pearson A, Roberts R, Tierney A,

Vaughan B 1984 A systematic approach to nursing care. Open University Press, Milton Keynes

Bradshaw J 1972 A taxonomy of social needs. Oxford University Press for Nuffield Provincial Hospitals Trust, Oxford p 69

Burgess W, Ragland F C 1983 Community health nursing; philosophy, process, practice. Appleton Century Crofts, Connecticut

Caplan G 1964 Principles of preventive psychiatry. Basic Books, New York

Caplan G 1974 Support systems and community mental health. Basic Books, New York

Clark J 1982a Development of models, and theories on the concept of nursing. Journal of Advanced Nursing 7: 129–134

Clark J 1982b A way to get organised; trying out principles in practice. Nursing Times, Community Outlook, October 11th pp 287–297

Clark J 1983 Integration and the future of health visiting. In: Owen G 1983 (ed) Health visiting. Bailliere Tindall, London, p 360–361

Council for the Education and Training of Health Visitors 1967 The functions of the Health Visitor. CETHV, London

Council for the Education and Training of Health Visitors 1977 An investigation into the principles of health visiting. CETHV, London

Council for the Education and Training of Health Visitors 1979 Principles in practice. CETHV, London

Dickoff J, James P 1968 A theory of theories. Nursing Research 17(3):197

Dubos R 1959 Mirage of health: utopias, progress and biological change. In: Ansen R N (ed) World perspectives. Harper and Row, New York

Dunn H 1959 High level wellness for man and society. American Journal of Public Health 49(6): 786–792

Dunnell K, Cartwright A 1972 Medicine takers, prescribers and hoarders. Routledge and Kegan Paul, London

Ebersole P, Hess P 1981 Towards healthy ageing. Mosby, St Louis, p 97–102

Helvie C 1981 Community health nursing: theory and process. Harper and Row, Philadelphia, p 99–101

Hockey L 1979 A study of District Nursing. The development and progression of a long term research Programme. Unpublished Doctoral Thesis, City University, London

Hobson W, Pemberton J 1956 The health of the elderly at home. British Medical Journal 1: 587–593

King I M 1981 A theory for nursing: systems, concepts, process. Wiley, New York

Lawton M P 1971 The functional assessment of elderly people. Journal of the American Geriatric Society 19:465

Luker K 1981 The role of the health visitor In: Kinnaird J, Brotherston Sir J, Williamson J (eds) 1981 The provision of care for the elderly. Churchill Livingstone, Edinburgh, p 157

Luker K 1982a Evaluating health visiting. Royal College of Nursing, London

Luker K 1982b Health visiting and the elderly; an attempt at process-outcome evaluation British Journal of Geriatric Nursing Sept–Oct: 5–8

McFarlane J 1977 Developing a theory of nursing: the relation of theory to practice, education and research. Journal of Advanced Nursing 2: 261–270

Maslow A H 1954 Motivation and personality. Harper and Row, New York

Maslow A H 1962 Towards a psychology of being. Harper and Row, New York

Mitchell P H 1977 Concepts basic to nursing, 2nd edn. McGraw Hill, New York

Murray R, Zentner J 1975 Nursing concepts for health promotion, 2nd edn, Prentice Hall, Englewood Cliffs, p 19

Neugarten B L, Havighurst R J, Robin B S 1961 The measurement of life satisfaction. Journal of Gerontology. 16: 134–143

Neuman B 1980 The Betty Neuman Health Care Systems model; a total person approach to patient problems In: Riehl J P, Roy C (eds) Conceptual models for nursing practice, 2nd edn. Appleton-Century-Crofts, New York, p 119–134

Neuman B, Young R J 1972 The Betty Neuman Model: a total person approach to viewing patient problems. Nursing Research 21(3): 264–269

Price I 1981 The nursing process. In: Illing M, Donovan B (eds) Bailliere Tindall, London, p 25–51

Raymond E 1983 Skills in health visiting. In: Owen G (ed) 1983 Health visiting. Bailliere Tindall, London

Riehl J, Roy C 1983 Conceptual models for nursing practice. Appleton-Century-Croft, New York

Rogers E S 1960 Human ecology and public health. MacMillan, New York

Roper N, Logan W W, Tierney A J 1980 The elements of nursing. Churchill Livingstone, Edinburgh

Roper N, Logan W W, Tierney A J 1983 Using a model for nursing. Churchill Livingstone, Edinburgh

Roy C 1970 Adaptation: a conceptual framework for nursing. Nursing Outlook 18(3): 42–43

Saxton D F, Hyland P A 1979 Planning and implementing nursing. Intervention: stress and adaptation applied to patient care, 2nd edn. C V Mosby, St Louis

Schmitz M 1983 The Roy adaptation model: application in a community setting. In: Riehl J, Roy C (ed) Conceptual models for nursing practice. Appleton-Century-Crofts, New York

Selye H 1956 The stress of life. McGraw Hill, New York

Smith J A 1983 The idea of health: implications for the nursing professional. In: Smith D, Ranshorn M 1983 (eds) Nursing education series. Teachers College Press, Teachers College, Columbia University, New York

Williams I 1979 The care of the elderly in the community. Croom Helm, London, p 41–42, p 110

Yura H, Walsh M B 1978 The nursing process, 3rd edn. Appleton-Century-Crofts, New York

FURTHER READING

Griffith J W, Christensen P J 1982 Nursing process: application of theories, frameworks and models. Mosby, St Louis

Knight J H 1974 Applying the nursing process in the community. Nursing Outlook 22: 708–711

Kratz C (ed) The nursing process. Bailliere Tindall, London

Kurtzman C 1980 Nursing process at the aggregate level. Nursing Outlook 28: 737–739

Revill S, Blunden R 1980 Goal planning with mentally handicapped people in the community; report on an evaluation of the use of goal planning techniques by health visitors. Report No 9, Mental Handicap in Wales, Applied Research Unit

Stoll R 1979 Guidelines for spiritual assessment. American Journal of Nursing 79:1574

6

Caring for the elderly within various community settings

As already indicated the effective health care of older people rests on two main components: carer competence and commitment, (whether they be lay, voluntary or professional carers), and organisational efficiency. Because professional ability, responsibility, accountability and commitment have already been discussed, this chapter focuses on some of the administrative settings within which health visitors may work, and the different forms in which care for older people may be organised.

The main purpose of the chapter is to emphasise the preventive and educative nature of the health visitor's work, irrespective of organisational patterns and to discuss the methods which health visitor practitioners may adopt in order to identify the vulnerable elderly who require their care. Only in this way can they assess health needs and provide older persons with necessary help. For these reasons surveillance and screening are highlighted, because of their importance in the health care of elderly populations. An epidemiological approach is adopted, because studying the distribution of health and disease within elderly populations, and discovering the prevalence of health problems within specific groups can point up areas for health visiting intervention. Some intervention strategies may then best be aimed at earlier age-groups. Although investigations may be conducted in different ways, the goal is always to identify causal relationships so that measures for promoting health and preventing disease can be developed.

However, inevitably the administrative structures within which health visitors work will affect their activities, facilitating or constraining these. For this reason some of the advantages and disadvantages of the different patterns are mentioned. The rapid growth of knowledge concerning health and disease, often leading to greater specialisation and consequent proliferation of services, makes it necessary for multi-disciplinary approaches to be made to the complex needs of individuals and communities, hence the chapter is also concerned with teamwork. Whilst it is not the purpose of this book to examine all the facets of multi-disciplinary and inter-disciplinary teamwork, reference is made to some of the different concepts of care which may be held by the various workers, and the value bases which may underlie their activities. Readers are urged to explore these issues further, in order to see how health visitors may collaborate more effectively with others in short- or longer-term programmes designed to benefit older people.

Care sectors

Within the present National Health Service framework, which operates at Regional, District and Unit level, care is organised in two sectors: *primary* and *secondary*. Primary health care services are usually generic and continuing; they represent the first point of contact individuals have with the health care system, and are the services most often utilised. They include midwifery, school nursing, health visiting and district nursing services; general practitioner services; community medical services such as family planning, maternal and child health, school health, and infectious disease control; dental, ophthalmic, pharmaceutical and chiropody services; and other supporting services such as physiotherapy, occupational therapy and speech therapy, where these paramedical activities are provided by Health Authorities. Although located within hospitals, Accident and Emergency services are also primary care services. Additionally occupational health services, which are currently outside the NHS and may well be used by older workers, and some environmental health services provided by local authorities, may also be regarded as primary. Of course not all these outlined services are necessarily appropriate for elderly people.

Secondary care services, therefore, are those hospital and specialist services to which persons may be referred for consultation and intermittent, specialised help. However, this is a somewhat artificial division, since in an integrated health service, staff from both sectors may mingle and certainly will liaise. This contact is likely to increase in the future, particularly as community gerontology teams increase, aiming to promote combined interest in work with the elderly; foster less conventional methods; define priorities; and integrate medical, social work and nursing care.

There is no qualitative distinction between the two sectors which should be regarded as complementary. Although until recently the primary services outside hospital were comparatively under-resourced, the avowed policies of successive governments have been to redress this imbalance (DHSS 1976). Time alone will show whether these claimed intentions become realities. Because of the expressed intention to increase community care as a major organisational method of treating and caring for older people, health visitors have a keen interest in, and responsibility for seeing that resources for the community services are adequate. However, it must be borne in mind that older people also make relatively heavy demands on secondary care services, and are likely to do so increasingly, as more persons achieve greater longevity. Furthermore, under policies of planned early discharge to community services, those remaining in residential care are likely to be the more heavily dependent elderly.

Current administrative structures

Health visitors are almost always located within the primary care sector, which means they form part of the community nursing services. They maintain their contact with clients and colleagues working in secondary care sectors, through formal liaison schemes, informal visits, planned meetings and case conferences, telephone communication, records and reports.

Joint study days and shared in-service courses also assist communication and understanding. In each of these activities it is important to recognise the part played by client/patients and their relatives, and to respect and appreciate the roles of the various workers involved in the care of older people.

Within the community nursing services health visitors form part of the line-management structure, being currently answerable to Community Nursing Unit Managers. This hierarchical pattern is similar to that prevailing in social work, but is in direct contrast to the more autonomous and horizontal organisation of general medical practice. Except where joint appointments prevail, it has the effect of requiring health visitor practitioners to surrender their direct client-service skills, if they wish to assume full-time teaching or managerial duties. Health visitor tutors then transfer to educational settings, whilst health visitor managers assume responsibility for the service, facilitating and supporting staff, the transmission and implementation of District Health Authority policies, the deployment of resources and the monitoring of standards. Whilst it can be argued that such structuring enables effort to be concentrated on either education and training, or efficient service-organisation, (each of which have important repercussions for the care of elderly people), some consider it negates professional autonomy, restricts interaction, affects innovation and may reduce both teachers' and managers' appreciation of the intensity of problems met with in field work practice. Another view is that this pattern could be interpreted as devaluing direct client-service skills, which would be highly detrimental to older people who require optimum-level competence from those who care for them. In order to minimise these possible detrimental effects, regular intra-disciplinary communication and consultation must be maintained and field workers urged to represent their views, encouraged to innovate and act as agents of social change.

Organisational patterns at field level

At field level health visiting is usually organised on either a geographic basis, or attachment to a general practice. The relative merits and demerits of each method are well documented and each pattern has its ardent supporters. In each

case the total population served forms the unit for determining staff establishments, although actual case-loads
frequently relate to extrapolated age-groups.

Geographically-based health visiting

This is the traditional administrative pattern. Health visitors
relate to a population which is geographically defined, and
within such an area assume responsibility for the care of the
elderly, either within a generic or a specialist case-load.
Although not exclusively so, the pattern tends to be more
common in inner-city areas, where there are many single-
doctor practices and often a multiplicity of health and socio-
economic problems. In more rural areas where this pattern
prevails, the 'patch' covered by general practitioners, district
nurses and health visitors, may well coincide. This co-termi-
nosity of catchment areas encourages teamwork, and has very
many advantages for co-operation.

Those favouring this traditional method of working contend
that it allows health visitors to identify more strongly with a
particular neighbourhood, thus making it easier for them to
recognise the prevailing culture patterns and discover the
indigenous and informal networks which sustain the elderly.
This is of great significance when it is realised that over 75%
of all health problems are dealt with directly, on a self-care
or lay-care basis. Under this pattern health visitors are more
likely to become familiar neighbourhood figures; they can
enter readily into community development schemes and it is,
therefore, possible that they are approached more readily for
ad hoc advice and help. Drennan (1984) discusses how the
health visitor complements the work undertaken with family
units, by extending her practice with community groups. This
form of action may be easier when undertaken within clearly
demarcated boundaries, where communities of interest are
apparent.

Working within a circumscribed locality may also afford
opportunity to observe older people more regularly as they
go about their daily activities, either at home, during shopping, when they are visiting friends, or attending clubs and/or
community centres. Such informal and unobtrusive observation may prove invaluable. Health visitor practitioners iden-

tifying with a defined area may also find it easier to locate, and hence visit and liaise with, staff in sheltered housing schemes, day centres, or residential accommodation for the elderly. Such staff can provide valuable information which can subsequently affect care, and in return may welcome guidance on the care of some older people with whom they are jointly involved. This can reduce the risk of fragmented service, as well as overlapping care. Facilitating and supporting each other in this way can mean that differing workers in the field of care for the elderly act as encouragement for one another. It can also mean that they spur one another on to action, which may then benefit their elderly clients. However, there is often increased difficulty maintaining contact with a number of different general practitioners and nursing colleagues, so there is a risk of giving conflicting advice. Furthermore, in spite of alignment and liaison schemes it is possible for health visitors to become rather professionally isolated, both from peers and other professional colleagues. Sometimes in such circumstances there may be a tendency for work to assume a particular emphasis, without being challenged. Also older people may fail to benefit from the pooling of knowledge and resources that a team of workers can provide.

Nevertheless many health visitors enjoy this geographic pattern of delivering care. They forge close and necessary contacts with social workers, since these colleagues are mainly organised through area-based social services teams, and also become involved with staff in voluntary organisations concerned with the care of the elderly. Thus they can maintain their essential health education and supportive and caring roles. Moreover, proponents of this method argue that small area statistics can be obtained from the Office of Population, Censuses and Surveys, which relate more closely to geographic or administrative areas, than to specific medical practices. This could make it easier to scrutinise the mortality and morbidity data for specific age-sex and ethnic groups, by disease category, and hence obtain incidence and prevalence rates, which indicate the patterns of health and disease prevailing within the population. In this way it is possible for practitioners to obtain an average risk estimate, for particular conditions and then relate this to the 'younger elderly', the 'older elderly', and 'the very old' his then enables health visitors to identify priorities of need within each group, so that they can find out the action which needs to be taken, in conjunction with others, to reduce disease and/or disability.

The study of family history, positive or negative factors in personal health history, and past and present lifestyles, thus makes it possible to adjust quantitatively, the average risk for the particular group, and then obtain a probable risk for an individual. Advocates of this method then use such person-alised probability estimates, when undertaking personal health appraisals, so that individuals can be shown how they can reduce *their* risks and increase *their* well-being and the probability of *their* survival, if they so wish. Many prognostic categories are now well recognised, having been derived from a number of retrospective or prospective research studies, population surveys, actuarial findings from life insurance companies, professional reviews, reports and/or controlled experimental research. Of course such personalised preventive care can be offered under any administrative pattern, providing data is easily obtainable from which to work out probable personal risks.

Whilst this form of health promotion and disease preven-tion is currently receiving more attention in the United States and Canada than it is in Europe, some health visitors are interested in developing the method. They are referred to Hall & Zwemer (1979), and to Table 6.1. which sets out some prognostic categories for some causes of death, which are currently constituting major causes of mortality amongst older people. Although it should be appreciated that at present there is insufficient evidence to confirm that risk reduction necessarily increases life expectancy and/or fitness, the assumption appears eminently reasonable. It gives a basis for one-to-one and group health education, provided it is not so zealously practised that it generates excessive anxiety amongst older people. However, the evaluation of such activities presents a challenge to health visitors, and to all those who are engaged in preventive health care. Of course there are those who argue that it may be easier to develop such personalised preventive care programmes within the ambit of the general practice team setting, where more than one worker may be involved with the client.

Table 6.1 Some prognostic categories for certain major causes of death amongst older people

Cause of death	Prognostic categories — some identified risk factors
Accidents	
Home	Alcohol habits — increased intakes Drugs and medications Mobility problems Reduced sensory acuity Stress
Motor vehicle	Alcohol habits Drugs and medications Reduced reaction-time Mileage driven per year Seat belt use
Arterio-sclerotic heart disease	Raised blood pressure Raised cholesterol levels Diabetes mellitus Exercise habits (reduced activity) Family history Smoking habits Weight — obesity
Cancer	
Breast	Family history Personal history of benign breast disease Pregnancy history Non-use of self-examination
Colon and/or rectum	Family history Prior polyp Undiagnosed rectal bleeding
Lung	Smoking habits
Uterus	Undiagnosed vaginal bleeding (post menopausal)
Cerebrovascular accidents	Raised blood pressure High cholesterol levels Diabetes mellitus Exercise habits (reduced activity) Smoking habits
Respiratory disease	
Bronchitis/ emphysema	Smoking history Occupational history
Pneumonia	Personal history of bacterial pneumonia Alcohol habits Smoking habits

Based on data derived from:

DHSS 1981, Prevention and health: avoiding heart attacks. HMSO, London

Donaldson R J, Donaldson L J 1983 Essential community medicine. MTP Press, Lancaster, p 61–164

Geller-Gesner Tables In: Hall J H, Zwemer J D (eds) 1979 Prospective medicine. Department of Medical Education, Methodist Hospital of Indiana, USA

Meanwhile, a number of the innovatory forms of care with older people are being developed by those who are working in geographic settings, frequently those health visitors who are specialising in geriatric, or rather, gerontological practice (Day 1981, Kewley 1983). Some of the most imaginative schemes being developed are brought about by those who are carrying out geriatric liaison duties, with hospitals staffs and those working in residential accommodation for the elderly. There is clearly much scope for work with the elderly in geographic placement.

General practice based health visiting

Under this system health visitors relate to a population who have registered with a general practitioner, or a group practice. Such schemes have been in existence since the mid-1950s and those who introduced them were enthusiastic about their potential. Since 1974 this pattern has been preferred DHSS policy (DHSS 1976, 1977). The teams, which are sometimes called primary health care teams, have been defined as:

> inter-dependent groups of general practitioners, secretaries, and/or receptionists, district nurses, health visitors, and sometimes practice nurses, and social workers and specialist staff such as community psychiatric nurses, who share a common purpose and responsibility . . . pooling their resources to provide an effective primary health care service.
>
> Harding Report, DHSS 1981

The beliefs underlying this pattern of work include the following:

1. Augmented care is potentially more comprehensive and continuing than that given by individuals.
2. Resources within teams are likely to be used more economically and rare skills utilised more appropriately.
3. Standards of care are likely to be raised, through discussion, informal learning and peer group influence.
4. Working together is likely to improve communication, raise members' morale, foster inter-dependence and encourage co-ordinated care.
5. Diversifying talents and skills is likely to increase job satisfaction.

6. Working together enables team members to deepen their awareness of their own roles, and respect and acknowledge the roles of others.

Although these ideals are sound, and many persons have argued logically and keenly for them, not all general practice based teams function at this level. Many health visitors have expressed considerable disquiet about this matter and other workers also appear somewhat disenchanted with the concept. There are several reasons for some holding less positive views. A number of teams have been brought into being without adequate preparation. Not all members have had prior consultation before the schemes were introduced, so not everyone has necessarily been committed to the concept. Environments have not always been conducive to collaborative work. Essential 'tools' such as age-sex registers, vulnerability indices and cross-referencing systems have not always been made available. The different premises underlying professional activity have not always been explored and acknowledged. Merely placing people together in an administrative structure does not constitute a 'team', and many so grouped are still discovering that the powerful forces mobilised within groups can have positive or negative effects, and that 'pulling together' is an art to be learned, often through conflict and disequilibrium, (Lonsdale et al, 1980, Dingwall 1982).

Improving the chances of team success

In an analysis of the advantages and disadvantages of teamwork one health visitor has identified some common barriers which stand in the way of effective team functioning (Hunt 1983):

- educational preparation of team members
- role ambiguity and incongruent expectations
- status differentials
- authority and power structures
- leadership styles.

Because teamwork is essential for the achievement of certain health and social services goals, particularly with the elderly, the acceptance of such barriers as 'inevitable' and the conclusion 'that teams do not work' would clearly be inappropriate. In consequence those interested in developing high level collaborative care for vulnerable goups such as older people, will doubtless wish to consider those factors which have been consistently identified as contributing towards effective team functioning. Not unexpectedly these include the following:

a. The equality of all team members should be recognised, all being regarded as partners in care; members of a whole range of services, all of whom may at different times serve as a point of first contact, or be the most appropriate person for consultation or referral.

b. Roles should be clarified so that they can be respected and recognised, mutual acknowledgement being made. Where role expectations are not clearly defined and communicated, role ambiguity, role conflict and sometimes role overload can occur. To avoid unnecessary waste of energy, role negotiation should be used to deal with any role difficulties. It is important that each team member feels confident in her own role, as well as appreciating her role limitations.

c. Team goals should be mutually determined. They should be clear, relevant and feasible. Each member should understand and assent to such team aims and objectives and should know what she has to do to achieve them.

d. Time must be made for talking together on both a formal and an informal basis. This is helped if members are housed under one roof; if meetings are scheduled; if feedback and interaction are encouraged; if leadership is apparent but not dominant; and if everyone recognises that re-negotiation is a continuous process.

e. Team members should be prepared to be flexible with roles, allowing working practices to sometimes overlap. However, this does *not* mean that roles are interchangeable.

f. Team members should have a firm commitment to the team and an understanding of team concepts.

Helpful activities are the sharing of post-basic education courses and in-service study and training. Many colleges have attempted to integrate learning between health visitors and social workers since the late 1960s. More recently with the move of district nurse and school nurse courses into Colleges of Higher Education, such shared learning has been extended. However, whilst learning together has done much to disabuse stereotypes and make for clearer understanding of roles and relationships, it would be unwise not to recognise the difficulties. Students sometimes have difficulty achieving role elucidation during education and training, because of their restricted knowledge of practice aspects. Learning is accomplished through building on the known and moving through to the unknown, therefore theory must be constantly related to practice before it becomes meaningful.

It is during the period of supervised practice when much assimilation and enlightenment is achieved and this is often the time when opportunities for shared discussion no longer exist. This suggests that students would probably benefit from a longer period of supervised practice, during which time they continued joint study days in order to have multi-disciplinary discussion. During this time they would be exposed to the intricacies of team care and would learn more about professional relationships. Another difficulty is that trainee general practitioners are rarely involved in joint learning in College courses. This places more onus on field work teachers, practical work teachers and trainers within general practice, to bring their respective students together in the working situation, in order that they may learn from each other.

Since the late 1960s there have been noteworthy attempts at the formal level to promote inter-professional learning. The Council for the Education and Training of Health Visitors, The Royal College of General Practitioners, The Council for the Education and Training in Social Work, and The Panel of Assessors in District Nursing promoted many joint conferences and seminars which stimulated local initiatives in co-operation in care. Even more emphasis on full inter-disciplinary education is envisaged in future (United Kingdom Joint Professional Committee for Primary Health Care 1983).

Nevertheless if older people are to benefit fully from the activities of the general practice based team, it requires highly motivated team members who are determined to create effective working groups.

The role of doctor in general practice

As the administrative setting relates to the practice population, the medical role is considered first, though this does *not* imply precedence. In fact, within the team, leadership should be shared, being varied in relation to particular goals. Doctors bring a wealth of clinical knowledge to the team. In the course of any one year they are likely to have contact with some 70% of the elderly who are registered with them and in consequence are in a strong position to carry out opportunistic as well as planned health education and practice prevention at all three levels. Furthermore they may well come across health and social problems requiring referral to other team members, who can more appropriately deal with them. Until fairly recently much of their medical training led them to perceive themselves as the first and probably the only entry for NHS care.

Much prescribed medical care is delegated to nurses in hospital, and in consequence they were unused to the idea that other workers, such as health visitors, district nurses, community psychiatric nurses or social workers might be the first point of client contact. For this reason many of them have had to unlearn notions about other workers being merely an extension of medical activity, in order to appreciate what they can offer and hence utilise this appropriately. Not all general practitioners are preventive-minded, and do not necessarily understand the difference between primary *health* work and medical activity. However, this is likely to change, as since 1981 it has been mandatory for all doctors entering general practice to have undergone 3 years post-registration vocational training, during which there is an educational emphasis on socio-medical aspects of care. This move away from the perception of the general practitioner as largely a reactive worker, has been given impetus by a Report emphasising prevention and anticipatory care (Royal College of General Practitioners 1983).

About 50% of all general practitioners work in group practices of between 2 and 10 members; some 20% are currently housed in health centres. Although when in group practice a senior partner wil be recognised, the autonomous and horizontal-type medical administration makes it difficult for some doctors to understand the vertical structure of nursing. This can sometimes create problems.

The majority of doctors have between 2000 and 2500 persons of all ages registered with them. Within such an average practice, approximately 350 persons would be aged 65 years or more, with approximately 120 of these being over the age of 75 years. In some areas of retirement choice, such as the south coast resorts, the proportion of older persons to younger ones may be very much higher, sometimes reaching 35–40% of the total practice population.

Unlike other team members, general practitioners are not state-salaried employees. They have a contractual arrangement with Family Practitioner Committees to provide a general medical service over a 24-hour period, daily throughout the year. As clinical medical specialists within a general practice setting they therefore have heavy clinico-legal responsibilities and, given present patterns of consultation over all age groups, are unlikely to be able to spend more than an average of 6 minutes with each person. This is a factor to be borne in mind, when realising that the very old are likely to require more frequent home visiting than other age groups, which likely entails extra travelling time. Furthermore the non-specific presentation of illness, which is a common feature of old age, may require longer time for diagnosis.

From Table 6.2 and Figure 6.1. it will be seen that on average 16% of the elderly aged 65–74 years and 19% of those aged 75 years and over, consult their doctor over a fortnight period, with the average pattern of consultation for each

Table 6.2 Average patterns of consultation with general practitioner by sex and age, 1982

Age groups (years)	No. of consultations per person per year		
	Males	Females	Total
0–4	7.2	6.4	6.8
5–15	3.0	3.0	3.0
16–44	2.2	5.2	3.7
45–64	4.1	5.1	4.6
65–74	4.9	5.5	5.3
75+	6.3	6.0	6.1
Average over all age groups	3.5	5.0	4.3

Reprinted from General Household Survey 1982. HMSO, London

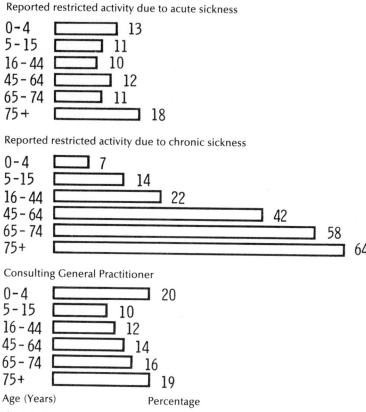

Reported restricted activity due to acute sickness

Reported restricted activity due to chronic sickness

Consulting General Practitioner

Age (Years)   Percentage

Fig. 6.1 Comparative picture of reported illness and the use of general practitioner services, within a 2-week period during 1982 (Based on data from The General Household Survey 1982.)

person being 5.7 per annum. Although the elderly are heavier utilisers of their doctor's services than most other age groups except very young children, their pattern of illness varies, with acute sickness occurring more frequently in the older group, but much restricted activity being due to chronic sickness. Caring for those with chronic illness and disability can be more challenging than dealing with acute and specific conditions, which are frequently self-limiting. It may also carry less job satisfaction, reminding doctors of their limitations and frustrating their efforts to cure. Familiarity with persons who have complaints of long standing may sometimes blunt one's perceptions of what might be done to help them, so it is

important for other team members to recognise these difficulties which doctors may face, and to support and encourage
them to provide more innovative forms of care. However, in
spite of this heavy work-load with older people and the
constant demands of other age groups, some general practitioners have initiated regular sessions for checking the health
of their apparently well elderly patients, by carrying out joint
programmes with district nurses and health visitors (Williams
et al 1972), Barber & Wallis (1976, 1982). In company with
many other studies these workers found a high incidence of
unreported need.

The role of district nurse

Over 60% of the work-load of district nurses is concerned
with the care of the elderly. As skilled independent practitioners they are:

> responsible for identifying the needs of patients in their own homes, and
> planning and providing appropriate programmes of nursing care. They
> advise patients and their families about the physical, emotional and social
> aspects of care, and assist in the promotion and maintenance of health
> by education and preventive techniques.
>
> Hockey Report: SHHD 1978

Thus, although their duties are largely oriented towards symptomatic and rehabilitative care, district nurses are increasingly
involved in preventive geriatric services, in the promotion of
self-help and the maintenance of optimum physical and
mental activity amongst persons in later life. Kratz (1980)
discusses the nature of district nursing functions within multi-
disciplinary teams, pointing out the opportunities which exist
for both role expansion and role extension. Furthermore it is
also important to realise that district nurses also work in
district nursing teams, with registered district nurses heading
up the work of enrolled district nurses, nursing auxiliaries
and/or bath attendants. Like ward sisters, registered district
nurses carry out assessment, planning, implementing and
evaluation activities. In addition to their clinical and supervi-
sory work they also liaise with hospital and residential homes
staff, and with a range of statutory and voluntary personnel.

Since 1982 the district nursing qualification has been
mandatory for all practising district nurses. Courses covering

an expanded curriculum have been sited within institutes of higher education, alongside health visiting, community psychiatric nursing and school nursing and social work courses. Already there is some evidence that this new form of preparation is generating enthusiasm, with students and qualifying staff, 'exercising their professional initiative and taking responsibility for maintaining standards of care' (Battle & Salter 1984).

The recommended ratio of district nursing staff to practice population is 1 per 2500. This also allows for a ratio of 1 district nurse to 1 general practitioner. At present, however, district nurses are carrying far heavier population case-loads than those recommended and the average ratio of district nursing staff of all grades to general practitioners is 1–1.7. Approximately 72% of district nurses when asked reported 'good' or 'very good' relationships with general practitioners. Where disquiet was expressed nurses were most concerned about a lack of reciprocity in relationships (Dunnell & Dobbs 1982, Phillipson & Strang 1984). However, some observers have expressed concern that this reasonably high level of reported rapport may be sometimes brought about by the acceptance of a more subordinate role.

Although the work of district nurses and health visitors may occasionally overlap, particularly with the elderly, the roles are distinct and complementary, as was recognised by the Briggs Report (Committee on Nursing 1972). Over 80% of district nurses report good rapport with health visitors, although this can represent superficial relationships, marked by an absence of conflict, which may not always be to the benefit of the team, or to elderly clients. Where good rapport exists there is likely to be greater co-operation. The true partnership of district nurses and health visitors can result in great strength, so that the elderly within the practice can be assured, not only of competent clinical nursing care when sick, but surveillance, support, sustaining and protection, as well as health education and preventive care, when well.

Within her work it is likely the district nurse will spend a high proportion of her time with elderly persons who have been referred to her from general practitioners, social workers, hospital staffs, wardens in sheltered housing and staff in residential establishments for older people. For some there will be a large element of prescribed care; in other cases there will be considerable scope for nursing initiative. Moreover she is more likely to be caring for those who are heavily dependent and for the very old. She is also involved in the care of the elderly who are terminally ill. Both district nurses and health visitors have a role in supporting and caring for relatives and family members, especially where these lay-carers are also elderly. However, district nurses are more likely to discover those who are caring for the severely handi-capped, the more disabled, less mobile or acutely sick elderly.

Like health visitors, district nurses often express their frus-tration over the lack of sufficient back-up services and the ever-increasing size of their case-loads, without necessarily matching resources. It is important therefore for health visi-tors to realise the physically demanding nature of the work, as well as the interpersonal, educative and organisational skills which district nurses must exercise. In this way they can facilitate their colleagues. Those wishing to examine further the role of district nurse within the primary health care team, particularly in relation to the care of the elderly, are referred to Illing & Donovan (1981), Baly (1981), and Kratz (1982).

The role of health visitor

Facets of the role of the health visitor with the elderly have already been discussed, but as the team's chief primary prevention worker, she too has a distinctive contribution to make. The strength of the health visitor's input lies in the continuity of her contact with families in both health and disease, and in the versatility of her duties, although unless great care is exercised the latter may constitute a weakness.

The functions of the health visitor have been generally defined as:

- prevention of mental, physical and emotional ill-health and its consequences
- early detection of ill-health and the surveillance of high risk groups
- recognition and identification of need, with the mobilisa-tion of appropriate resources where necessary

- health teaching
- provision of care: this includes support during periods of stress and advice and guidance in cases of illness, as well as in the care and management of children.

The health visitor, is however, not actively engaged in technical nursing procedures.

CETHV 1967

Whilst not all of these functions apply to the elderly, most do. Critics of this pattern of field-work organisation argue that the health visitor, who is general practice based, increases the secondary and tertiary prevention components of her role to the detriment of primary prevention. They see a possibility of a shift of emphasis within her work, towards the medical model, instead of the health-related model which best befits her. Conversely, those who are proponents of the general practice based pattern, point to the deepening of the role which can occur where the health visiting practitioner has access to all age groups. They emphasise the scope for health promotion and disease prevention, which a well-run practice can offer. Where mortality and morbidity statistics are available for the practice population, it is possible to carry out epidemiological investigations, as with a geographic placement, and to apply the search principle to the identification of health needs amongst the elderly clients, who do not necessarily refer themselves. Of course age-sex registers which are kept up-to-date are essential tools for this task, but not all general practitioners recognise this and therefore do not always co-operate in making them available. It must be acknowledged, however, that not everyone registers with a general practitioner, and that, therefore, some of the most vulnerable members of society may be 'lost', unless flexibility can be extended in the provision of care. This is one reason why it is so essential that any health visitor who is general practice based, maintains a community dimension to her role.

Nevertheless, there is evidence which suggests that the self-initiating nature of the health visitor's work, and the major educative thrust she adopts, may be less readily understood than the more overtly displayed clinical skills of doctors and nurses, who tend to share activities more often, within the framework of the medical model. In consequence facets of the role, such as client-advocate, or community health worker, may be less readily perceived. Research shows that the different value bases between doctors, nurses and health visitors may be an important contributory factor in explaining the varied perceptions and expectations of the team (Gilmore et al, 1974, Dingwall & McIntosh 1978).

Another factor which may affect relationships, is the lower ratio of health visitors to doctors. Currently this stands at 1:2.4 nationally, which means that health visitors cannot always give sufficient time to deepening rapport, or expanding their role within the practice team, however much they might wish to do so. Moreover, there is some evidence to suggest that health visitors generally tend to prefer scheduled team meetings, in addition to ad hoc and informal contact, so that team goals can be mutually determined and evaluated, as well as team problems discussed. Doctors and district nurses, on the other hand tend to rely more on informal contact (Gilmore et al 1974).

Within the team all members have a mutual responsibility to support their colleagues and help them derive the utmost benefit from team membership. As health promoters health visitors have a particular interest in identifying the ways in which other team members may be facilitated. Applied to the care of the elderly, this means becoming conversant with the volume of colleagues' work-loads; appreciating their expectations and aspirations; recognising their disappointments and frustrations and respecting their methods of work and their goals of care. In this way health visitors can act as enablers.

Because case-finding and surveillance is such a strong feature of the role of the health visitor within general practice settings, this topic is dealt with separately, later in the chapter. It forms a major example of team activity. Other main health visiting tasks stem from the many referrals which are increasingly made by the families of older persons, as well as by voluntary services personnel and colleagues in other statutory services. Some health visitors have also established consultation sessions within normal 'surgery' hours, so that those who wish for help can gain easy access to them. Such sessions also allow doctors to refer their patients for health visiting help, during their one visit. Whilst supportive home visits and health teaching are given to elderly clients direct, and/or to their families who care for them, a large element is also concerned with educating community groups. Particularly close liaison is necessary with community psychiatric nurses, who may be providing specific follow-up care for those elderly persons who have experienced psychiatric illness. Caring for the mentally frail is however a marked component of health visiting.

Dealing with socio-economic difficulties which older people frequently experience, is another role aspect. Whilst many of these problems can be handled through discussion within the family context, others may require referral to a range of different colleagues. There is thus a wide-spread role set. Possibly the care of the elderly is one of the main areas for health visiting and social work co-operation, and the degree of contact may be considerably enhanced when health visitors are able to carry out their case finding work, through the medium of the age sex register.

The role of social worker

In some districts social workers also form part of the nuclear team within general practice, although they still remain members of their own area social work team. Whilst they continue to have responsibility for a range of recreational and social facilities for the elderly, such as the provision of clubs, places in Day Centres, recuperative holidays, short-term admissions and accommodation within residential homes, their contribution also includes support and counselling for those clients who are blind, deaf and/or physically handicapped, mentally disturbed or in danger of physical and/or mental abuse. They are thuse valuable resources in any scheme of health and social care for older people.

Ford (1980) points out that the main contribution of social workers lies in dealing with social relationship problems which may or may not relate to medical conditions. Clare & Corney (1982) and Rowlings (1981) have given notable accounts of their work, which tends to increase with the elderly when they are attached to health centres. Like their colleagues, social workers and their assistants face many pressures, so that much of their work also becomes crisis intervention.

Several writers have suggested historical reasons for a relatively low priority social workers have with the elderly, but a more pragmatic reason may be that they have many statutory duties with other age groups, particularly in the field of child care. In consequence they have not always been able to devote the time to older people which demographic trends indicate they should. Goldberg & Connelly (1982), whilst critical, suggest that there are signs of more imaginative involvement with older age groups, particularly in relation to admissions and discharges from hospital, mobilising resources, conducting assessments, providing direct case work and dealing with social problems within family settings.

Relationships between social workers and other members of the general practice team have sometimes been rather uneasy, but joint education is helping to improve this situation. Although there may at times be some fear of overlap between the roles of health visitor and social worker, they are in fact complementary. Whilst at present it would be euphoric to infer dramatic changes of emphasis in a service which has limited resources in relation to the demands made upon it, there are signs that social work is developing both a preventive dimension and an increase in community work. Thus in future both health visitors and social workers can look forward to increasing co-operation in the development of self-help groups, group counselling and pre-retirement preparation. It does, however, require a very positive effort to be made by all team members in promoting conditions in which constructive relationships can flourish, so that the quality of life for older people can be improved. Within the closer contact of the general practice team it may possibly be easier to achieve this.

Some impression of the current demands made by the elderly on certain health and social services is shown in Table 6.3. It will be noted that as with district nursing and health visiting, the percentage of persons using certain social work services increases steadily with rising age (Crosbie 1983, Marshall 1983).

The wider team

There are many others with whom the nuclear team must liaise

Table 6.3 Use of some health and social services by elderly persons, within a 1 month period prior to interview for the General Household Survey, percentages shown by sex and age

Services used	Sex	Age groups using services (%)				
		65–69	70–74	75–79	80–84	85+
District nurse or health visitor	M	2	4	4	11	12
	F	2	4	11	15	18
NHS Chiropodist	M	3	5	8	8	8
	F	4	8	15	14	18
Home help	M	2	3	2	15	15
	F	2	5	14	21	30
Luncheon clubs	M	2	3	2	2	6
	F	2	3	4	8	9
Day Centre	M	2	3	4	2	6
	F	4	5	7	5	8
Meals-on-wheels	M	1	1	1	5	5
	F	1	1	2	3	11

Data obtained from General Household Survey 1982. HMSO, London

if they wish to offer a comprehensive programme of care to the elderly. These include community-based psychiatric staff; consultant geriatricians and hospital nurses in geriatric settings; nurse specialists such as those involved with stoma care or care of the terminally ill; occupational, speech and physiotherapists; health education officers, home helps and those in day and residential units catering for the elderly. Whilst in some areas health care planning teams have developed, there is much greater scope for collaboration and joint planning in future.

SCREENING AND SURVEILLANCE WITHIN THE TEAM SETTING

Screening of the elderly began shortly after the Second World War when Sheldon (1948), using the ration card register as a means of identification, interviewed a random sample of old people in their homes in Wolverhampton to assess their physical and mental status. He found a high proportion of unmet needs, with locomotor, dental, hearing and visual problems predominating. Mental health and general levels of nutrition were, however, quite good. Anderson & Cowan (1955) also examined persons who were able to attend a health centre near Glasgow. They found many had obesity, hypertension, pain and dyspnoea of effort, all the more noteworthy since their group were ambulant and motivated to attend the sessions. Later Williamson and his colleagues (1964) carried out a full physical and psychiatric examination of elderly persons in three general practices in Scotland, and demonstrated the frequency of multiple disabilities. Men had a mean of 3.26 problems, of which 1.87 were unknown to their general practitioners, whilst women had 3.42 problems, of which 2.03 were also unknown. Problems included poor mobility, visual and hearing defects, heart and gastrointestinal conditions, and disabilities of the respiratory, central nervous and urinary systems. They also found a high incidence of psychiatric morbidity, including a 10% incidence of depression, with half the cases unknown to their general practitioners. This high proportion of unreported illness has been subsequently confirmed by several studies, including Barber & Wallis (1976) and Abrams (1978, 1980).

Unreported illness has thus become known as 'the iceberg of morbidity', with the submerged portion of the iceberg showing a characteristic pattern, with the bulk of 'unknown' conditions being urinary tract disorders, locomotor difficulties, foot problems, dementia and depression. It is clear, therefore, that as self-referral of the elderly is insufficient to ensure comprehensive health coverage, some system of earlier detection must be instituted, if diagnosis and treatment are to be offered, and crisis situations avoided. This of course assumes that if disorders or disease states are identified and treated, the person will ultimately benefit — a belief inherent in the medical model which some have questioned (Luker 1981).

In earlier life the application of secondary prevention methods in the form of screening may lead to early detection and possible cure. However, in old age there is less scope for cure, so the emphasis must rest on the implications of the detected conditions for physical, mental and social functioning. For this reason there has been an attempt recently to differentiate between '**screening**' and '**case-finding**'.

'Screening' is defined as

> the seeking out of persons with *no* overt symptoms, and asking them to undergo examination to see if any disease is present.
>
> DHSS 1976

'Case-finding' is considered to be

the detection of overt but unacknowledged or disregarded symptoms.
Williamson 1981

Both of these activities may be used for the elderly, although the latter is more common.

Some attempt to identify pre-symptomatic disease *is* carried out for older people, such as biochemical assays of thyroid function, or blood glucose. Sometimes multiphasic studies are made, but while such biochemical profiles of elderly may show unsuspected disease, there is little correlation between the results and subsequent causes of death (Murray & Young 1977). Some of the problems in identifying pre-symptomatic disease stem from difficulties in determining 'normality'. For instance, screening for anaemia, which is defined as a value less than 12 g/Hb/100 ml, is of limited use, since vascular and psychomotor symptoms do not appear until values of about 8 g/Hb/100 ml are reached. Similarly, in screening for hypertension, there are difficulties in deciding what levels of systolic pressure to accept as 'normal', and then in determining how best to treat elderly persons who are symptom-free. Drug-induced hypotension can itself lead to poor cerebral perfusion and subsequent problems. Furthermore, many biochemical values derived from population studies have been obtained from younger groups, and have less applicability to older people, amongst whom only limited investigations have been conducted.

'Reference values' for many biochemical and haemotological variables are therefore not yet known for the elderly, although an important subsidiary aim of the 1972/73 and 1977/78 Nutrition Surveys, sponsored by the DHSS, was to try to establish these (Exton-Smith 1981). However, this does not mean that screening should *not* be underaken for the elderly; rather that it should be regarded with caution, with the understanding that it is more problematic. On the other hand screening for hearing loss or visual impairment, such as glaucoma or cataract, appears eminently worthwhile.

Since health visitors frequently undertake certain forms of screening in their own work, as well as participating in screening programmes with others, they should be aware of the underlying principles, otherwise much time, trouble and expense may be used to little effect. Almost 20 years ago, validation of tests showed that health visitors could detect physical disabilities efficiently and psychiatric morbidity moderately well (Williamson, Lowther & Gray 1966). Since then, improved education in the field of mental health and gerontology, should have considerably enhanced their skills.

The principles of screening

The principles of screening relate to the disease; to the test to be applied; and to the proposed treatment. The disease or condition to be searched for should be an important health poblem, for both the individual and the community. Its natural history, including its development from the latent to the manifest stage, should be fully known. Factors should be identified which will determine response to treatment.

Screening tests should be, simple, acceptable, accurate, cost-effective, precise, sensitive and specific (Donaldson & Donaldson 1983). Tests which involve simple observation, with little or no undressing, such as tests of hearing, sight, or venepuncture, are more likely to be associated with a high degree of co-operation, whereas painful and time-consuming tests are less likely to be accepted.

The cost of a screening programme must be related to the benefit expected to follow from early detection of any disease. The test must be precise, and give reliable, consistent results. For example the problem of obtaining reliable blood pressure readings, due to subject and observer factors, are well known.

Screening tests must also be sensitive and specific. Sensitivity means the ability of the test to give positive results in clients with the disease being screened for. Specificity, however, means the ability of the test to give negative results, in healthy individuals without that disease. Ideally the screening tests should give true positives and true negatives only, i.e. both specificity and sensitivity will be 100% each. However, this will only be achieved when the normal and the diseased populations are widely separated according to the test used (Fig. 6.2). Unfortunately, in real life, the situation is seldom so clear-cut, because the normal and diseased populations have test values which overlap. Consider, for example,

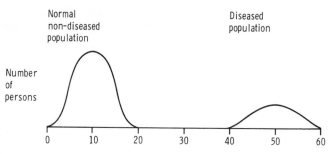

Fig. 6.2 Hypothetical screening test

the measurement of intra-ocular pressure in order to screen for simple glaucoma, where there is an over-lap between people with non-glaucomatous eyes and those with glaucomatous eyes (Fig. 6.3).

Those with intra-ocular pressure values below 22 mmHg will all have normal eyes. Those with values above 26 mmHg will all have glaucomatous eyes. However, for those with values of between 22–26 mmHg it is not possible to say to which group a particular person belongs. The degree of sensitivity and specificity of the test will be varied depending on which screening value is chosen. Thus if the values of 26 mmHg and over are used the test is 100% specific. All persons with

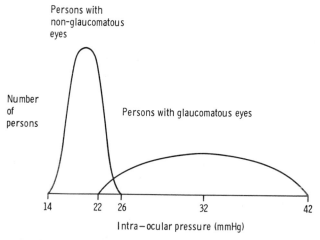

Fig. 6.3 Specificity and sensitivity of tests for simple glaucoma, (hypothetical values)

normal eyes will be excluded and, therefore, there are no false positives.

However, this is at the expense of excluding some people with values of 22 mmHg, or more, but below 26 mmHg, who *may* have glaucomatous eyes, and who therefore, form a 'false' negative group. Conversely if the value is set at 22 mmHg and above, the test becomes 100% sensitive. All the persons with abnormal eyes have been included, but this is at the expense of including a few people with normal eyes, who now form a 'false' positive group. Clearly, very careful judgment has to be exercised in determining the values which will be used for demarcation purposes, so that individuals are not 'missed cases' on the one hand, nor exposed to needless anxiety and the risk of hypochondria on the other.

There is little point in screening persons for any condition, unless the treatment for the condition is available, acceptable and can influence the course and prognosis of the disease in a favourable direction. This is of paramount importance with the elderly. A high detection rate can swamp existing treatment facilities, causing frustration and distress. Curiously enough, perhaps, some persons who have agreed to be screened may refuse the treatment offered. For instance, some clients have refused chiropody, and others oral iron therapy for anaemia. Follow-up surveys after screening studies have shown reductions in the number of disabilities, though the effect on the quality of life has not been indicated. However, it is interesting to note that a trial of multiphasic screening of middle-aged persons in South-East London found that 9 years after the initial screening there was no significant difference between the control and the screened groups in any of the measures of outcome (South-East London Screening Study Group 1977).

The organisation of screening and case-finding in general practice

Programmes of detection, based on general practice, are very effective ways of recruiting clients, since studies have shown a response rate of some 80–90%. Possibly this is because older people are more aware of the value of health. However, it is also important to consider the vulnerable section of the population who are non-responders. Before embarking on such programmes, the aims and objectives of the exercise should be clarified. All team members should be committed to the idea, since it has been shown that work-loads increase considerably, at least initially, and particularly for the nurse members and health visitors (Barber & Wallis 1978).

It is essential to decide beforehand what will be done about any disabilities found; who will carry out which particular activity; who is responsible for ensuring that action actually occurs; and what criteria will be used to evaluate process and outcomes. Where decisions made by the team will have implications for others, e.g. laboratory technicians, it is essential that they are involved in early planning, or schemes may be wrecked and relationships jeopardised. Sessions may be arranged at a health centre, clinic, surgery, day centre, residential accommodation or in the client's own home. Adequate time must be allowed to put clients at ease, conduct necessary tests, provide for record-keeping, give associated health teaching and ensure reciprocal communication. Most teams arrange for health histories to be taken beforehand.

Many teams concentrate on the groups of older persons assumed to be at highest risk. These vulnerable groups have been identified by several writers and researchers, including Williamson (1981). The Black Report also stressed social class-related inequalities in health, thus indicating vulnerability (DHSS 1980). Table 6.4 gives the commonly accepted list, as priority-rated by Taylor et al (1983). However, it should be noted that these researchers found these categories *less* efficient as an identifying tool than initial screening letter, as described by Barber & Wallis (1976 — details given below).

Case-finding programmes usually follow six stages:

Stage 1 Identification of clients
Vulnerable clients are discovered using the chosen reference-frame, such as an age-sex register or vulnerability index.

Stage 2 Initial assessment
This is often conducted by the health visitor, sometimes using a client self-administered mental and physical health status questionnaire. It may include taking a health history and will include subjective and objective ratings. These will seek to

Table 6.4 Potential high risks groups among elderly persons, ranked in piority order

Category 1 Elderly potentially at highest risk
Divorced/separated
Recently discharged from hospital
Recently moved/relocated
The very old (80+)

Category 2 Elderly potentially at medium risk
Recently widowed
Living alone
Poor
Social class V category

Category 3 Elderly potentially at lowest risk
Isolated persons
Single persons
Childless

Based upon data given by Taylor R, Ford G, Barber H 1983 The elderly at risk. Research Perspectives on Ageing, 6: Age Concern Research Unit, Mitcham

determine presenting problems if any; levels of functional ability; simple tests of hearing and vision; and information about socio-economic and environmental circumstances.

Most health visitors adopt a scoring method for determining levels of the client's functional ability and independence: this may include ranking on either a 'health' or an 'independence' continuum.

Record cards should be systematic, easy to complete and preferably in a form suitable for computerization.

Stage 3 Follow-up assessment
An examination by the general practitioner is then arranged. Blood tests and other clinical procedures deemed relevant are carried out. District nurses often participate in these tests.

Stage 4 Planning care
Standard care plans are then related to clients'/patients' needs, and individualised. Programmes of action are devised with client consent and participation, depending on the findings of the examination, and any screening conducted.

Stage 5 Implementation of planned programmes
Where defects are found, specific treatments will likely be offered. Action should be monitored at each stage to check that it is goal-related. Surveillance will almost certainly be

continued, even if no specific disorders are discovered. Health education will be related to findings, and to relative risks client may run (Table 6.1).

Stage 6 Evaluation
Specific pre-determined criteria should be used to determine client/patient outcomes, as well as appraise the processes used. Where screening has been incorporated, the 'detected' group may be longer-term evaluated against the 'control' group.

An alternative approach to detecting vulnerable elderly

With the resources now available, screening and case-finding on the comprehensive basis just described, whilst probably desirable, may pose difficulties for some general practice based teams. If such programmes are to realise their potential they must be ongoing. However, with the many other demands made upon staff, they may be sacrificed to expediency or pared to a minimum; this often means they then become ineffectual. In consequence, some teams have reverted solely to the use of opportunistic screening and case-finding, which defeats the purpose of a comprehensive preventive service, which depends upon surveying the whole field at risk. A simple and quick method of detecting those elderly persons most likely to benefit from health visitor assessment and subsequent general practitioner examination would therefore prove helpful.

One team has devised a method which was been successfully used in a Glasgow practice, at Woodside Health Centre (Barber & Wallis 1976, 1978, and Barber et al 1980). They use a simple postal questionnaire as a basis for further investigation and follow-up (Table 6.5). When tested the questionnaire was found to have a response rate of 81%, a sensitivity of 0.95, and a specificity of 0.68. The predictive value was 0.91. Thus any person answering 'Yes' to any of the questions would be given priority in subsequent assessment. It is estimated by these researchers that the use of this procedure reduces the workload of assessment by 20%.

This approach represents one tried method of helping teams tackle the difficult question of where to begin with the

Table 6.5 Postal questionnaire as sent out to selected high risk groups of elderly from Woodside Health Centre, Glasgow (accompanying letter not shown)

Name
Address

	Please circle the answer applicable to you	
e.g. Do you live on your own?	Yes	No
Do you live on your own?	Yes	No
Are you in the position of having *no* relatives on whom you can rely on for help?	Yes	No
Do you need regular help with housework or shopping?	Yes	No
Are there days when you are unable to prepare a hot meal for yourself?	Yes	No
Are you confined to your home through ill health?	Yes	No
Is there any difficulty or concern over your health you still have to see about?	Yes	No
Do you have any problem with your eyes or eyesight?	Yes	No
Do you have any difficulty with your hearing?	Yes	No
Have you been in hospital during the past year?	Yes	No

Thank you for answering these questions. Would you please return this form to me at the surgery? A stamped addressed envelope is enclosed.

Reproduced by kind permission of Dr J H Barber and Miss J Wallis H V

systematic screening, case-finding, assessment and surveillance of elderly persons.

SUMMARY

This chapter began with a consideration of some organisational patterns for the delivery of health care for the elderly. After briefly contrasting geographic and general practice team based health visiting, the emphasis has been towards the structure, function and dynamics of the latter team, as the officially 'preferred' pattern of administration. The respective contributions of some team members have been discussed in the light of prevailing patterns of reported illness, consultation trends and the use made of health and social services. The merits of screening and/or case-finding for the elderly have been considered, against recognised principles and as a prelude to surveillance, treatment and care. Some pointers concerning the organisation of such screening and/or case finding programmes have been outlined, including reference to one practical and research-tested approach, which appears to facilitate identification of vulnerable elderly. Whilst mention has been made of research findings which show the effectiveness of health visitors in assessment and identification of recognised and unacknowledged health needs of the elderly, the need for improved education, especially in relation to psychiatric care and the developmental stages of ageing, must be stressed. Furthermore the qualitative aspects of care, through health screening and surveillance of the older practice population, have not yet been established, and this represents a challenge to each member of the general practice team. Whilst emphasising the need for health visitors to retain a community dimension to their role in general practice, the main tenor of this chapter has been the need for positive attitudes and collaboration in care for the elderly.

REFERENCES

Abrams M 1978 Beyond three score years and ten. First Report on a Survey of the Elderly. Age Concern, Mitcham

Abrams M 1980 Beyond three score years and ten. Second Report on a Survey of the Elderly. Age Concern, Mitcham

Anderson W F, Cowan N R 1955 A consultative health centre for older people. Lancet 2: 239–240

Baly M 1981 (ed) A new approach to district nursing. Heinemann. Medical, London

Barber J H, Wallis J B 1976 Assessment of the elderly in general practice. Journal of the Royal College of General Practitioners 26: 106–114

Barber J H, Wallis J B 1978 The benefits to an elderly population of continuing geriatric assessment. Journal of the Royal College of General Practitioners 30: 428–433

Barber S, Wallis J B 1982 The effects of a system of geriatric assessment and screening on a general practice work load. Health Bulletin 40(3): 125–132

Barber J H, Wallis J B 1982 The effects of a system of geriatric assessment in preventive geriatric care. Journal of The Royal College of General Practitioners 30: 49–51

Battle S, Salter B 1984 The reality of practice. Journal of District Nursing June: 16–21

CETHV 1967 The functions of the health visitor. The Council for The Education and Training of Health Visitors, London

Clare A W, Corney R H 1982 Social work and primary health care. Academic Press, London

Committee on Nursing 1972 (Briggs Report). Report of the Committee on Nursing. Cmnd 5115 HMSO, London

Crosbie D 1983 A role for anyone? A description of social work with the elderly in Area Offices. British Journal of Social Work 13: 123–148

Day L 1981 Health visiting the elderly in the 1980s. Health Visitor 54 (December): 534–538

Department of Health and Social Security 1976 Prevention and health: Everybody's business. HMSO, London

Department of Health and Social Security 1980 (Black Report) Inequalities in health. HMSO, London

Department of Health and Social Security 1981 (Harding Report) The primary health care team. Report of a joint working group of The Standing Medical Advisory Committee and The Standing Nursing and Midwifery Advisory Committee. HMSO, London

Dingwall R 1982 Problems of teamwork in primary care. In: Clare A W, Corney R H (eds) Social work and primary health care. Academic Press, London

Dingwall R, McIntosh J (eds) 1978 Readings in the sociology of nursing. Churchill Livingstone, Edinburgh

Donaldson R J, Donaldson L J 1983 Essential community medicine. MTP Press, Lancaster, p 144–154

Drennan V 1984 A new approach. Nursing Mirror 159(14) October 17 HVA Supplement, p x

Dunnell K, Dobbs J 1982 Nurses working in the community. OPCS, HMSO, London

Exton-Smith A N 1981 Issues for research in ageing In: Kinaird J, Brotherston Sir J, Williamson J (eds) The provision of care for the elderly. Churchill Livingstone, Edinburgh, p 184–195

Ford 1980 The social worker. In: Barber J H, Kratz C R 1980 Towards team care. Churchill Livingstone, Edinburgh, p 65–78

Gilmore M, Bruce N, Hunt M 1974 The nursing team in general practice. CETHV, London

Goldberg E M, Connelly N 1982 The effectiveness of social care for the elderly. Heinemann, London

Hall J H, Zwemer J D 1979 Prospective medicine, 2nd edn. Department of Medical Education, Methodist Hospital of Indiana, 1604 North Capital Avenue, Indianopolis

Hunt M 1983 Possibilities and problems of inter-disciplinary teamwork. In: Clark J, Henderson J (eds) Community health. Churchill Livingstone, Edinburgh, p 233–241

Illing M, Donovan B 1981 District nursing. Bailliere Tindall, London

Kewley J 1983 New ideas in caring for the elderly. Health Visitor 56 (December): 443

Kratz C 1980 The district nurse. In: Barber J H, Kratz C R (eds) Towards team care. Churchill Livingstone, Edinburgh p 49–64

Kratz C R 1982 Community nursing-prescription for excellence. Nursing Times April 21:677

Lonsdale S, Webb A, Briggs T (eds) 1980 Teamwork in the personal social services and health care. Croom Helm, London

Luker K (1981) The role of the health visitor. In: Kinnaird J, Brotherston Sir J, Williamson J (eds) The provision of care for the elderly. Churchill Livingstone, Edinburgh

Marshall M 1983 Social work with old people. Macmillan Press, London

Murray T S, Young R E 1977 A laboratory survey in a geriatric population. Update 14: 191–196

Phillipson C, Strang P 1984 Health education and older people: the role of paid carers. Health Education Council in association with Department of Adult Education, University of Keele

Rowlings C 1981 Social work with elderly people. Allen & Unwin, London

Royal College of General Practitioners 1983 Promoting prevention. Royal College of General Practitioners, London

Scottish Home and Health Department 1978 (Hockey Report) District nursing in Scotland. HMSO, Edinburgh

Sheldon J H 1948 The social medicine of old age. Oxford University Press, Oxford

South-East London Screening Study Group 1977 A controlled trial of a multi-phasic screening programme, in middle age: results of the South-East London Screening Study. International Journal of Epidemiology 6: 357–363

Taylor R, Ford G, Barber J H 1983 The elderly at risk. Research perspectives on ageing 6. Age Concern Research Unit, Mitcham

United Kingdom Joint Committee 1983 (Council for the education and training of health visitors: Panel of assessors for district Nurse Training: Royal College of General Practitioners: Central Council for the Education and Training in Social Work) Statement on the development of Interprofessional education and training, for members of Primary Health Care Teams. London

Williams E I, Bennet F, Nixon J V, Nicholson M R, Gabert J 1972 Sociomedical study of patients over 75 in general practice. British Medical Journal May 20: 445–448

Williamson J 1981 Screening, surveillance and case-finding. In: Arie T (ed) Health care of the elderly. Croom Helm, London

Williamson J, Lowther C P, Gray S 1966 The use of health visitors in preventive geriatrics. Gerontologia Clinica 8: 362–369

Williamson J, Stokoe I H, Gray S, Fisher M, Smith A, McGhee A, Stephenson E 1964 Old people at home; their unreported needs. Lancet i (May 23): 1117–1120

FURTHER READING

World Health Organization 1977 Working group on prevention of mental disorder in the elderly. WHO, Copenhagen

7

Health promotion
in later life

Retirement can be the passport to freedom — the gateway to opportunity — but the extent to which such a possibility becomes a reality depends on a number of factors, not least of which is good health. This chapter therefore adopts a positive approach to health, believing that its promotion is both a legitimate and a desirable health visiting activity at all ages, but particularly in middle and later life. Promotion is an active, go-getting word, which conveys the thought of advancement, progression, elevation and enterprise. In the business sense the term is used to describe the vigorous pursuit of a campaign in which the attributes and purported benefits of a particular product are presented to the public, in the hope that they will be convinced and become purchasers. Similar notions prevail with health promotion, for it is through the strategy of health education that the practitioner seeks to convince individuals, groups and communities that health is a fundamental right, a desirable, personal and social goal and that *it is achievable*.

The World Health Organization, through their now famous Alma-Ata declaration (WHO 1978), re-affirmed their intent to make health a valued asset for everyone; their slogan 'Health for all by the Year 2000' showed the vigour with which they intended to pursue their global strategy. For too long negative attitudes on the part of many professional workers towards health education, and the tendency to medicalise problems, has meant that people have grown to feel they are powerless to control their ageing process. One result has been for them to hand over their health problems to professional persons, particularly doctors, and expect to be prescribed 'a pill for every ill'. The idea of active participation in promoting and maintaining one's own health in middle and later life is, however, beginning to gain a little ground. If the health visitor is to capitalise on these emerging trends, and vigorously to attempt to 'sell health', she needs both the energy of the entrepreneur and the zeal of the reformer.

Helping persons and communities to move forward and upwards in health terms is a two-pronged activity, covering both personal and environmental measures. Personal change is encouraged through health education, with its major components of health teaching, health counselling and occasionally selective behaviour modification. Environmental improvements, however, depend for success upon ecological safeguards and hazard control; for these to be effectively achieved, social and economic measures have to be taken, which may in turn require political decisions. Thus health visitors find they are not only actively engaged in programmes themselves, but participating also with many other disciplines in order to meet goals.

Some may question whether health promotion in later life is a worthwhile exercise. Certainly it is best undertaken from the earliest years, but there are certain phases of the life-span when particular events occur, which cause individuals to reflect on their situation, possibly re-appraise their health status and behaviour, and move towards improved lifestyles. Retirement is one such time; harnessing the potentially new motivations is therefore a major health visiting task, which utilises all the indentified health visiting principles.

Retirement can be considered from three viewpoints:

1. as a significant event
2. as a social status
3. as a developmental process
   (Streib & Schneider 1971, Murray et al 1980)

Nevertheless, within each of these perspectives, health visitors will have to adapt their approaches to individuals, according to the communities in which their clients live, and within the lifestyles they adopt.

Retirement as a significant event

The connotations of the term 'retirement' are many and varied. For some it means 'a moving on', for others 'standing down', a few may react negatively and regard it as a situation of retreat, whilst those more positively inclined may see it as a chance to 'do their own thing'. Thus some look forward eagerly to the event, whilst others perceive it as bringing loss and social distress. Hemingway is reputed to have thought it to be the vilest word in the English language, and indeed it can sometimes propel persons from familiar roles and comfortable routines into states of role confusion and des- equilibrium, thus posing threats to physical and mental health.

Successful negotiation of this transition depends on many factors, including personality attributes, personal perceptions and beliefs about work and worth; socio-economic circum- stances; physical and mental well-being; and the attitudes of significant others and society. Most importantly, it depends on adequate preparation.

Preparing and planning

Because retirement heralds the onset of a further develop- mental phase, which can last for as long as 40 or more years, one might expect that it would be anticipated and prepared for over a long time. Paradoxically however, although we spend some 15–20 years preparing for adulthood and the world of work, few people give more than scant attention to how they will spend their latter days, until they are within immediate sight of pensionable age. Nevertheless, it is during the active phase of later middle life, when family and work roles have mostly been carved out, that thoughts can best be directed to planning for the years of increased leisure and change. Furthermore, the period 45–64 years represents a time when mortality and morbidity risks increase steeply, indicating that health visiting contact might profitably be directed not only to younger adults, but also to this middle-aged group.

Apart from the pressures of time, which may render it difficult for health visitors to spend much time with those in middle life, some practitioners express concern about how best to make contact with clients in these vital years. Some health visitors overcome this by running 'drop-in clinics', in which they offer older adults a health advisory service, covering such topics as diet, exercise, weight control, relaxation, stress management, smoking control, counselling on personal health problems and the wise use of leisure. Others, working together with general practice team members, use their age-sex register to identify potential clients, and then issue personal invitations to attend for screening and health counselling programmes (see Ch. 6). Whichever of these two methods is adopted, it is important that positive concepts of health are presented, so that individuals do not become preoccupied with morbidity, but have their attention focused on their *health potential*, seeing it in terms either of development, independence or adaptation, as was discussed in Chapter 5.

Additionally many health visitors are now working more closely with occupational health nurses, realising that, by such liaison, both become better informed and thus are able to give more personalised and scientifically sound help to clients and their families. Hopefully this is an area which will rapidly develop as health visitor practitioners take the initiative in collaborative care.

Another avenue of contact is provided when health visitors participate in organised pre-retirement courses, which may be offered by forward-looking and thoughtful employers, Colleges of Further or Higher Education; the Workers Educational Association; or the Pre-Retirement Association. However, such contact, whilst more useful, is often made quite late in the pre-retirement phase, thus offering less scope for anticipation, education and change. Of course a great deal of contact is already made through the many self-help groups in which older adults engage, as well as through home visiting, sometimes initially directed at other age groups such as young children. Health visitors have long been aware that their initial reasons for contacting persons in their own home, or at clinics, give scope for further encounter: but although the opportunities are manifold, and most practitioners are aware that taking advantage of them is their responsibility, such activities are often 'officially ignored' and thence are not perceived as legitimate and purposeful health visiting functions. This is a sphere where clarification is urgently required, since one visit to a home may mean that a number of persons receive health education, including those who are facing retirement as a forthcoming and significant event.

During this preparation for retirement, clients should be encouraged to think ahead, plan their financial affairs, consider their living and housing arrangements, and legal requirements and their hobbies and interests. Hobbies should be creative rather than competitive and ideally individuals should try to obtain some of the needful tools and materials for these whilst they are still earning. Older people often show great potential in leisure pursuits, and so some interests of a sporting nature are strongly advised. In addition it is helpful if household furnishing, bedding and floor coverings are appraised and renewed where necessary. Entering retirement in as well-planned and well-equipped a manner as possible can prove a great boon later on. Comfort (1977) captures some of the sense of excitement associated with preparing and planning for this phase of life, when he describes retirement as 'entering a second trajectory, for which older people need to plan and get on a launching pad.' It is clear he sees them shaping society to expect every senior to have an active and fulfilling retirement career. Already there are signs that some pensioners groups are eagerly seeking this kind of active involvement in controlling the ageing process, and in determining their own affairs. Health visitors are well placed to help generate and sustain such self-help and enthusiasm.

Preparing significant others

Another important facet of health promotion in the pre-retirement period, is the preparation of significant others, be they spouses, family members, relatives or friends, because their attitudes can profoundly affect the way impending retirers perceive themselves and their future. For some women who have not engaged in the direct labour market, the concept of retirement has little personal meaning. Because they continue to have many active roles, interests and responsibilities, and do not alter their lives profoundly, nor undergo any marked status change, they may find the retirement of a spouse, relative or friend a disruptive event. This in turn can cause mutual distress. Such reaction may be particularly marked where couples have had widely segregated conjugal roles and different daily living patterns. As one woman pithily remarked: 'I married my husband for better or worse, but not to have to get lunch for him every day.'

Anticipatory guidance is a familiar health visiting technique which has much to offer in such circumstances, since it has both educative and facilitating elements. Through focused discussion it is possible to explain how those contemplating, or experiencing employment loss, may feel and act, so enabling others to appreciate their outlook and hence prepare themselves to react favourably to the mutual adjustments required. Of course many significant others look forward eagerly to the retirement of their spouses, relatives or friends, finding the post-retirement years · ones of enrichment.

The time of retirement

Some employers, mindful of the effect of 'retirement shock', have introduced flexible policies, whereby older employees can have a phased 'wind-down', through part-time work, job-sharing or planned early leaving. This gradual tapering off can help to promote positive adaptation, allowing employees to see the event of retirement as the culmination of one progressive, sequential career, and the entrance to another. This perception is much helped if the financial accompaniments of the change are high. However, for those in whom the work ethic is deeply ingrained, or who regard retirement as a loss of valued social contact, or for whom the future seems but a dreary prospect, of dependence on limited financial resources, the moment of severance from employment can be very traumatic. Even the rituals associated with leaving can heighten pleasure or increase despair, depending upon the way they are perceived. The traditional gift of a time-piece may be unintentionally cruel for some retirers, whilst others may be given mementoes which remind them of achievements, or presents which encourage them to look forward to the future. In the matter of customs and conventions associated with retirement, health education can play a part in creating more positive attitudes, and demonstrating these through appropriate symbols. For instance, one health visitor got the message when her leaving gift turned out to be a tricycle!

There are however, many other complex factors associated with the event of retirement. Recent social upheavals resulting from mass unemployment and/or occupational redundancy have introduced new dimensions into the issue, sometimes rendering it highly disruptive. Furthermore, in future health visitors may well be meeting older people who have not worked for many years before reaching official pensionable age; for such persons the accepted notions of retirement will be irrelevant. For these many different reasons, health visitors as a collective body need to be particularly alert to the ways they can help favourably to influence policies affecting the health of persons in later life. Already research studies are demonstrating the profound effects loss of employment status is having on physical and mental health, not only for those directly involved, but for their families as well (OPCS 1984, Nuffield Centre 1984).

Promoting self-esteem

One way in which health visitors can help to counter the adverse effects of enforced retirement for individuals is to promote self-esteem. The maintenance of a positive self-concept is essential for morale and hence well-being in body, mind and spirit.

Encouraging some older people to recount their past achievements, may foster their sense of identity, whilst showing interest in any displayed symbols of success, retirement gifts or cards, may help to strengthen continuity. However, it is important to stress identity apart from the work-role and to emphasise the many opportunities to contribute to society which exist in the present. As part of the raising of consciousness, it is necessary to elicit seniors' perceptions of themselves, discover their usual coping strategies and discuss their future expectations, as preludes to assisting them realistically to appraise their skills, talents and interests. Only then is it possible to suggest ways in which these might be channelled to provide social usefulness and to obtain personal satisfaction.

A range of activities should be encouraged to cater for physical, mental, emotional, social and spiritual needs. Cicero knew the value of such wide-ranging interests in later life. He engaged in horse-riding, kept busy in farming, gardening and tending his vineyards, met frequently with friends to converse over meals and participated freely in debates and civic affairs.

> 'I study Greek literature,' he said. 'I am examining the secular and pontifical law, and daily I practise the habit of the Pythagoreans, running over in my mind all I have said and done. In my old age these are my mental gymnastics, these the race-courses of my mind.'
>
> Falconer 1923

Self-regard can be enhanced with encouragement of appropriate attention to personal appearance and the maintenance of heterosexual social relationships. Other vital elements are maintaining hope, and the sense of feeling needed and cared for; being able to communicate freely with others and having a sense of control over one's personal affairs.

Case study

John S., a recently retired bachelor, had become down-cast and somewhat slipshod in personal habits when a health visitor, who knew of his talent for photography, put him in touch with a local, mixed, community group, where the members were keen to learn about this hobby. His outlook brightened once his knowledge and skills were utilised; his personal appearance improved and by the end of the year John was eagerly planning to help the group mount an exhibition of their work.

Retirement as a social status

Retirement denotes a new social position, a changed status, which is officially marked by entitlements to specific contribu-

Table 7.1 Normal retirement age for women and men for selected countries

Country	Normal retirement age	
	Women	Men
Denmark	67	67
Greece	57	62
Norway	70	70
Switzerland	63	65
UK	60	65
USA	65	65
USSR	55	60

Based on material in The ageing — Trends and policies, United Nations, New York, 1975.

tory benefits. Although many countries use this device to mark this particular social state administratively, the age they select for official retirement age varies (Table 7.1).

However, there are other factors which can affect retirement age. These include the type of occupation undertaken, the harshness of weather or climate, the working conditions, and the years of service given, e.g. athletes, gymnasts, footballers and tennis players often 'retire' before they are 40, some taking up subsequent careers in other fields. Conversely, judges are not forced to leave work until they are 75 years old, whilst some doctors, politicians and business personalities, as well as self-employed persons in trade, industry or the arts, do not retire at all. Similarly, housewives are denied this opportunity to cease work.

As part of this status transition, there can sometimes be an increased emphasis on parent-child relationships, with subtle changes in the giving and receiving of help. This may be very evident where those who have just retired themselves find that they are still carrying responsibility for the care of their own aged parents. Sometimes considerable curbs may be placed on the activities that those just retired can engage in, because of the demands of the very old. Where this causes hurt or resentment it is important for health visitors to try to suggest positive ways of resolving the difficulties, as part of an overall strategy of health promotion for both parties. The tyranny of over-dependent elderly can constitute a very real risk to well-being for some in later life.

For some who have retired, there may be a greater chance to derive increased pleasure from grandparenting. Understandably, geographic or social mobility can affect the frequency and quality of contact between the generations, but at different times grandparents can act as confidants; representatives of family history and identity; reservoirs of family wisdom; sources of additional fun or treats; surrogate parents; or complementary bankers! Encouraging positive interaction between grandparents and grandchildren thus aids mutual well-being.

Once former roles have been relinquished, however, most people find it helpful to forge new ones quickly. Some do this by finding avenues of community service. This may involve acting as sources of local or social history, such as working as guides in museums or places of historic or artistic interest, or helping local school children discover their heritage. Some assist in hospitals, canteens or local homes for the old or handicapped or in shops for various charities. Others like to help in play-groups and creches, youth clubs or community centres, where they may be utilised as story-tellers, games partners, toy repairers and maintainers, craft teachers and/or general helpers. Sometimes individuals need a nudge to help them to find such a niche, or organisers requiring helpers may welcome suggestions about where to seek potential recruits. The notion of 'foster grandparenting' is as yet little exploited, but older people have much to offer in this role, if carefully selected. They may need to be taught to give supplementary care to children with special needs, such as those in long-stay hospitals, residential schools or homes, where contact with families may be limited. Moreover, there are a number of children suffering impairments or social deprivation who are living in their own homes. They and their parents, often welcome the friendly contact and wise counsel that an older person can give, as well as the practical help that might be possible from time to time. This is a sector of activity which is ripe for development, requiring great tact and judgment. However, it is important to try to ensure that older people undertake such community service *by choice* and not from a mistaken idea that 'retired persons owe the community some do-gooding'. Such attitudes fuel ageism and detract from dignity.

Apart from the many voluntary schemes in which seniors can engage, there are a plethora of self-help groups or recreational clubs. There is also great scope for the marketing and bartering of skills. In some communities these exchange schemes already exist, with those good at carpentry, home decorating or gardening, helping others in return for services like cooking, sewing, washing or shopping. However, it frequently requires someone to act as a catalyst before others recognise what they can do to create mutual support systems. As part of their general health-promoting activities, health visitors often need to assume this role, thus making a substantial contribution to the personal and social well-being of the retired.

Of course there is also the aspect of encouraging the community to recognise and meet the special needs of its senior citizens, through the provision of appropriate leisure facilities, sports amenities, educational courses, special interest sessions, social centres and clubs. Many commercial enterprises are now aware of the newly retired as a potential market for special holiday ventures, or as house purchasers. Care must, however, be exercised when encouraging specific status recognition of older people, to avoid creating a 'ghetto mentality'.

Maintenance of income

Fundamental to successful retiring, and affecting health and social status and well-being in later life, is the possession of an adequate income. Social policy advisors often recommend an income of 80% of previous earnings, if lifestyle is not to be too severely disrupted. Unfortunately, although more are now retiring on occupational pensions, few attain these recommended levels and many fall far below this. Some seniors face grave financial difficulties, although they may try not to make these manifest. Townsend (1979) found, in his sample of persons experiencing poverty, that over one-third were in the older age range. Fixed incomes and the erosion of savings by inflation create anxieties for many older people, who may therefore welcome unobtrusive guidance on budgeting and measures to increase income.

Income represents far more than just having the money to buy the basic necessities of life and health. It means a measure of independence and the ability to give to others, as well as to fulfil some of the dreams which could not be realised during working life. It also represents security against a future which may sometimes seem threatening and unsure. Although health visitors are not expected to know all the intricate details of a complex social security system, they have a responsibility to act as advisors on welfare rights, and are often required to be advocates, hence they must appreciate the principles underlying relevant policies, and should certainly know where to go to get help. In discussing these general principles below, specific details of monetary allowances are *not* given; this is because detailed amounts quickly become outdated, and, at the time of writing a major review of the entire benefits system is being undertaken.

Retirement pension

One of the main sources of income maintenance in later life comes from retirement pension. Most of these pensions are contributory, being paid either on a personal contribution record or that of a spouse or former spouse. A few pensions are non-contributory; they are paid respectively to those who were already of pensionable age on 5th July 1948, or who are now aged 80 years or over and have no insurance record. Married women, living with their husbands, do *not* receive the full amount. At present the basic retirement pension approximates to 25% of the average national male manual wage. Some people may, in addition, receive earnings-related benefit, although the full impact of this scheme will not be felt until the mid 1990s. Rates for pensions are subject to regular review and updating, and appropriate leaflets are available from the Department of Health and Social Security, or from Citizens' Advice Bureaux or Post Offices. Where there is any doubt, health visitors should go direct to such local sources in order to ensure that any advice they give is both current and appropriate.

Some, who may have to take early retirement before reaching pensionable age, may suffer considerable financial disadvantage. It is therefore important to be aware of the different ways in which such clients can receive aid, e.g. where individuals have taken 'voluntary retirement' they may, under certain circumstances, be eligible for unemployment benefit for a period. They should be referred to the local employment office or Citizens' Advice Bureau for personal guidance. Individuals forced to retire early through sickness or incapacity, who are already in receipt of invalidity benefit, may opt to continue this for the first 5 years of retirement. Although the amount is usually lower than the alternative retirement benefit, it is non-taxable, unlike retirement pension; hence it may confer a small advantage on the recipient.

Males, aged 60–64 years, who are disabled and in receipt of statutory sick pay, may be able to retire and apply for a non-taxable Job Release Allowance. This is a recent arrangement and it is not certain how long it may remain operational, but again advice can be obtained from the Department of Health and Social Security (DHSS) or Citizens' Advice Bureaux. However, even with state retirement pension, or these other benefits, it is estimated 72% of disabled seniors and 64% of non-disabled seniors were living at, below, or just up to 40% above the official poverty line in 1981 (DHSS 1983, Disability Alliance 1984).

Supplementary Benefit is intended to act as a 'safety net' for those whose incomes fall below a prescribed level. Approximately 2 million persons aged 65 years and over currently receive this benefit, i.e. about 1 older person in 4. The benefit may be a replacement income, or be a smaller amount to 'top up' other income to a specified level. However, it is estimated that 25% of those who are entitled to claim do not do so, whether because of ignorance, pride, a sense of stigma, or unwillingness to become involved with a government agency. At present older persons are automatically assessed for longer-term benefit, which is paid at a slightly higher rate than the ordinary benefit. Such benefit is means-tested and savings of up to £3000 may be disregarded. In addition, there are small extra allowances for those who are blind; need additional heating; require special diets; are on home dialysis or have to pay laundry costs or employ domestic help other than that provided by a local authority. Single payments may be made in respect of essential equipment such as beds, bedding, cookers, heating appliances or fireguards.

As many of these benefits are discretionary, and the onus

to claim rests with the claimant, it is necessary for health visitors to liaise closely with DHSS or Welfare Rights staff, to ensure correct uptake. The Child Poverty Action Group and The Disability Alliance both issue helpful general information, and publish handbooks which give details of national welfare benefits. More recently the DHSS has set up a free telephone advisory service, which is advertised in each locality; this provides tailored advice before a claim is presented. The purpose is to try to encourage reluctant individuals to seek help and at the same time reduce the number of potential refusals. Some older people require assistance with the completion of the necessary forms and, if their claims are rejected, may need help to lodge an appeal. Once more the local Citizens' Advice Bureau or the Welfare Rights organisation can help to determine if an appeal is indicated, and the best grounds on which this might be made.

Housing benefit

Housing costs and rates swallow up a large proportion of income, so that many older people may need help to meet these charges. From April 1983 the former rent rebates, rent allowances and rate rebate schemes were abolished and replaced by two forms of housing benefit:

1. certificated housing benefit
2. standard housing benefit.

The former is paid to those qualifying for supplementary benefit, the latter to those whose means-tested income is below certain levels, but which does not entitle them to supplementary benefit. The onus to decide which benefit to claim rests with the claimant, but recent research suggests that many older people who are currently claiming standard housing benefit would be better advised to ask for supplementary benefit (Kerr 1983). Seniors should therefore be encouraged to seek guidance about the most advantageous arrangement for them, *before* lodging their claim with either the DHSS or the Local Authority.

Other budgeting ideas

Seniors may welcome information about the monthly budget

schemes which are operated by the electricity, gas and telephone services. Certain fuel tariffs may also confer advantages, so clients should be advised to consult with their gas or electricity showrooms about this. Earnings are the most obvious way of increasing income, but for the first 5 years after pensionable age, are subject to the earnings rule. It is helpful if health visitors check the current amount which can be earned before reduction of pension occurs. Of course all paid employment is subject to income tax, although after age 65 small concessions *may* apply. For some people annuities may prove helpful. These are mostly paid for the remainder of a life-time, subject to a lump sum investment, or pledged collateral such as a house. They are best considered when one is much older, as the return tends to be higher then. Since there is an element of speculation in this arrangement, clients should be advised to seek legal advice before commitment.

RETIREMENT AS A DEVELOPMENTAL PROCESS

As a developmental process, retirement moves on from the impact of the actual event, through adjustment to changed social status, to a daily dynamic adaption to changing personal and environmental demands. The major developmental tasks include: learning to cope with altered and frequently lower income levels; maintaining adequate nutrition, sometimes within the limits of lessened physical capacity; solving issues such as transport, housing, cleaning and household management; and ensuring adequate personal and environmental safety measures. Other tasks are learning to get the maximum benefit from each day of life, dealing with health problems as they arise, and making the necessary preparations for a good death when it comes. Assisting seniors to achieve these tasks in a positive fashion is a health visiting responsibility; it is much facilitated if there has been active involvement in the earlier years and if predictive judgment has been exercised, so that problems have been anticipated and either avoided or reduced as far as possible. All too often the crisis work which confronts health visitors today could have been prevented, had there been improved communication and earlier intervention. This is why it pays dividends to make contact with older people in the pre-retirement period, stimulate them to exercise informed control over their own ageing, and maintain supportive contact with them as they grow inevitably frailer, so that they will take the initiative in calling for help at the first signs of distress.

Nutrition in retirement

Good nutrition is basic to good health at all ages, but is particularly important in later life. The nutritional needs of the elderly differ little from those of younger persons, but certain points need to be considered, since they modify advice. For instance the four major principles of diet still apply, namely that food taken should be:

- physiologically appropriate
- nutritionally adequate
- psychologically appealing
- socio-culturally acceptable

However, changes in energy output may modify calorie requirements. Additionally, alterations in the gastrointestinal tract may affect chewing, swallowing and digestion, whilst co-existing disease and/or drug therapy may affect absorption and excretion.

Table 7.2 gives recommended allowances for major nutrients, describes major sources and offers some comment pertinent to needs. However, it is important to bear in mind that, like all standardised tables, such details only apply to the older population as a group, and group solutions often do not match individual requirements. Advice will therefore have to be tailored to individuals within these broad considerations.

An intake of 1800–2000 kilocalories for women and 2100–2400 for men usually suffices, but factors to consider include desirable body weight in relation to height and build; energy output; climate and season; and any existing health problems. As protein requirements remain relatively high, in order to maintain nitrogen balance and maintain vital processes, between 10 and 12% of energy intake should come from foods of high biological value. These can be met from such items as lean meat, poultry, fish, cheese, eggs, milk,

Table 7.2 Some nutritional requirements and considerations in later life

Nutrient	Recommended daily amounts Men		Women		Comment	Major food source*
	65–74	75+	55–74	75+		
Energy (kilocalories)	2400	2150	1900	1680	Compiled from 10–12% protein; not more than 35% fat: balance from carbohydrate foods	
Fibre (g)	30	30	30	30	Provides bulk: prevents constipation: aids satiety; favourably affects colonic transit-timing	Whole grain products. Legumes; fresh fruit vegetables
Protein (g)	60	54	47	42	Repairs cells. Maintains vital functions: enzymes: Is affected by prolonged heat (denatured)	Eggs; cheese; fish; legumes; milk; nuts; whole grains
Thiamin (vitamin B1) Also known as Aneurin (mg)	1.0	0.9	0.8	0.7	Facilitates energy release from CHO. Easily lost in cooking. Is water soluble	Eggs; fortified flour; milk; offal; whole grains and yeast products
Riboflavin (vitamin B2) (mg)	1.6	1.6	1.3	1.3	Maintains health of mucous membrane. Unstable in light and heat: water soluble	Eggs; liver; kidney; cheese; marmite; yeast products and potatoes in season
Nicotinic acid (Niacin) = vitamin B3 (mg)	18	18	15	15	Utilises food energy. Keeps nervous tissue healthy. Gross deficiency linked with dementia, digestive upsets and dermatoses	Cheese; eggs; fish; whole wheat grains; milk; some vegetables
Pyridoxine (vitamin B6) (mg)	2	2	2	2	Manufactures amino acids. Utilises essential fatty acids	Widespread in many foods. May be inactivated by certain drugs eg. Isoniazide

Table 7.2 Contd.

Nutrient	Recommended daily amounts Men 65–74	75+	Women 55–74	75+	Comment	Major food source*
Folate (folic acid) (µg)	300	300	300	300	Helps to prevent megaloblastic anaemia. May help to protect against dementia.	Bananas; bread; offal; oranges; whole grains; raw green leafy vegetables
Vitamin B12 (Cyanocobalamin) (µg)	3	3	3	3	Needed for cell division. Erythrocyte formation. Healthy nerves	Liver and other animal protein
Ascorbic acid (vitamin C) (mg)	30	30	30	30	Oxidises rapidly. Water soluble. Easily lost in heat and in alkalis	Citrus fruits; blackcurrants; tomatoes; potatoes in season (N.B. highest Aug–Sept lowest March–May)
Vitamin A (µg) Retinol equivalent	750	750	750	750	Anti-infective action. Promotes healthy skin and epithelial tissue: Intake often inadequate: can be toxic	Fish liver oils; fortified margarines; eggs; liver; milk (variable amounts); cheese; carrots; green leafy vegetables; apricots
Vitamin D (Calciferol) (µg)	10	10	10	10	Needed for bone mineralisation. Thought to protect against osteoporosis: intakes often low. Produced by action of sunlight on ergosterol in skin, if exposed	Fatty fish; fish oils; fortified margarine; milk and dairy products; liver; ovaltine
Vitamin E (Tocopherol) (international)	100	100	100	100	Acts on skin to aid elasticity and is thought to improve health of collagen. Thought to be an anti-ageing factor. Oxidises very rapidly	Vegetable fats; sunflower and sesame seeds; nuts; whole grain cereals

Sodium (g)	4 4 4 4	Needed for many enzymes and for electrolyte balance. Often taken in excess in old age due to sensory losses. Intakes should be reduced when water retention is present and may be restricted when hypertension is diagnosed/treated.	Added to many processed foods. Amounts not always quoted on labels. High amounts in bacon, butter, canned vegetables, cheese some treated cereals, kippers and sausages. Often found in association with high sugar content of processed foods
Potassium (g or mmols)	2.5–6 g daily for all (= 65–200 mmols)	Intakes often very inadequate in old age. Deficiency leads to muscle weakness: poor grip: mental confusion and heart failure. May also be associated with depression (Davies 1981)	Fruit, especially bananas and oranges. Vegetables, especially potatoes. Marmite: herrings: legumes: offal: milk: tomatoes and tomato juice but note this is also high in sodium content
Certain other trace elements are also very important for the elderly particularly:-			
Cobalt	Exact requirements not known at present	Needed for healthy blood and nerve cells to act with vitamin B12. May be deficient in Vegans: those without intrinsic factor and post-gastrectomy patients.	Present in liver; fish; cheese; egg; barmene.
Iodine	Exact amounts not known	Required for healthy function of thyroid gland. ? helps to prevent myxodema	Sea food; vegetables grown in soil with iodine present. Iodized salt

Table 7.2 Contd.

Nutrient	Recommended daily amounts Men 65–74	Men 75+	Women 55–74	Women 75+	Comment	Major food source*
Zinc	Exact amounts not known Thought may be 15 mg				Required for healthy enzyme functioning. Absorption is affected by a high fibre intake so zinc intake adjusted accordingly	Present in most protein foods. Therefore increase protein intake for those on high fibre diets
Water (pints)	3–4	3–4	3–4	3–4	Needed for body fluids and vital enzymes. Often inadequate intakes in later life and risk of dehydration	Water. Some in other foods such as fruits and some vegetables, but these amounts should be ignored in calculating intakes

* Major sources given represent those regarded as inexpensive in relation to food value. When advising on nutritional intakes for older people consider cost in relation to benefit, choose foods in season, easy to obtain and prepare. Advise on storage and cooking, so that food values can be conserved as far as possible.
Table is based on data obtained from DHSS 1979b, Davies 1981 and Ebersole & Hess 1981

nuts, legumes and whole-grain cereals. With an increasing proportion of the population becoming less meat orientated, and bearing in mind certain social or religious taboos, it is necessary to be very flexible in advice. Where certain foodstuffs have limited protein value, i.e. they do not contain all the essential amino acids, it is necessary to recommend complementing items, so that the diet is balanced in protein content. Other factors to bear in mind include availability of foodstuffs; cost in relation to value; digestibility, any food allergies; and, of course, personal preferences. Alerting signs of hypoproteinanaemia include senile pruritus; slow healing wounds; fatigue and oedema.

It is important to follow recent recommendations that fat intake should not exceed 35% of total energy needs, and that a higher proportion of polyunsaturated to saturated fatty acids should be included (COMA 1984). For many people this may mean an overall reduction in their fat intake and an adjustment in the content. However it is also necessary to ensure adequate intakes of the fat-soluble vitamins, especially for vulnerable groups. Vitamin A continues to be required to meet demands made on epithelial tissue, to aid body resistance against infection and to maintain functional light-dark adaptation. Vitamin D is also needed to maintain the strength of bones and teeth. Although the chief source of vitamin D is the action of ultraviolet light on the skin, it is important to appreciate that latitude, the angle of the sun during exposure, and the amount and duration of such exposure are limiting factors. Some elderly housebound people have limited opportunity for such skin exposure, and in any case ageing skin and the atrophy of sebaceous glands probably affects ergosterol manufacture. Thus, whilst it is important to encourage older people to take full advantage of sunlight, attention *must* be paid to dietary intake. In practice this means encouraging seniors to eat fortified, polyunsaturated margarines; fatty fish, fortified evaporated milk; cold pressed oils such as sunflower and safflower oil; and eggs and other dairy produce in moderation. Unfortunately, some elderly people are fearful of the bones in fatty fish, or may find some varieties of this, and liver, too strong in taste; many still regard butter as socially superior to margarine, whilst others cannot be bothered to shop or cook very much. Thus people living alone, who do not feel it is worth troubling about meals, may be vulnerable even when other aspects of their circumstances would not cause one to consider them so. It is worth bearing in mind that osteomalacia has been found to be present in approximately 4% of elderly admitted to hospital. Furthermore the high accident rate amongst older people, particularly females, renders them at great risk of bony injury, which a diet high enough in vitamin D may help to counteract.

Fibre-rich carbohydrate foods, such as whole-grain cereals, bran, bread, fruit and vegetables, should be increased in line with energy requirements, to compensate for lower sugar intakes and reduced fat content. These will also help to avoid constipation and improve colonic transit-time, thus possibly helping to reduce the risk of malignant disease, although the latter is not proven. An intake of 30 g of fibre daily is recommended (NACNE 1983, Wenlock et al 1984). It may mean exercising considerable ingenuity to persuade some older clients to re-orientate their eating habits in this way, but it is well worth trying. This is another reason for endeavouring to lay down patterns of healthier eating in earlier life.

By following such advice older people should ensure an adequate amount of essential minerals and other elements, the intake of which is of such importance. Although generally no gross nutritional deficiencies have been detected in later life, the studies which have been carried out have been limited and have not always explored associated socio-economic status. There is some evidence to suggest older persons are at risk of sub-deficiency states, especially in relation to thiamin, riboflavin, folic acid and ascorbic acid (DHSS 1979a, 1979b, Davies 1981). As these particular vitamins are both heat- and light-sensitive and water soluble, it is possible that prolonged storage and faulty cooking methods contribute to high wastage. Less mobile old people may have difficulty in obtaining fresh foods, especially when they rely on small corner shops, with slower turnover of stock. There is also a tendency for older males, especially those living alone, who have been unaccustomed to preparing their own meals, to adopt 'tea and toast' regimes to their detriment. 'Widower's scurvy' is a known syndrome.

Older people should not increase their salt intake unduly, although altered taste often leads them to do so. Fluid intake should also be maintained at about 3–4 pints daily, with more in cases of constipation. Potassium intakes are sometimes low, and need to be assessed, particularly where individuals are taking prescribed diuretics. Alcohol ingestion should be tactfully determined; not more than 30 g per day is advised for men and 23 g for women; it should be remembered that half a pint of beer, one measure of spirits or one average glass of wine, port or sherry provides approximately 10 g of alcohol. Where obesity is present, diet is usually restricted to 1000 calories daily, but of course proportionate amounts of protein, fat and carbohydrate are advised, and mineral and vitamin intakes remain the same. If there is any doubt about them being included, a supplement may be recommended.

Assessing nutritional status

Assessing and monitoring nutritional status in later life is an important part of health promotion. Factors to consider when undertaking this include:

- client's knowledge about food values and sources
- levels of motivation towards food intake
- ethnic and cultural beliefs and practices
- socio-economic resources and specific food budgets
- availability of foodstuffs; access to shops and markets; freshness of supplies
- transport facilities in association with mobility
- means of food storage, preparation and cooking, and methods of cooking used
- life-time and present patterns of eating and drinking, including the timing of meals in relation to body rhythm and activity
- socialisation — if meals are taken on a solitary basis, or in company
- degree of control older people can actually exercise over the food they receive, especially if they are living with others, or receiving meals-on-wheels, or eating in luncheon clubs or restaurants
- levels of physical, cognitive, emotional and social health.

Measurement of individual nutritional status can be assessed by noting height, weight, general appearance,

Table 7.3 A guide to desirable weights in later life *

Height (in bare feet)			Weight (without clothes)				
Ft	in	cm (nearest equivalent)	st	lb	st	lb	kg (nearest equivalent)
Men							
5	0	152	8	4 –	9	1	53–58
5	1	155	8	7 –	9	4	54–59
5	2	157	8	10 –	9	7	55–60
5	3	160	8	13 –	9	10	57–62
5	4	162	9	2 –	9	13	58–63
5	5	165	9	5 –	10	2	60–65
5	6	168	9	8 –	10	5	61–66
5	7	170	9	11 –	10	8	62–67
5	8	173	10	0 –	10	11	64–69
5	9	175	10	3 –	11	0	65–70
5	10	178	10	6 –	11	3	66–71
5	11	180	10	9 –	11	6	68–73
6	0	183	10	12 –	11	9	69–74
6	1	185	11	1 –	11	12	70–75
6	2	188	11	4 –	12	1	72–77
6	3	191	11	7 –	12	4	73–78
Women							
4	9	142	7	0 –	7	11	44–49
4	10	145	7	3 –	8	0	46–51
4	11	147	7	7 –	8	4	48–53
5	0	151	7	10 –	8	7	49–54
5	1	152	7	13 –	8	10	50–55
5	2	155	8	2 –	8	13	52–57
5	3	157	8	5 –	9	8	53–58
5	4	160	8	8 –	9	5	54–59
5	5	164	8	11 –	9	8	56–61
5	6	165	9	0 –	9	11	57–62
5	7	168	9	3 –	10	0	50–64
5	8	170	9	7 –	10	3	60–65
5	9	173	9	10 –	10	6	62–66
5	10	175	9	13 –	10	9	63–68
5	11	178	10	2 –	10	12	64–69

* This weight range is for medium to large frames, as judged by shoe size. For small frames deduct 5–7 lb (2–3 kg) from medium weight. However it is important to realise this is only a general guide which does not cater for specific individual factors.

colour, skin texture, muscle tone, the state of mucous membranes, and general vitality. Anthropometric measurements, such as mid-arm circumference, and skin-folds, either taken from the triceps of the non-dominant arm, or the tip of the scapula, are also helpful. These take 2 minutes to perform, using skin calipers; they provide the most accurate measurement of body fat density and muscle mass, and are useful for base-line and comparative purposes. Height and weight should be compared with standard tables, such as that given in Table 7.3, and anthropometric data assessed against measurements such as shown in Table 7.4.

Where clients are willing and able to co-operate, the most systematic approach is to obtain a 7-day diary of what is eaten, when, where and how. However, whilst this will provide clues about qualitative and quantitative aspects of the diet, it will not indicate *why* seniors eat what they do, and these are the all-important motivations. Whenever possible, those requiring help with meals should be encouraged to attend luncheon

Table 7.4 Anthropometric measurements in later life

Method of measurement	Standard measurement		Usual range for older people	
	Male	Female	Male	Female
Triceps skinfold thickness Measured over loosely hanging, non-dominant arm, by standard millimetre skinfold calipers, approx 1½ cm above mid-arm point. Gently lift skinfold and maintaining grasp read to nearest millimetre 2–3 seconds after releasing caliper extender. Usual to take average of 3 such readings. This estimates subcutaneous fat reserves.	12.5 mm	16.5 mm	7.4–11.5 mm	9.9–13.6 mm
Mid-arm circumference Measured at point midway between acromial process of scapula and olecranon process of elbow, on posterior aspect of arm. Use a non-stretchable tape; bend elbow to 90°: palm upwards. Read to nearest fraction of a centimetre, using no force. This estimates skeletal muscle mass (protein portion) Sometimes the mid-upper arm muscle circumference is measured as well or the subscapula skin fold.	29.3 cm	28.5 cm	17.4–26.3 cm	17–25.8 cm

Drawn from data from (i) Jellife D B 1966 The assessment of the nutritional status of the community WHO Geneva
(ii) Ebersole P, Hess P 1981 Towards healthy ageing. Mosby, St Louis p 124–125

clubs, rather than have meals-on-wheels at home, as the former caters for exercise and socialisation as well as nutritional complement. Of course for some very old and frail seniors such advice is unsuitable. However, even they can receive nutritional education.

Some may question if it is desirable, or possible, to attempt nutrition education for the elderly. However, Davies & Holdsworth (1982) and Holdsworth & Davies (1982) have shown that profitable changes *can* be brought about. For this reason health visitors should take every opportunity to stress good dietary intake, sound cooking and storage procedures. It is, of course, also essential to check that those *caring* for the elderly are fully conversant with their nutritional needs.

Healthy habits

Apart from dietary advice, persons experiencing the developmental process of retirement will benefit from personalised information on exercise, sleep, elimination, personal hygiene habits and sexual adjustment (see Table 2.1). Walking, cycling, golfing and swimming are particularly helpful activities in later life and can be safely continued by the majority of people into ripe old age. To obtain maximum benefit such exercise should be undertaken in full sunlight, whenever possible. Seniors should also be encouraged to balance work and play; to cultivate the art of relaxation, visual imagery and/or meditation for 15 minutes twice daily; and to take regular holidays. Mental attitudes are believed to have a strong influence on somatic states; negative attitudes to stress predispose to chronic heart and circulatory disorders, migraine, digestive upsets and skin conditions. Therefore, all action aimed at adverse stress control may be deemed beneficial.

Dental health is a basic need that may become neglected with advancing age, limited mobility or debilitating illness. Where older people have preserved their teeth, regular oral hygiene and dental check-ups should be conscientiously continued. Brushing correctly after meals, and using dental floss and/or toothpicks to remove the debris that collects round teeth and soft tissue, should be followed by rinsing. A soft, round-bristled toothbrush minimises the risk of gum trauma, and where there is difficulty with dexterity, some older people find it helpful either to use a child's size tooth-brush, or to glue a small soft rubber ball or handle grip to an ordinary size brush. Many old people are currently, however, edentulous. Whenever possible they should be fitted correctly with dentures, for both masticatory and cosmetic reasons. Advice should be given on their appropriate daily care, and it is wise to mark the dentures indelibly on their under-surface so that, should the older client subsequently be admitted to hospital, they can easily be identified.

Feet influence the physical and psychosocial well-being of individuals significantly, affecting mobility and amiability. Many older people suffer soft tissue complaints: corns, callouses, toe-nail disorders and/or bunions. Without treat-ment these can become disabling, thus threatening inde-pendence. Daily cleansing, encouraging maximum movement, wearing well-fitting footwear and guarding against trauma and infection, are essential areas of advice. Regular chiropody can be a very worthwhile investment, and is a service to be invoked for many seniors. Particular attention may need to be paid to those who suffer from diabetes mellitus, cardiac or renal disease, peripheral vascular and neurological disorders, the sequelae of cerebro-vascular accident, or arthritis (King 1978).

Whenever possible seniors should be encouraged to reduce or abandon smoking. Apart from the known harmful effects on respiratory, cardio-vascular and digestive systems, recent research suggests an association between smoking and bone de-mineralisation which, given a generation of higher-smoking females, might indicate even higher fracture rates among women in the future (Mellstrom 1982, WHO 1982).

Other protective measures. As infections can create considerable morbidity, personal hygiene advice and immu-nisation has a place in the care of older people. Vaccination against known influenzal viruses should be offered, especially to vulnerable seniors, and active immunisation against tetanus should be regularly maintained, especially as many older persons enjoy gardening and horticulture. For those holi-daying abroad the usual recommended vaccinations against enteric disease and malarial prophylaxis apply. Where people are likely to make long-distance journeys by air it is wise for them to check with their doctor that there are no contra-indications. Those suffering from respiratory disorder may experience oxygen deficit at certain altitudes, and so may need to ascertain if their intended destinations are appropriate. All older people should be advised to exercise their feet and legs during flights, not only by stretching and walking at intervals, but by 'walking' for approximately 10 minutes in every hour, whilst sitting still. This heel-to-toe mechanism activates the calf-muscle pump and reduces the risk of oedema.

Safety education

Safety education is an integral part of health promotion at any age, but its significance for older persons is highlighted by the mortality and morbidity statistics, which show accidents to be a prime cause (Table 7.5). Although seniors constitute a reasonably safe group of motorists, slowed reaction times and sensory deficits do render them vulnerable to road traffic accidents, especially as pedestrians and cyclists. It is important for health visitors to reinforce the highway code and to encourage older people to wear light-coloured and/or protective clothing when exposed to risk.

Home accidents among the elderly are, however, a major problem, as although older people have fewer accidents than do children, they are often more serious. Home accidents currently account for approximately 4000 deaths per annum, and a further 100 000 cases of injury. The latter statistics may well be under-represented, as minor cases of injury often go unreported. Not unexpectedly, fatal cases prevail in those aged 75 years or more; the higher numbers of female deaths probably reflects their greater longevity (Table 7.6).

Most accidents are a combination of human error and environmental hazards, but human frailty assumes even greater significance in later years. Falls are by far the most frequent cause of death and injury amongst seniors, as can be readily seen from Table 7.6. Falls occur most frequently on steps, stairs and in the living-room. Health visitors are, of course, aware of the different pathological causes of instability in the elderly which may predispose to falling and are, therefore, particularly likely to counsel those suffering from

Table 7.5 Average pattern of fatal and non-fatal home accidents occurring in any one year in UK.

Fatal accidents (Total 6500)

Age-group	0–14	15–64	65–74	75+	Total
Sex					
Male	230	1060	430	880	2600
Female	170	740	570	2420	3900
Age-group total	400	1800	1000	3300	6500
% of total	6%	28%	15%	51%	100%

Non-fatal accidents, involving a visit to a Hospital Accident and Emergency Department (Total 1 000 000)

Age group	0–14	15–64	65–74	75+	Total
Sex					
Male	250 000	220 000	20 000	10 000	500 000
Female	190 000	240 000	30 000	40 000	500 000
Age group total	440 000	460 000	50 000	50 000	1 000 000
% of total	44%	46%	5%	5%	100%

Based on data supplied by The Royal Society for the Prevention of Accidents (1983). Home and Leisure Safety: for Pre-Retirement Course Organisers, p 6–8

Table 7.6 Average pattern of fatal home accidents occurring within any year in the population aged 65 years and over, in UK shown by type of accident

Age group	65–74 M	F	75+ M	F	Total M	F	
Type of accident							
Falls	250	350	700	2150	950	2500	
Fire, flames etc.	70	100	110	220	180	320	
Poisoning	30	50	25	25	55	75	
Suffocation and choking	40	50	20	60	60	110	
Other causes including excessive cold	30	40	30	90	70	120	
Total	420	590	885	2545	1315	3125	(4430)

Based on data supplied by The Royal Society for the Prevention of Accidents (1983) Home and Leisure Safety, p 6–8

visual deficits, dizziness, basilar artery insufficiency, or proneness to postural hypotension. Additionally, mobility problems arising from arthritis or neurological difficulties often precipitate tripping, whereas the side-effects of certain drugs, such as sedative and anti-hypertensive agents, should not be under-estimated. Mitchell (1984) considers 'sway' to be a contributory factor in falls amongst elderly females; so education about gait could be helpful (see Ch 2).

The primary aim of health visitors within general safety education is to encourage a combination of hazard-free surroundings and safe personal habits. It is, therefore, important to correct any sensory deficits as far as possible, and to remind seniors of the importance of good lighting, especially as there is a tendency for older people to try to economise by using low-wattage bulbs. They also tend to undertake do-it-yourself activities, for which they are often inadequately equipped. Older people should be encouraged to conduct a comprehensive assessment of possible home hazards, whilst they are active enough to remedy them. Any necessary re-positioning of shelves, window catches, door bolts and letter boxes should be carried out soon after retire-ment. Waist-level shelves for milk deliveries are considered a good idea, avoiding the risk of sudden dizziness from stooping. Although some seniors scorn the use of walking-sticks, a stout umbrella or shooting-stick can prove very useful. Gray & McKenzie (1980) give a number of helpful tips about walking aids, including the use of a stick strap to facilitate movement. Their book may prove helpful reading for carers of the elderly. Bath aids, safety rails, firm banisters and raised toilet seats are other devices for aiding safety. Some older people prefer to come downstairs backwards, but whichever way they choose, they should always be encouraged to check-count the number of steps, and to take especial care if suffering poor vision, or wearing bi-focal spectacles.

Preparing for action in the unfortunate case of falls is another essential part of health promotion and safety education. Seniors should be taught mat exercises and how to rise if un-injured. They should be encouraged to work out a suitable alarm system beforehand, so that they can summon help quickly in the event of an accident. The danger of hypothermia after falling should be discussed — another reason for emphasising the need for adequate safe house-heating, especially during very cold spells. Where individuals have conditions which may threaten consciousness, are taking specific drugs, or have known allergic responses, they should be encouraged to wear a medic-alert bracelet or carry a card to inform others.

Fire safety

It is always wise to reinforce teaching about fire hazards, especially if such dangers are apparent during visiting. Seniors should be encouraged to have fire-smothering blankets handy, and to position pan handles safely, as well as taking care when using tea towels and oven gloves. Fire-guards often become 'bones of contention' when seniors feel cold, but they should be fitted, and all electricity wiring and appliances should be regularly checked. This can prove difficult when seniors have limited income and the property they live in is old. Sometimes grants may be available from Local Authorities for improvements, or from voluntary societies. Particular attention should be paid to those who tend to be forgetful and leave saucepans on stoves until they boil dry or to older persons who smoke.

Case study
Lydia Brown, aged 83 years, was a diabetic who knew that others disapproved of her smoking, so she always kept her cigarettes hidden under the mattress, and only smoked secretly when in bed. She became very unnerved and spent several weeks in hospital after burning her hands badly because she fell asleep whilst smoking.

Of course, all the important aspects of poisoning risks which apply generally, also apply to the elderly, but because of sensory deficits and the risk of confusion over medicines and such substances, extra care needs to be taken. Flood precautions should also be checked. Another aspect is to ensure that older people are protected against criminal damage and violence. They should be advised about suitable security measures, such as locks and window-bolts, and cautioned not to admit unauthorised persons into their premises, nor to entertain persons who cannot produce accredited evidence of their identity. Pocket alarms should be carried. However, it is important not to arouse fear unnecessarily, nor to underestimate their confidence so that they become over-suspicious, or obsessive about security to the detriment of the quality of their life. Further help on safety education in retirement can be obtained from The Royal Society for the Prevention of Accidents, whose address is given in Appendix 6.

Housing

Choosing with whom to live and where, is one of the most important tasks of later life. Very frequently decisions are made in the immediate post-retirement phase, and they have to be altered when frailty increases. Currently some 50% of elderly people are owner-occupiers, and although often regarded as comfortably off, may be unable to deal adequately with repairs and maintenance costs. Before deciding to 'stay put', such home owners should be encouraged to assess the state of their housing, identifying what needs to be done, particularly in relation to basic amenities. Some local authorities offer grants for renovations and repairs, and special schemes are available through such organisations as The Anchor Housing Trust, Age Concern or Shelter. Advice can also be taken from local Housing Aid Centres, or Citizens' Advice Bureaux. Some owner-occupiers who feel they can no longer sustain responsibility for maintenance, either sell their property to a Housing Association, or operate a gifted housing arrangement such as that run by Help the Aged Housing Trust, whereby they are given guaranteed accommodation for the rest of their life. Great care, however, should be exercised before this step is taken, and sound advice should always be sought from an independent solicitor.

Some elderly people decide to move to new homes, whether in the country, at the seaside or in a designated 'retirement area'. Such migration may have a marked effect on the recipient area, as well as the elderly who move. Karn (1977) found that the majority of elderly migrants tended to be childless, with fewer younger relatives to help them, so health and social services in such localities were severely stretched. It is always wise to suggest that persons contemplating a move to their 'retirement dream area' spend some time reading through local accounts of the services available, and checking on specific local difficulties. They should try to spend at least one winter month in their 'retirement dream area' before deciding what it is really like. They should check if the topography, climate, noise levels, air, pollution, transport facilities, accessibility to shops, churches and other social amenities are suitable. The nearness of the location to family, friends, or other supports should also be carefully considered. It is all too easy to become enamoured of a new area without working through possible eventualities. A couple contemplating a move should think well how each would cope if they should lose their partner.

Council tenants now have a right to buy their homes at a discount price, but the advantage of this for the older person is less obvious, especially if little renovation has been carried out. Repairs and improvements may be dealt with fairly quickly as tenants, and transfers to more suitable property can usually be arranged. However, rents may rise steeply and thus wreck budgeting plans, unless offset by housing benefit. Where tenants are living in private property they may face problems relating to security of tenure, rent controls and getting repairs done. Sometimes they may need special guidance about enforced leaving, or harrassment. Special needs may be presented by those elderly who live in tied accommodation, or those who are homeless. Other seniors who may require particular consideration are those living in high-rise flats or isolated dwellings, where loneliness may be intense; those in areas where vandalism is rife, or where crime rates are high; or those who are undecided about moving in with relatives. In the latter case health visitors may find themselves acting as advisers for both parties. As it is likely that there may be benefits and stresses for each, it is wise to outline in general terms the possible advantages and disadvantages derived from such proposals, and to encourage free communication between both parties, in order to try to ensure beforehand maximum space, privacy, comfort and independence for each. However, it is unwise to give definitive opinions, and both parties should clearly understand that any decisions made must be their own.

Sheltered housing

Although sheltered housing may be an answer for a number of older people, it is not necessarily a universal panacea. There may be no balance between the ages of residents, nor their levels of dependence, so that wardens may sometimes find themselves facing heavy demands from frail, sick or handicapped old people. Furthermore some schemes tend to isolate the elderly from the rest of the community. However, some sheltered housing schemes can contribute to a sense of community, particularly where there is regular interaction between residents, supervising warden and nearby neighbours. There is a great deal of scope for developing this type of housing and for health visitors to exploit such complexes for a whole range of health education purposes. However, this requires considerable tact and a great deal of preparatory communication with residents and with wardens. Wardens often have very ambiguous role responsibilities and frequently welcome support (Butler et al 1983, Heumann & Boldy 1982, Phillipson & Strang 1984).

PROMOTING HEALTH IN BEREAVEMENT

One of the most frequent happenings which health visitors may encounter when helping people in later life, particularly the very old, is bereavement. This is because over 70% of all the deaths that occur in the United Kingdom, do so in those aged 60 years and over; the major causes being heart and circulatory disorders; cerebrovascular accident; trauma and respiratory disease. Thus death of contemporaries can be a fairly common experience for older people. Furthermore, at the turn of the century, when present-day seniors were born, families were larger, so many older people have several siblings and other relatives, rendering them vulnerable to repeated losses. As with retirement, bereavement may be studied as an event, a status and a process, with each phase calling for particular knowledge and skill, in order that intervention may be effective. Figure 7.1 deals particularly with health visiting care at the individual level.

It may seem strange to speak of promoting healthy bereavement, but that is exactly what health visitors seek to achieve, recognising that death, grief and mourning are an inevitable part of life. Death is almost always a blow bringing with it anguish and sorrow. In its wake can come shock, numbness, denial, anger, guilt, intense sadness and eventually accept-

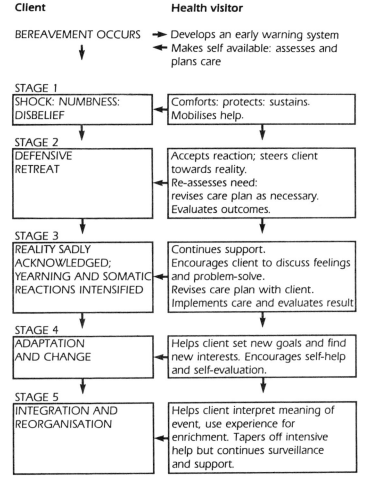

Fig. 7.1 The crisis of bereavement and health visitor intervention (crisis intervention model after Caplan 1964, 1974; see Appendix 3)

ance and readjustments (Fig. 7.1). For conjugal pairs the pain of separation may be very great, depending on the length and quality of the relationship, and its intensity as other options have diminished. For older people there is also the unlikelihood of replacement. Raphael (1984) gives an in-depth review of the literature relating to bereavement, pointing out that elderly marital pairs often have such closely interwoven lives that the loss of the one may cut across the other's very existence.

For these various reasons it is helpful if there has been a period of health visiting contact prior to the death, because this means a relationship which can be built on. Coping strategies may then be known and, if the death was expected, the practitioner may have been involved with the dying person, known some of their attitudes and wishes, and possibly may have helped the remaining seniors to dissipate some of their grief beforehand, and brace themselves for the inevitable. Sometimes, when illness has been prolonged and pain distressing, the end comes as a relief, however tinged with sadness. Sudden death, however, intensifies all the reactions and may cause great physical as well as psychological disturbance. Where the senior was very dependent on the dead person, or had ambivalent feelings about them, signs of upset may be exaggerated. The most adaptive responses to mourning are found where seniors have a strong personal belief system; supportive people around them; activities to fill the void; and a chance to establish new and meaningful roles and make new ties.

Bereavement as an event

Initial help should be of a comforting and strengthening nature. Since numbness, shock and disbelief tend to predominate at first, seniors may welcome practical assistance in letting family and friends know of the event. They also often appreciate practical guidance on procedures such as registering the death and contacting the funeral director to make needful arrangements. If inquests have to be held, there may be a need for explanations about procedures, and perhaps added support, especially if older people are alone.

Attention to basic needs, especially safety, *must* be considered, since elderly bereaved persons may disregard these in their grief. Spiritual counsel is often valued, but should be mobilised only at seniors' request, though suggestions of such help often need to be made. It is at times like this that an appreciation of cultural and ethnic differences is particularly important. Being aware of what death means to specific groups, and understanding their rituals and ceremonies, are all ways of offering silent support. Grief reactions vary considerably; some groups mourn overtly, whilst others withdraw, or aim to 'keep a stiff upper lip'. Each may require different handling.

The symptomatology immediately accompanying bereavement has been well documented. Cardinal signs include disturbances of sleep, appetite and weight, digestive and elimination upsets, and liability to sudden panic attacks. Depression is common (Parkes 1972). Underlying the elderly bereaved persons's distress is a sense of threat to the life of the survivor, a fear of being left alone, and a prominence of helplessness and dependence. It is important for health visitors to appreciate the welter and depth of these feelings, in order to be able to offer the understanding support which is required.

Bereavement as a status

The recognition of widowhood is formalised by the state, through the issue of widow's benefit. Older females form the greater proportion of all widows; they may welcome advice about obtaining such allowances and other sources of help available to them. Organisations such as Cruse provide immense support for widows and widowers, but there is sometimes a tendency for other bereaved relatives or friends to be left outside such groups, whereas they too may be grieving deeply. Health visitors may therefore find that bereaved support groups, open to all ages and held on a general basis, meet needs in many localities. It is perhaps at this level that the *community* aspects of the health visiting role become most apparent. Educating the community to understand and help bereaved persons is part of this role.

Bereavement as a process

Once shock has given way to denial, there is need to give seniors space to 'collect themselves'. This stage of denial is often accompanied by rationalisation or projection, sometimes amounting to frank hostility. It may be necessary to explain this mechanism to significant others, who could otherwise feel hurt and distressed.

As reality dawns on the bereaved individual, sadness usually deepens and somatic complaints predominate. Medical aid may need to be invoked, but seniors also respond to empathetic listening, extra comfort measures and kind concern. They may find great solace in other family members, friends or pets; in reiterating the history and qualities of the dead person; and in cherishing their possessions. Throughout the period, bereaved seniors need help to realise that their reaction to grief and loss are normal, so that they can learn to accept them and gain from them; can treasure memories without wholly dwelling on them; and can learn to develop new interests and activities. Thus, even in mourning, there is scope for health education at both personal and group levels.

Epidemiological studies indicate that the impact of bereavement on health and mortality lasts for a considerable period after the event of the death. Parkes et al (1969) showed an association between cardiovascular deaths and bereavement amongst widowers, and Maddison & Viola (1968) traced the health patterns of widows in the first year after death of their spouses, finding increased morbidity and mortality. Thus there is evidence that the bereaved elderly increase their utilization of health care services, mainly between the 5th and 8th month after bereavement (Raphael 1984). This may suggest when health visiting contact may most profitably be intensified.

Using findings such as these, health visitors would offer intensive initial support, followed by continuing help, education and surveillance, particularly between the 4th and the 9th month, after bereavement with such supportive help gradually being tapered off as independence is fully restored. Since anniversaries of deaths, especially the first, are poignant times for bereaved persons, older people in particular may value unobtrusive visits at such times. Keeping careful records so as to identify such occasions is part of efficient health visiting (see also Kübler-Ross 1969, 1975).

SUMMARY

In this chapter retirement has been viewed as an event, a status and a process. The objective has been to show how fulfilling the latter years can be if individual groups and communities adopt healthy lifestyles and are helped to achieve their potential in all planes of development. The significant aspect of the health visiting role has been emphasised as helping individuals and communities to take a positive approach to their own ageing, seeing this as a vital part of the cycle of life. Whilst such a role has caring and supportive elements when displayed at the individual level, its thrust is largely educative. It is therefore particularly demonstrated at the community level, where instigating, interpreting and teaching functions predominate.

It has been suggested that this area of health visiting work is currently underdeveloped, but that there is great scope for extension. In future it is likely that persons who have benefited from the improvements in health care, education and social welfare and from the general socio-economic changes, including a greater use of leisure, will move into the last long phase of human development in a fitter state than some elderly do today. If this is the case, health visitors may well find they have greater opportunity to fulfil their preventive functions instead of so often being forced to give reactive care. Given effective health promotion it may well be possible that future generations of seniors may be able to say with Cicero:

Nothing is more enjoyable than an active and leisured old age.
Falconer 1923

REFERENCES

Butler A, Oldman C, Greve J, 1983 Sheltered housing for the elderly. Allen & Unwin, London
Comfort A 1977 A good age. Mitchell Beasley, London, p 181–190
Committee on Medical Aspects of Food Policy 1984 Report of the panel on

diet in relation to cardiovascular disease. Report on Health and Social Subjects 28. HMSO, London

Davies L 1981 Three score years and then? Heinemann, London

Davies L, Holdsworth D 1982 Pre-retirement education in a longitudinal survey, through periods of pre- and post-retirement. Gerontology Nutrition Unit, Queen Elizabeth College, London

DHSS 1979a Nutrition and health in old age. Report on health and social subjects, No. 16, HMSO, London

DHSS 1979b Recommended daily amounts of food, energy and nutrients for groups of people in the United Kingdom. Report on health and social subjects No. 15. HMSO, London

DHSS 1983 (SR 3) Analysis of Family Expenditure Survey, 1981. HMSO, London

Disability Alliance 1984 Disability rights handbook. Disability Alliance, London

Falconer W A, 1923 Translation of Cicero, De Senectute. Heinemann, London

Ebersole P, Hess P 1981 Towards healthy ageing Mosby, St Louis

Gray M, McKenzie H 1980 Take care of your elderly relative. Allen & Unwin, London, p 71–76

Heumann L, Boldy D 1982 Housing for the elderly. Croom Helm, London

Holdsworth D, Davies L 1982 Nutrition education for the elderly. Human Nutrition: Applied Nutrition 36: 22–27

Karn V 1977 Retiring to the sea-side. Routledge & Kegan Paul, London

Kerr S 1983 Making ends meet. Occasional Papers on Social Administration No. 69. Bedford Square Press/NCVO, London

King P A 1978 Foot assessment of the elderly. Journal of Gerontological Nursing 4 Nov–Dec: 47

Kübler-Ross E 1969 On death and dying. Collier-MacMillan, London

Kübler-Ross E 1975 Death: the final stage of growth. Prentice Hall, Englewood Cliffs, New Jersey

Maddison D C, Viola A 1968 The health of widows in the year following bereavement. Journal of Psychosomatic Research 12: 297–306

Mellström D 1982 Tobacco smoking, ageing and health among the elderly. Age and Ageing 11:45

Mitchell R G 1984 Falls in the elderly. Nursing Times. January 11: 51–53

Murray R, Huelskoetter M, O'Driscoll 1980 The nursing process in later maturity. Prentice Hall, Englewood Cliffs, p 137–156

National Advisory Committee on Nutrition Education 1983 Proposals for nutritional guidelines for health education in Britain. Health Education Council, London

Nuffield Centre of Health Services Studies 1984 Unemployment, health and social policy. Nuffield Centre, 71–75 Clarendon Road, Leeds

Office of Population Censuses and Surveys 1984 Unemployment and mortality. Unpublished report, quoted in The Guardian, September 17, 1984

Parkes C M 1972 Bereavement: studies of grief in adult life. Tavistock, London

Parkes C M, Benjamin B, Fitzgerald R G 1969 Broken heart: a statistical study of increased mortality amongst widowers. British Medical Journal 28: 3–6

Phillipson C, Strang P 1984 Health education and older people. The role of paid carers. The Health Education Council, in association with the Department of Adult Education, Keele University p 93–110

Raphael B 1984 The anatomy of bereavement: a handbook for the caring professions. Hutchinson, London

Streib G, Schneider C 1971 Retirement in American Society: Impact and process. Ithaca N Y, Cornell University Press

Townsend P 1979 Poverty in the United Kingdom. Penguin, Harmondsworth

Wenlock R W, Boss D H, Ageter L B 1984 New estimates of fibre in the diet in Britain. British Medical Journal 288: 1873

World Health Organization 1978 International Conference.on Primary Health Care. Alma Ata declaration. WHO, Geneva

World Health Organization 1982 Epidemiological studies on social and medical conditions of the elderly. Euro Reports and Studies 62. WHO, Copenhagen

FURTHER READING

Anchor Housing Trust 1981 The Anchor guide to staying put in retirement. Anchor Trust, Oxford

Casey J 1983 Your housing in retirement. Age Concern, Mitcham DHSS 1978 A happier old age. HMSO, London

Dickman S R 1979 Nutritional needs and effects of poor nutrition in elderly persons. In: Reinhardt A M, Quinn M D (eds) Current practice in Gerontological Nursing. Mosby, St. Louis, p 74–87

Donaldson R J, Donaldson L J 1983 Essential community medicine. MTP Press, Lancaster.

Gray J A M 1982 Better health in retirement. Age Concern, (England)

Health Education Council 1984 A Programme of Education for Health in Old Age. HEC 1984

Latto S 1983 Extra care for frail elderly tenants. In: Glendenning F (ed) Accommodating frail elderly people. Beth Johnson Foundation Publication, in association with the Beth Johnson Housing Association and University of Keele, Adult Education 1983

Pincus L 1981 The challenge of a long life. Faber & Faber, London

Tinker A 1983 Housing elderly people. Public Health 97: 290–295

Yurick A G, Robb S S, Spier B E, Ebert N J 1980 The aged person and the nursing process. Appleton-Century-Crofts, New York

8

Illness in old age

While undoubtedly the primary role of the health visitor is prevention of ill health, it is obvious that in her work with old people she will have to advise on, manage or contain some situations which have got beyond the preventative stage. Her role will become that of detector, carer, co-ordinator or even troubleshooter. It is, therefore, appropriate that the health visitor should know how illness in old age differs from that of younger people, and have some knowledge of the causes and management of common medical problems in the elderly.

HOW ILLNESS DIFFERS BETWEEN YOUNG AND OLD

Case study

Mr T. was an 80-year-old widower who lived alone. Gradually he did less and less for himself and eventually the house and garden became neglected. His appetite and weight deteriorated. His memory was blunted and he lost confidence in his ability to be self-caring. Depression set in. Arrangements were made for him to have a home help, meals on wheels, and a district nurse. The opinion of a geriatic physician was sought when Mr T. became virtually immobile and incontinent. Examination and investigation showed that the patient had parkinsonism, myxoedema and osteoarthritis, and was also suffering from polypharmacy.

He made a good recovery following physiotherapy and amendment of his drug treatment. Later he had a successful home visit and returned to his home mobile and self-caring. Although no social services were required, the health visitor was asked to watch his progress.

Illness in the young often presents rapidly, the history is easy to obtain and symptoms frequently point to disease in one body system. However, the elderly, especially those over 75 years, often have multiple system diseases, disorders or disabilities; the history is often difficult to obtain, the signs and symptoms are altered and presentation of disease is frequently non-specific. Frequently they are prescribed a multitude of drugs which cause problems of compliance and adverse drug reactions. In addition, the isolated, housebound and elderly confused person can present major management problems in community care.

Multiple diseases

It is classical medical teaching that a patient's signs and symptoms should be integrated into one disease entity. This approach frequently fails in the 'old' elderly (over 75 years) who often have multiple acute and chronic disorders, e.g. a chest infection with heart failure superimposed on long standing features of arthritis, obesity, diabetes, leg ulceration and a stroke. Unfortunately, the signs and symptoms of new disorders and diseases may be wrongly attributed to pre-existing conditions, e.g. the aches and pains of osteomalacia may be attributed to osteoarthritis.

The history

Although it may be difficult to elicit, an accurate history of events leading up to the illness is absolutely vital, since it may strongly influence both treatment and management. The health visitor can be of considerable help if she passes on to the doctors any useful information from neighbours, friends, relatives, social workers, or meals-on-wheels or home help supervisors.

She should also use her eyes when visiting an elderly person. For example, a well-kept room suggests that the person has been well until recently, or equally, has had effective back-up help, whereas an untidy house with accumulation of newspapers or unopened milk bottles suggests some degree of confusion or self-neglect, and smells may indicate incontinence. The presence of walking aids, raised toilet seats or chairs, a bed downstairs, a key hanging on a string inside the front door — all suggest impaired mobility.

Signs and symptoms

It is perhaps not so well recognised that pain threshold raises with age. Many elderly people with an acute myocardial infarction, a perforated peptic ulcer, or even a fractured neck of femur do not complain of pain.

Fever is less common in the elderly and the patient's temperature often cannot be used to assess the progress of an illness. Indeed a potentially febrile illness may be associated with hypothermia.

Presentation of disease

Symptoms in the young are usually obvious, discrete and point to a specific disease process. Symptoms in the elderly, on the other hand, are often non-specific, vague and ill-defined. Common presentations include toxic confusional state, failure to thrive, or 'he's gone off his feet, doctor, and taken to bed', or 'collapse'. Direct questioning may not clarify the issue, but the health visitor, by simple observation, can often establish the diagnosis or which body system is involved.

Adverse drug reactions

The Royal College of Physicians (1984) has recently emphasised that the incidence of adverse drug reactions, such as confusion, incontinence, falls or dizziness, rises with age.

Although the elderly have received great benefit from the pharmacological revolution — L-dopa in the treatment of parkinsonism is an excellent example — they frequently suffer from being given too many drugs with resulting poor compliance. Indeed, one professor of geriatric medicine has said that his greatest therapeutic triumphs are achieved by stopping drugs given by other doctors. Consequently, the alert health visitor can do much to help prevent iatrogenic ill health.

The frail elderly at home

Quite often the physically and mentally frail wish to remain at home, although they find it hard to manage, even with maximum community support. Sometimes they are quite unrealistic about their capabilities. The health visitor has a vital role in monitoring the situation, ensuring that all necessary help is provided, and quality of life maintained. Relatives and neighbours who act as 'carers' must also be supported.

COMMONER ILLNESSES IN THE ELDERLY

Confusional states

Case study

Mrs W. was a confused 83-year-old lady who was brought to the casualty department by the police. She had been found wandering in the street at night, dressed only in her night clothes. She was hypothermic and, because of the confusion, was quite unable to give any account of herself or her illness. No relatives or friends came with her. Later it became clear that until recently she had been quite well and capable of looking after herself. This suggested that she was suffering from a toxic confusional state.

Confusion in old people may be due to a toxic confusional state or dementia, or a combination of both. It is absolutely essential to distinguish between the two conditions, since a toxic state is treatable and reversible, while a dementing

process is often irreversible and presents more of a management problem. Unfortunately, there is a very regrettable tendency to equate confusion in the elderly with dementia, which
results in failure to search for a treatable cause.

Toxic confusional states (acute brain failure)

The history of the illness enables a toxic confusional state to
be fairly readily distinguished from dementia; in the former
there is a short history of sudden onset of mental changes,
whilst in the latter there is a long history with slow onset. Old
people with a toxic state may show fluctuations in their mental
state, sometimes appearing lucid, sometimes very confused.
They may be restless, aggressive, sleepy, have reversal of
night/day sleeping pattern and experience visual hallucinations. Sometimes a client is not as confused as relatives
allege. This may be due to a change in the level of tolerance
of the carer. The degree of confusion can be assessed by
using a mental test questionnaire (see appendix at end of
chapter).

There are many causes of transient toxic confusional states,
the most common being:

infections
drugs
heart failure
metabolic disturbance, e.g. diabetes
change of environment
constipation
(bereavement)

and which the health visitor may be able to recognise by using
her eyes intelligently. An infection is perhaps the most
common cause. A chest infection is suggested by rapid
breathing associated with a cough productive of infected
sputum — chest pain may not be a feature. Urinary infection
may be suggested by smell and history of frequency. Dysuria
per se may not be a symptom. Cellulitis, particularly of the
skin of the legs will be seen as a reddened, hot area which
may be associated with blistering and which occurs in heart
failure, or with pre-existing varicose or traumatic ulcers.
Drugs are an all too frequent cause of confusion or halluci-

nations. There is evidence that the ageing brain becomes increasingly sensitive to the effects of drugs which act upon it — therefore the health visitor should look particularly for evidence of use of hypnotics sedatives, tranquillisers, anti-depressants and anti-Parkinsonian drugs. The fact that the person has taken the drug for a long time does not necessarily exclude it from consideration. Heart failure may be suggested in a person who is becoming increasingly short of breath on exertion, has swelling of the ankles and is unable to lie flat in bed. The diagnostic trap is that prolonged periods of immobility can produce dependency oedema.

Other causes of confusion are less easily recognised, but knowing that the client is a diabetic can be useful. Changes of environment or constipation can cause temporary confusion, but this occurs mainly in those patients whose mental reserve is already limited. Confusion after bereavement may not be a true reflection of the situation — the surviving spouse may have been supported by the one who has died, and who successfully covered up or concealed the fact that the survivor's mental state was impaired.

Treatment of toxic confusional states is the treatment of the precipitating cause which in most cases is fairly straightforward and may be managed at home. Patients will need sympathetic handling, bright lights should be avoided, and carers will need much patience. If patients have to be moved to hospital, they must be given adequate explanation and friends should accompany them.

Dementia (chronic brain failure)

Clients with a dementing illness have a slow onset of memory loss which is of long duration, usually over many months or years. Only a few cases can be treated and reversed; in the majority the best that can be done is to support both client and carer. The most common causes of dementia are:

senile dementia of the Alzheimer type	(50%)
multiple infarct dementia	(20%)
mixed senile and multi-infarct	(20%)
others including:	
vitamin B deficiency	
hypothyroidism.	

Research into the causes of dementia continues apace, but no effective treatment is currently available.

It is difficult to establish accurate statistics for the prevalence of dementia due to diagnostic problems. However, approximately 5% of those aged 65–74, or 10% of those aged over 75 years are affected. This increase with age, linked with the rapid increase in the number of old elderly, has led to the expression 'the silent epidemic'. To health visitors, with their epidemiological approach, such statistics mean that more than half a million demented old people are being cared for at home. Furthermore, about 45% of affected men and 10% of affected women are living with their elderly spouse. Other family members give resident care to about 30% of sufferers, but the remainder live alone until their state has so deteriorated as to necessitate institutionalisation. Three out of four of those old people who live alone in a demented state are supported by relatives, friends and/or neighbours, who may plead with the health visitor to 'do something' to relieve the socio-psychological problems produced by the elderly person (Hirschfield 1978, Gurland et al 1983, Gilhooly 1984).

The majority of cases of senile dementia are of the Alzheimer type, the aetiology of which is unknown. It affects more women than men. The brain shows signs of atrophy with proliferation of senile plaques and neurofibrillary tangles. There is a marked deterioration of the cerebral cholinergic pathways involved in memory. Deterioration is progressive with marked short-term memory loss, with some preservation of long-term memory. Those affected may try to cover up by confabulating. Abstract ideas become difficult to understand, initiative and motivation are blunted, the capacity to make decisions is reduced and the person's previous personality is exaggerated with the client becoming more absent-minded and self-centred. Paranoid delusions can occur which can be most vexatious to the relatives. The person can become restless and start to wander, easily getting lost due to memory loss. The vocabulary becomes restricted, reduced in words and becomes simpler. Depression with anxiety and hypochondriasis may develop, personal hygiene and care tend to deteriorate. Life expectancy for those who become dependent is said to be about 2 years, but skilled nursing can prolong life considerably.

Multi-infarct dementia is more common in men and starts at an earlier age than senile dementia. It is caused by small multiple brain infarcts occurring over many years. The onset may be abrupt with clouding of consciousness due to the infarct. As this resolves there is some degree of recovery until the next incident occurs, when a further mental deterioration develops, but without full recovery. This produces the so-called step wise deterioration in mental state. The personality is often well preserved and the patient can be all too well aware of the mental changes, thus becoming depressed. Emotional lability is common. Paranoia may develop.

A few causes of dementia, such as hypothyroidism and Vitamin B_{12} deficiency are potentially reversible. These are easily detected by simple specific blood tests. Treatment can result in some improvement, particularly in those with vitamin B_{12} deficiency. Normal pressure hydrocephalus is recognised clinically by an ataxia/apraxia of gait, incontinence, and mental confusion. The diagnosis is easily confirmed by the non-invasive computerised axial tomography (CAT). Treatment is by insertion of a shunt.

Many demented people can, for most of their life, be managed at home where the surroundings are familiar. However, carers who have an elderly relative at home can find their task very wearing, both physically and mentally, due to symptoms such as night wandering, incontinence, sleep disturbance, unaesthetic, bizarre or dangerous behaviour, gross disturbance of mood and constant demands for attention. Indeed dementia often causes greater strain for the carers than does physical disability, thus leading to a breakdown of health and placing a strain on family or marital relationships, especially when children live in the household. However, where the elderly spouse is the carer there may be often a greater demonstration of acceptance. Clearly health visitors must be aware of the many problems posed by dementia so that they can intervene early in a situation and prevent crises when relatives will say 'enough is enough'.

It is important to realise that the closer the carer is in emotional terms to the sufferer, the more distressed he or she is likely to become at the personality disintegration of the loved one. Help may be needed to handle this emotional situation, especially if decisions about institutional care have to be made. Great comfort may be derived from attending support groups with those in similar situations and reading the publications of the Alzheimer's Disease Society (1984) (see Appendix 6).

It is essential that caring relatives and friends receive the maximum support from the primary health care team, hospital and social services as well as any monetary benefits to which they or the sufferer may be entitled. Meals-on-wheels, home help, care attendant, district nurse, community psychiatric nurse, luncheon clubs, day attendance at a day centre or hospital, the continence service and intermittent relieving admissions to hospital or welfare home can all be valuable. Drugs may be used to treat depression or reduce wandering, which is best prevented by ensuring that the client has an interesting day time occupation which tires him or her out. No specific drug treatment for dementia exists at present. Permanent institutional care is reserved for those who cannot manage at home. Those with minimal behavioural disturbance may be admitted to a welfare home, while the very disturbed may need admission to a psychogeriatric unit.

Communication techniques and very simple reality orientation measures can help the quality of life of demented elderly people. They can be encouraged to keep diaries and calendars up to date, and helped to put days and time within a meaningful context, e.g. 'Today is Tuesday and Mrs Green is coming to tea' or 'As it is Thursday, you must get ready to go to the Day Centre.' Other helpful measures include using photographs and mementoes to aid reminiscence, labelling objects, doors and pictures clearly and adopting simple colour coding schemes. It is wise to suggest that the affected client wears an identity necklace or bracelet, giving the person's name, address and telephone number as a precautionary measure against wandering away from home.

Those who are confused may not bother, or may be unable to manage their financial affairs. Demands for payment of rates, electricity, gas or telephone bills will all be ignored and the person will be in danger of having all forms of power and heating cut off. Initially, if the person has a bank account, it may be possible to arrange payment by standing order or by payment of small regular monthly amounts, and relatives may find it helpful to assume the power of attorney. However, the client has to be aware of the implications and agree to the suggested arrangements.

For the very confused it may be necessary to use the Court of Protection. Here relatives or social workers make an application to the Court for it to take over the financial affairs of the client. The Court will ask for a medical certificate confirming the mental state and if this is accepted, it will take over the finances and appoint a relative to do the 'donkey work'. If a suitable person is not available, or is unwilling, the Official Solicitor will take over the function. The caring relative is responsible to the Court for what he does, and therefore the mechanism is not a blank cheque for wild spending. The whole procedure can be reversed should the person's mental condition improve. For clients in Scotland, an approach should be made to the Court of Session in Edinburgh. Sometimes it may be necessary to arrange compulsory admission of an elderly person. The new Mental Health Act of 1983 has changed some of the previous regulations (1959). The current situation is as follows:

Section 2. Admission for assessment (previously Section 25). The maximum period of detention is 28 days. The criteria is (a) the patient is suffering from mental disorder of a nature or degree which warrants his detention in hospital for assessment and subsequent treatment if necessary and (b) he ought to be detained in the interests of his own health and safety or with a view to the protection of others. Application is made by an approved social worker or nearest relative, based on the written application of two registered medical practitioners who must state that the current criteria for assessment are satisfied. One of the practitioners must be approved by the Secretary of State for Social Services as having special experience with diagnosis and treatment of mental disorders.

Section 3. Admission for treatment (previously Section 26). The maximum period of detention is 6 months, renewable for a further 6 months and then for periods of 1 year at a time. The criteria are (a) a patient suffering from mental illness which makes it appropriate for him to receive medical treatment in hospital to alleviate or prevent deterioration of the condition, (b) for the patient's health and safety and protection of others. Application and recommendations involve two registered medical practitioners (similar to Section 2), and an approved social worker or nearest relative.

Section 4. Admission for assessment in cases of emergency (previously Section 29). The maximum period of detention is 72 hours. The criteria is that it is of urgent necessity for the patient to be detained, and compliance with the provision for admission for assessment would involve undesirable delay. The procedure involves recommendation by one medical practitioner (e.g. the general practitioner) and an application by an approved social worker or nearest relative.

On occasion the health visitor may face the situation where an elderly patient is quite unrealistic about his or her capabilities of managing at home even with maximal community and social service support. This may be a suitable occasion for the use of Sections 7–10 of the new Health Act — Reception into Guardianship (previously Sections 33, 34). The criteria are (a) the person should be suffering from mental illness or severe mental impairment and (b) it is in that person's interest or for the protection of others that he or she be received into guardianship. The procedure involves two registered medical practitioners and an application by an approved social worker or nearest relative. The effect is that the guardian then has the power to require the patient to live in a specified place or to attend specified places for treatment. The maximum period of detention is 6 months extendable for a further 6, and then for periods of 1 year at the time.

Self-neglect

Case study

Mrs E.M., aged 68 years, was admitted with a history of increasing weakness, anorexia and loss of weight for several weeks. She had become a recluse since the death of her husband 15 years earlier, and had never invited anyone into the house until she became ill. It was found to be exceedingly dirty with thick layers of dust on all flat surfaces. Some 30–40 full milk bottles lined the walls of the front hall, and there were many piles of newspapers in the hall and in other rooms of the house. In the bedroom clothes were dropped when discarded, and were never picked up; consequently it was necessary to walk on a thick layer of clothing in order to get to the bedside.

The condition of self-neglect is now increasingly recognised, and the features are well described (Clarke et al 1975). Characteristically, these clients of the health visitor are of above average intelligence, but are unkempt, dirty and often incontinent. They live in what others consider squalid surroundings, and are often well known to the social services. Their clothing and bed linen have usually not been cleaned for a long time, the house is dirty and items, particularly newspapers, are kept, never to be discarded. Poverty is usually not a problem, although the client may appear penniless. They will tend to feed themselves out of tins, or live on tea and biscuits. Admission to hospital is usually associated with a high mortality rate.

Two other groups of people who may neglect themselves are chronic alcoholics and paraphrenics. Chronic alcoholics are unable to control the amount they drink, which can lead to malnutrition, vitamin deficiencies, paranoia and dementia. Alcoholism is developing when clients tell lies about alcohol intake, avoid the topic, take drinks earlier and earlier in the day, and give excuses to explain the situation. Paraphrenia is late onset schizophrenia which classically occurs in elderly isolated females. Such a client is often suspicious of close neighbours and fears they are spying on her. Thinking is disordered and difficult to follow. Some clients may be mute and others hyperactive, and show incongruity between feelings and experience.

Caring relatives and neighbours can find it very difficult trying to help those who neglect themselves, particularly if the person is 'awkward minded', eccentric and cantakerous. Goodwill is soon lost and a crisis situation will soon develop, particularly if some illness intervenes or support is withdrawn.

Health visitors can be faced with difficult ethical and management problems when the person appears ill, is failing to thrive and is clearly not coping but equally refuses admission either to an old people's home or to hospital. If the person is mentally clear and is adamant that admission is unacceptable, then it is reasonable to continue to care for that person at home with as much care as can be given and readily accepted. Unfortunately, if death occurs at home, there is often much ill informed criticism of the caring services, when they have often done their best to help within the limits that the patient would allow.

There may be situations, however, when although the person is mentally clear, compulsory admission to hospital is considered necessary. This involves the use of Section 47 of the National Assistance Act of 1948 or the 1951 Amendment. This allows the District Medical Officer, together with the general practitioner or geriatrician to move the person in need of care and attention from his or her home if it is thought to be in the interest of the patient, or would prevent injury to the health of, or serious injury to, other people'. A person 'in need of care and attention' within the meaning of the Act, is one suffering from grave, chronic illness . . . or being aged, infirm or physically incapacitated, living in insanitary conditions, and unable to devote to him or herself, or is not receiving from others, proper care and attention. The 1948 Act requires an application to a Magistrate's Court, with 7 days notice being given to the patient. The 1951 Amendment allows direct application to a magistrate and removal of a patient without delay. Accommodation in hospital or in a home must be available.

Discharge of these patients can be a problem. Neighbours may resist, because they have found the new situation more acceptable. Much depends on the attitude of the old person — if he or she is pleasant, there will doubtless be a willingness to try again.

Falls

The incidence of falls rises steeply with age and is more common in women. However, it is not often appreciated how frequent falls are in the elderly. It is calculated that in the UK 3 million falls occur in old people in the community in a year. While less than 2% result in actual injury, this will include 30 000 cases of fractured neck of femur. Unfortunately, over 3000 deaths occurs directly as a result of the fall. Many elderly people lie on the floor for several hours before being found, and about half of these patients will die within 6 months. Most falls occur inside the home, especially in the living room and on the stairs, and happen when the person is moving from chair, wheelchair toilet or bed. They are particularly common among the socially isolated, the depressed and demented. Though falls may not result in injury, they frequently induce a fear of falls in the person concerned who loses confidence and refuses to leave the house or even to walk at all.

The health visitor should try to find out why a person has fallen:

- environmental factors, e.g. loose mats, poor lighting, polished floors
- physiological/ageing process, e.g. reduction in balance control
- medical disease
  - cardiovascular system, e.g. postural hypotension, cardiac arrhythmias
  - central nervous system, e.g. parkinsonism, stroke, poor eyesight
  - locomotor system, e.g. arthritis
  - early phase of acute illness
- drugs
- local causes, e.g. painful feet

Some of the causes are quite easily preventable or treatable. Unfortunately, it is often difficult to obtain a clear accurate history or to interview a useful witness, but it must be remembered that falls can be a non-specific indicator of impaired health and therefore the causes must be identified if at all possible.

Accidental falls due to environmental problems account for almost half the causes. The elderly may trip over loose carpets or wires, slip on well polished floors, or fall on steep stairs without adequate hand rails or lighting. Poor eyesight and ill fitting footwear will compound the situation.

Control of posture deteriorates with age due to cerebellar degeneration and impaired proprioception, and results in delayed assimilation of postural information. Reaction times increase and an elderly person who stumbles may not be able to correct the situation quickly enough. General ill health and inability to concentrate compound the situation.

Cardiovascular disease is a potent cause of falls. Normally the tendency for the blood pressure to fall when a person moves from a horizontal to a vertical position is very rapidly corrected. This self-correcting mechanism may be impaired in the elderly and produce postural hypotension. It can be aggravated by drugs which affect blood pressure, e.g. anti-hypertensive agents, L-dopa, tricyclic antidepressants, phenothiazines and diuretics. Cardiac arrhythmias, particularly bradycardia, or tachycardia are also important causes of falls. Often the diagnosis can only be made with a 24-hour ambulatory ECG. Some falls are due to vertebrobasilar insufficiency which produces impairment of blood supply to the brain when the head is tilted sharply upwards or sideways.

Central nervous system diseases frequently impair mobility which can affect balance. Thus patients with parkinsonism or a stroke may find it difficult to make sudden or quick alterations in the direction of walking, and when these are attempted falls can result. Disease of the labyrinth of the ear or its central connections are not common in the elderly, but can cause vertigo and resulting falls.

Arthritis and muscle weakness will also make it difficult for the elderly to maintain proper balance. The situation may be compounded by painful foot conditions, such as corns or ingrowing toenails, and by the early phase of an acute illness.

Drugs which cause postural hypotension or excessive sedation can easily cause falls. The hangover effect of some hypnotics are well known. Alcohol can also blunt postural control, while long acting hypoglycaemic drugs, such as chlorpropamide, can cause falls due to low blood sugar levels.

The health visitor can help in management/prevention by noting how, when and where the falls tend to occur (see Ch. 7). She can note the number and type of drugs the person has been prescribed and can check compliance. She will be able to check for evidence of impaired mobility, painful feet and environmental problems. She will be able to advise about lighting, positioning of furniture and carpets and avoidance of polished floors. It may be helpful to bring the bed downstairs and have a bedside commode. Ramps over steps may be needed, or extra handrails on the stairs. The district physiotherapist may be able to give 'mat exercises' to restore the patient's confidence in getting off the floor without assistance. The local authority may be able to fit an alarm system to bring assistance when needed.

Many of the factors which cause falls also produce poor mobility. Their recognition is important since inability to move about the house or get out of it can seriously impair quality of life.

Hypothermia

Hypothermia, i.e. a deep body temperature of less than 35°C, has only been relatively recently recognised as a problem in the elderly. It occurs when heat production, generated by conversion of food to energy, is exceeded by heat loss from skin and expired air, a situation which can be precipitated by an acute or chronic illness. It generally occurs in elderly people who are not in good health. Hypothermia has been found in 3.6% of elderly patients admitted to hospital and in 10% of the elderly living at home during the winter months, and it contributed to the deaths of 3–4 people every day during the winter months in the UK in 1981.

Hypothermia is due to:

- cold environment
- impaired thermoregulation with age
- secondary precipitating causes
  infections, poor mobility, falls, fractures, endocrine disorders, diabetes, uraemia, drug side-effects, previous episode of hypothermia, dementia or depression.

A recent study of people aged over 65 years living at home showed that three-quarters of them had a room temperature less than 65°F, which is the minimum temperature recommended in the Parker Morris report on council housing and less than the recommended minimum of 70°F suggested by the DHSS. Thus hypothermia can so easily develop if an elderly person clad only in night attire falls to the floor at night and is not found for many hours.

Increasing age is associated with reduced efficiency of thermo-regulation, the shivering action is muted, the basal metabolic rate does not rise with cooling, loss of body subcutaneous fat reduces insulation and there is defective venous constriction (see Ch. 2). In addition, the elderly are less aware of temperature changes, and have reduced sensitivity to cold. Young people can detect mean temperature differences of about 0.8°C, whereas the elderly can only differentiate between mean temperature differences of 2.5°C, while some cannot perceive differences of 5°C. Consequently old people may wear inadequate clothing, have inadequate heating or room insulation. Lack of finances may be a contributing factor.

There are many secondary precipitating factors for hypothermia. Any severe illness due, for example, to infections or heart failure, which causes a toxic confusional state and lack of awareness of surroundings, may result in a fall in body temperature, especially if the environment is cold. Any disability or disease of the brain, cardiovascular or locomotor systems, which limits mobility or can precipitate falls is a potent risk factor. Drugs which slow mobility (e.g. sedatives or tranquillisers), impair consciousness (e.g. hypnotics) or impair shivering (e.g. phenothiazines) are potentially dangerous for the elderly. Falls and subsequent inability to get up may have been due to a fracture. Patients who are demented or depressed may not realise the house temperature is low. Those people who have had a previous episode of hypothermia are particularly at risk.

Hypothermia is easily diagnosed once the diagnosis is suspected. A quick test is to assess the anterior abdominal wall temperature. If this feels cold, the person is cold. A rectal temperature will confirm the situation. A hypothermic person often looks myxoedemic. The face is pale and puffy, cerebration is slow and the voice husky. Consciousness is impaired below 32°C and patients are usually unconscious with temperatures less than 27°C. Tone of the muscles is increased and the reflexes are depressed and relax slowly. The pulse is slow and the blood pressure low. The abdomen may look distended. The lower the temperature, the greater is the risk of cardiac arrest.

The health visitor will not necessarily be involved with the treatment of hypothermia. However, hospital admission should be considered for patients with a temperature of less than 35°C, although some patients with temperatures down to 35°C can be managed at home, provided adequate precautions are taken. All hypothermic patients should be removed from the cold environment and then allowed to warm up slowly, usually by being wrapped in a 'space blanket'. Rapid external rewarming in the elderly can cause an after drop of temperature and circulatory collapse. Rapid intense rewarming, e.g. by cardiac bypass or rebreathing technique, is not often used in old people.

The health visitor is mainly concerned with preventing hypothermia. Firstly she must be able to identify those 'at risk', i.e. those living alone, the frail, the housebound, the depressed and the confused. Then she can help to ensure that clients maintain an adequate environmental and body temperature, giving advice on how to reduce draughts and heat loss, insulating lofts and hot water tanks. An old person may need to live in one heated room to save fuel.

Advice about avoiding falls and the use of adequate clothing may be necessary. It may be possible to obtain suitable local authority financial heating and insulating grants, and to have the advice of gas and electricity board advisory team, as well as the local branch of Age Concern.

Incontinence of urine

Incontinence of urine is the unintentional and involuntary passing of urine in an inappropriate place or at an inappropriate time twice or more in the past month. It can be a major problem in the care of the elderly, and may become 'the final straw which breaks the camel's back'. It is an illness, or a symptom of an illness, which, if not curable, can often be improved and certainly the management can be made more satisfactory. The incidence varies with the population studied. A recent community survey (Thomas et al 1980) showed that 6.9% of men and 11.6% of women over the age of 65 were incontinent. Not surprisingly, the incidence is over 50% in long-stay institutions.

Physiology of micturition

Normal micturition control depends on two intact levels of nerve function (Fig. 8.1). At the lower level is the local parasympathetic reflex arc which connects the bladder to the

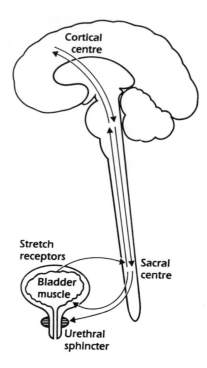

Fig. 8.1 Neurological control of micturition

spinal cord (sacral centre). At the higher level is the frontal cortex which permits voluntary control to be exerted over the reflex arc via its connections with the spinal cord. As the bladder fills, sensory impulses pass from stretch receptors along the afferent arc to the spinal cord, where motor impulses are sent along the efferent arc to the bladder detrusor muscle, causing it to contract, while relaxing the muscles of the external sphincter and pelvic floor. The desire to pass urine is usually felt when the bladder contains 350 ml, but micturition can be inhibited by voluntary will exerted from the frontal cortex.

Increasing age is associated with functional changes which affect bladder function. The elderly find it increasingly difficult to inhibit the reflex and postpone micturition. Eventually the old person may only be able to delay passing urine for a few minutes.

Types of incontinence

Incontinence may be either transient or established.

1. Transient
   — acute illness
   — drugs
   — constipation
   — infection of the urine

2. Established
   — disorder of nervous pathways
   a. uninhibited bladder (neurogenic bladder)
   b. autonomous bladder
   c. atonic bladder
   d. reflex bladder
   — unstable bladder
   — stress incontinence
   — outflow obstruction.

Transient incontinence may occur as part of an acute illness such as toxic confusional state or acute cerebrovascular accident, especially if the person is admitted to the strange environment of a hospital. Drugs are an important cause of temporary incontinence, e.g. loop diuretics such as frusemide, given to patients with poor mobility, or sedative drugs which impair sensory input to the frontal cortex. Anti-cholinergic drugs, e.g. tricyclic antidepressants such as imipramine, may cause retention of urine with overflow which can be potentiated by constipation. Temporary incontinence can result from constipation or when increased sensory input to the sacral reflex arc occurs, e.g. from cystitis, atrophic urethritis associated with atrophic vaginitis, or local lesions of the bladder, such as a stone or a tumour.

A person has established incontinence when the problem persists after acute conditions have been treated. The cause may be due to disorders of the nervous pathways to the brain or the bladder. Various types of neurogenic incontinence are described, of which the most common type in old age is the neurogenic bladder. In this situation damage to the frontal cortex, as in dementia or strokes, results in loss of ability to inhibit reflex bladder contractions, although sensation of bladder retention is retained. There may be urge incontinence when the person's desire to pass urine is almost immediately followed by the passage of urine. The other types of neurogenic bladder are less common in the elderly; autonomous, when there is destruction of the second to fourth sacral segments in the cauda equina, as in spinal cord tumour causing ineffective bladder contractions; atonic when the afferent part of the reflex arc is damaged, as in diabetes, causing retention with overflow; and reflex when the connections between the reflex arc and the frontal cortex are severed as in spinal injury, causing an unstable bladder which empties reflexly.

Bladder disorders may cause incontinence. The commonest problem in the elderly is the unstable bladder, which is characterised by uninhibited bladder contractions, occurring at any stage of bladder filling, and can follow coughing, laughing, getting out of bed or standing up, resulting in total bladder emptying. Elderly people with unstable bladders have frequency, nocturia and urgency, but are not always incontinent. However, they are predisposed to urge incontinence, nocturnal incontinence, and stress incontinence. In men obstruction to urinary outflow due to an enlarged prostate can cause an outflow obstruction.

Stress incontinence is a distinct different condition and separate from the unstable bladder. The history in both has similarities, but in stress incontinence a small quantity of urine is squeezed out of the bladder due to an increase in intra-abdominal pressure and an inefficient urethral closing mechanism. It is most common in multiparous women and those with uterine prolapse.

Management of incontinence

The health visitor may well be asked to advise relatives of clients with persistent incontinence. There are many ways in which she can help and attention to the following management points is essential:

1. Encourage optimism
2. Charting of incontinence
3. Habit training and avoiding constipation
4. Odour
5. Care of skin

6. Clothing
7. Physiotherapy
8. Appliances
9. Access to toilet/commode
10. Drugs
11. Catheter.

Above all she must be optimistic since much can be done to improve the patient's quality of life and self-esteem. She must treat her client — not just the wet bed. Initially it is useful for the times of micturition and incontinence to be charted, since it can help to establish the type of incontinence, the timing of habit training and indicates the most suitable appliance. Habit training can be a successful technique, which not only involves the client being taken to the toilet regularly, even when not requested, but also means trying to help the client understand the mechanism of the disturbance of bladder function. The bladder fills at a rate of about 100 ml/hour during the day and if the client cannot hold more than 250 ml of urine before micturition, then the right time for toiletting is every two hours. Over a period of time it will generally be possible to extend the time of visits to the toilet.

An accurately completed continence chart will help to establish the appropriate frequency of toiletting for that particular person. However great patience is required, especially with those people who pass urine just after visiting the toilet. Regular toiletting fails where the bladder capacity is so small that it is exceeded if urine is allowed to collect for only 2 hours. At night urine formation is reduced in volume, which will help control of incontinence, but fluid restriction after 6 p.m. may be needed. Naturally all clients should be advised to avoid constipation.

Probably nothing is more disturbing to client morale than the smell of stale urine. This problem can be reduced by changing soiled linen and placing in a bucket containing disinfectant; preventing the urine becoming concentrated by ensuring adequate fluid intake; rapid treatment of urinary tract infections and cleaning carpets as soon as they are soiled. Proprietary aerosol or solid block room deodorisers are often extremely helpful.

Care of the skin is helped by preventing it being in

prolonged contact with urine, and ensuring it is kept clean and dry. Clients should be able to wear indoor clothing during the day, and all clothing should be machine washable. Various types of specialised clothing are available (see Disabled Living Foundation address in Appendix 6).

Physiotherapy can help to improve mobility to and from the toilet and improve pelvic floor tone. Exercises to improve pelvic muscle power are given in three stages and need to be practised conscientiously for 6 months. Stage one involves the client sitting or standing and pretending that she is trying to avoid diarrhoea by tightening the ring of muscle around the anus. Stage two involves sitting on the toilet, passing urine and attempting to stop the flow in mid-stream by contracting the muscles around the urethra. Stage three involves the client sitting or standing, tightening the muscles around the anus then the urethral muscles and then both together. All exercises should be practised several times daily.

The health visitor must also look for difficulties experienced by clients reaching the toilet in time. If the toilet is upstairs and the patient is slow, a downstairs commode may be necessary. Male urinal bottles, especially with non spill valves can be helpful. Alternatively, extra rails for the stairs and a raised toilet seat may be needed. Clients may also experience problems when looking for public toilets if they do not know where they are; they may need to plan shopping to ensure they are always near a toilet.

Incontinent clients may be prescribed drugs with an anti-cholinergic action, which suppress bladder contractions (e.g. emepromium bromide or tricyclic antidepressants). However, they are often ineffective and are not without troublesome side-effects.

Relatives will often need advice about absorbent appliances which are mainly of two types: insert pads, and sheets or underpads. Unless overloaded, all will absorb fluid without becoming wet. The time an appliance will last depends on its absorbent capacity and the rate of urine formation. If a person forms 100 ml/ urine per hour during the day, it will take 3 hours to saturate a 300 ml capacity pad. Oversaturated pads can disintegrate and/or cause skin rashes. Insert pads are worn between the legs and are held in position by pants or retained in a special pouch either inside or outside the pants.

Most protect against mild or occasional incontinence, and are usually not recommended for night use, although some (Molnlycke pants) can be used over the 24-hour period. Most types hold 250 ml urine and therefore 2-hourly changing is usually necessary. The retaining pants may be disposable or reusable, and made of plastic, elastic, netting or paper.

Absorbent appliances for beds or chairs are of two main types: thin underpads or large sheets. The thin disposable underpads have limited absorbent capacity — 350 ml or 650 ml depending on size. They tend to disintegrate when wet and are best for clients who are only mildly incontinent. Alternatively washable absorbent draw sheets can absorb up to 3 litres of fluid without soaking the bed. These sheets are comfortable to lie on, are economical in use, the surface remains dry and there is no disposable problem. However, there is a high initial purchase cost, they become heavy when wet and are unsuitable for households without laundry facilities. At least three sheets are required per person — one in use, one in the wash, one drying.

Ultimately, catheter drainage may be suggested for those where other methods have failed. Used with discretion, it can alleviate much discomfort and improve morale. The drainage bag should be concealed as a leg bag or in a sporran bag, rather than carried for all to see. The health visitor must be sure that the client or the relatives is able to empty the catheter bag. Unfortunately, catheters are associated with urinary tract infections, and can be pulled out.

Faecal incontinence

Though faecal incontinence is less common than urinary incontinence it, too, can produce a crisis situation. It is found in 22 people per 1000 population over 65 years and many of them receive no help from health or community services. There are three principal causes: faecal impaction, neurological disease and diarrhoea.

Faecal impaction

This is a sequel of constipation, where there is a slowing of the passage of intestinal contents, which allows time for excessive removal of fluid. The hardened faeces impact in the rectum and colon, and are 'lubricated' by excessive mucus secretion. The patient becomes unaware of the mass in the rectum and loses the sensation of 'call to stool'. The faeces above the impaction become liquefied by bacterial action and pass around it, presenting at the rectum as spurious diarrhoea. If the situation is allowed to continue, and especially if antidiarrhoeal preparations are given, the patient becomes more constipated, resulting in anorexia and vomiting, and even restless behaviour. Pressure of the distended rectum on the bladder neck can precipitate urinary incontinence. The condition is simply diagnosed by rectal examination.

Treatment may require manual removal of faeces, suppositories or enemata. The bowel will need re-education by ensuring that the diet contains adequate roughage/fibre as in fruit or bran. The effect varies with the size of the fibre particle — the larger the particle, the greater the faecal weight due to water retention. A side-effect of bran is flatus. Patients can be given Fibogel, a colloid agent which makes the motion easier to pass; Senokot, a muscle stimulant of the large bowel, or Bisacodyl which causes large bowel peristalsis.

The elderly require re-education about the use of laxatives to avoid abuse leading to diarrhoea, dehydration and severe electrolyte upset. Excessive laxatives, in the presence of obstructive bowel pathology, can result in perforation. Excessive use of liquid paraffin can result in leakage of fluid faeces from the rectum, malabsorption of vitamin D and, if small amounts are retained in the pharynx, spill over can occur into the lungs, causing pneumonia. It is not really necessary to arrange weekly bowel clearance, as the Victorians seemed to think.

Neurogenic cause

Normally, eating food initiates the gastrocolic reflex which moves intestinal contents along the colon to the rectum. This produces a sensation of the need to defaecate. This can be postponed by voluntary inhibition until convenient, but if ignored for long periods, results in constipation. Voluntary control, however, can be lost in patients with gross senile dementia — a situation analagous to that of urinary incontinence. The situation is usually treated by a planned routine of regular evacuation of the bowel.

Diarrhoea

Patients with severe diarrhoea, which can follow from purgative abuse, may temporarily lose adequate sphincter control with resulting incontinence. The treatment will be that of the cause with possible use of constipating agents. Spurious diarrhoea is found in patients with carcinoma of the rectum or protocolitis.

Abuse of the elderly

Case studies

Mrs D. was 75 years old and very severely incapacitated by extensive rheumatoid arthritis. She frequently refused to come into hospital to give relatives relief, since she feared being abandoned. Eventually she did agree and she was then abandoned. She literally turned her face to the wall and died within 3 days.

Mr M. was 83 years old, cantankerous, confused and frequently liable to hit out at or scratch those who cared for him. One day the caring nurse threatened to break his arm if he struck her again. He did, so she did.

Mrs H. was 84 years old and lived in the small front bedroom of the house belonging to her daughter and son-in-law. She was admitted to hospital with a stroke and made a total recovery within 3 weeks. The relatives refused to have her back again and eventually she was found accommodation in a warden-controlled flat, to which all her furniture was moved. It later transpired that she and her son-in-law, although living in the same house, had not spoken to each other for 10 years.

This problem is receiving increasing, if grudging, recognition since its early description in the 1960s. It should be remembered that 40% of the over 65s are supported by caring relatives and American evidence is that about one-quarter of these are at risk from battering. Situations which are likely to predispose to abuse are:

1. where the family was initially loving and caring, but this relationship has broken down when the old person develops mental and physical disabilities or the carer herself becomes ill
2. where the elderly person has not been taken in willingly, but as a result of a crisis
3. where the family atmosphere is violent and antagonism exists between family members before the senior comes to stay
4. where the old person is very demanding
5. where the carers are rather immature, the housing situation is poor, and there are financial problems.

Several types of abuse are recognised. Firstly, there may be real physical attacks such as pinching, physical restraint or threats of physical assult, coupled with screaming attacks at the old person. Secondly, granny may be neglected, with the carer refusing to supply meals. Thirdly, the client may be abandoned in hospital or a home. Fourthly, there may be exploitation for gain and lastly, there can be social abuse.

It is unusual for battering to be admitted and the elderly person is often most unwilling to speak of the problem to others. However, the alert health visitor can get clues from both history and observation of the client and the family. There may be a story of repeated falls to explain multiple bruises and the carer may frequently visit the GP with problems of 'nerves'. There may be deep bruising on the inner aspects of the arms from rough handling, or straight horizontal marks across the tops of the thighs from restraining tables. The health visitor should enquire how the elderly person came to stay, whether her health or that of the carer has changed recently, what effect her arrival has had on the family accommodation, and finances, how often the carer manages to get out by herself and does she experience any problems, particularly recent ones in looking after the elderly relative. It would be useful to assess the quality of communication between members of the family. Tactful enquiry will probably show that there are precipitating factors on both sides and that the carer has been under great stress (see Ch. 9).

Management by the health visitor will often need great tact and understanding. A multidisciplinary case conference may be necessary. If specific problems such as incontinence or nocturnal wandering can be identified, appropriate help can often be arranged — home help, care attendant, district nurse, advice about financial grants, relief admissions or attendance at a day centre. Changes in accommodation usually will take a long time to arrange. The health visitor must avoid taking sides.

MEDICATION FOR THE ELDERLY

Although drugs have brought great benefit to old people, adverse drug reactions are important causes of illness in the elderly. Not only are the elderly prescribed proportionally more drugs than younger people, but studies in the UK, USA and Sweden have shown that the incidence of adverse drug reactions rises with age. A survey of admissions to geriatric units in the UK shows that 1 in 10 were admitted solely or partly because of adverse drug reactions. Not all the patients recovered — indeed the mortality due to drugs also rises with age. Two groups of drugs caused nearly two-thirds of all reactions; those which act on the cardiovascular system (e.g. digoxin, diuretics and hypotensive drugs) and those which act on the central nervous system (e.g. hypnotics, tranquillisers, antidepressants and anti-parkinsonian drugs).

Adverse drug reactions are due to excessive prescribing, coupled with inadequate review of long-term medication, inadequate clinical assessment, altered drug metabolism (pharmacokinetics) and altered target organ sensitivity (pharmacodynamics) which occur in old age, and impaired compliance. The most important factor is excessive prescribing. Doctors are keen to treat disabilities which affect old people, but this may result in an old person being prescribed 10–12 different drugs, which makes it difficult for the patient to remember how and when to take the medicines.

An additional problem is that drugs which are prescribed

during the acute phase of an illness may no longer be needed in the later convalescent phase. However, to stop drugs which have already been prescribed requires a time-consuming routine for assessing their need. It is often quicker for the doctor to complete a new prescription form. Inadequate clinical assessment can occur when symptoms are treated rather than the disease, because history-taking and examination are very difficult and time-consuming. Dependency oedema of the feet due to immobility, for example, may be assumed to be due to congestive heart failure. If diuretics are given, incontinence can result.

There is now ample evidence that the way drugs are handled/metabolised in the elderly is less efficient than in younger people. The principal factors are a decrease in renal function and impaired liver function (Ch. 2). Consequently drugs are less efficiently detoxicated and excreted. Thus a standard adult dose of a drug will last longer and be more effective in the older person.

Another problem is that the ageing brain is more sensitive to drugs which act upon it, compared with the brain of younger people (increased target organ sensitivity: altered pharmacodynamics). Therefore hangover effects of hypnotic drugs and minor tranquillisers are often more prominent, and confusion following the use of antidepressants and anti-parkinsonian drugs are quite common.

Impaired drug compliance is a major problem in old people: as many as three-quarters of elderly people make errors in their prescriptions, a quarter of which are potentially dangerous. There are three main causes: first, the person may make a positive decision to stop taking medication because of lack of, or persistence of, symptoms; early response to treatment, or side-effects. In addition, those with impaired eyesight may not be able to read the label, while the confused elderly may fail to remember how and when to take the tablets.

Second, the doctor and/or the nursing staff may give inadequate explanations about how to take the medication , e.g. nearly half of a group of patients failed to take off the wrapping from suppositories before insertion. The doctor is also responsible for completing adequately the prescription form which the patient will take to the chemist for dispensing.

Inadequately completed forms may result in the chemist putting the instruction 'To be taken as directed' on the bottle. One ill elderly lady seen recently had a bottle of 0.25 mg digoxin tablets which were to be taken as directed. She was taking them three times a day.

The third factor in the compliance equation is the medication and its container. Drugs which are unpleasant to take, cause side-effects, or are difficult to swallow may not be taken. Old people often have difficulty in opening drug bottles, especially the recently introduced child resistant containers, e.g. the clicloc, pop loc and snap safe bottles. Neither do they find it easy to use blister or bubble packs.

Patients who do not comply accurately with their medication are likely to keep or hoard the medication. Recent 'Dump' campaigns have shown the size of the problem — two and a quarter tons of medicines were returned in Glasgow. In 1979 one-third of a million tablets and capsules were returned to Birmingham, but this was considered to represent only 3% of the potential total! Over 70% of the drugs were more than 1 year old. The dangers of hoarding are that drugs will be shared or used inappropriately. New supplies of medicines may be confused by the patients with older stocks already in the house. Although most drugs have a long shelf life, some do not, e.g. trinitrin tablets deteriorate within 2–3 months.

Health visitors must be aware of the need for accurate prescribing and compliance so that they can take advantage of their close and understanding relationship with their clients to help them as necessary. They should be alert to the problems of overdosage and adverse effects on the one hand, and those of inadequate therapeutic effect or lack of compliance on the other. They should be aware of methods of improving compliance by reinforcing verbal instructions and using written instruction cards. Medication aids, such as the Dosett box, can be used to good effect. They should ensure that the labels on the drug containers are legible, the directions are understood and the patient can open the bottle.

Patients with special medical needs

Health visitors may be asked to advise not only their elderly clients with special problems or needs, but also their caring relatives, friends or neighbours. The post myocardial infarction patient, those whose mobility is limited by a stroke, parkinsonism or chronic obstructive airways disease, and the elderly diabetic are among those who commonly seek advice.

The post myocardial infarction patient

Patients discharged home after a myocardial infarction may still be worried and fearful about their future, even when counselled by hospital staff. While there is no doubt that a heart attack is a serious illness, many people are able subsequently to lead an active life. The greater the degree of independence the person achieves after the event, the better the life expectancy. Therefore clients should be encouraged to be optimistic about the future and persuaded to lead as normal a life as possible.

The client can undertake many simple measures himself. Since excessive weight causes the heart to carry out extra and unnecesary work, weight should be reduced sensibly and slowly to the normal range. Fats and sugar should be taken in moderation. If a diet is advised to lower the blood cholesterol levels, it should be adhered to. Alcohol can be taken in moderation. Cigarette smoking should cease — abrupt cessation is probably easier for the patient than drawn out reduction in the number of cigarettes smoked. Exercise is clearly important. Going for walks is good to start with and should be started 4–6 weeks after the infarct; however care should be taken to avoid sudden severe exertion in the early days. The client is the best judge of his or her capabilities, and time will show what can be achieved. Some clients may not find it physically easy to cope at home. Here the health visitor must be able to assess the situation and call in what extra help is needed. She should also ensure that those clients who are on medication know how and when it is to be taken. Advice about when to resume sexual activity may also have to be given: it is usual to wait 6–8 weeks after return home or since the attack.

The bronchitic patient

The physical problems of chronic bronchitis and emphysema

will be well established and irreversible by the time patients become elderly. Indeed few patients with chronic obstructive airways disease survive to become aged. The disease is due almost entirely to cigarette smoking, especially cigarettes with high tar content, with the possible contributory factors of air pollution or dusty atmospheres. The disease causes bronchial narrowing and production of excess white or grey sputum, resulting in dyspnoea and a persistent cough. The lung tissue itself is damaged, causing reduced blood oxygenation.

Health visitors must help the client to get the best quality of life possible. Cigarette smoking should stop, unless perhaps it is the only pleasure the patient has. Clients should be warned of the dangers of crowded public areas where the chance of picking up a chest infection is increased. The advisability of anti-flu vaccines should be considered. Excess weight serves no useful purpose and should be lost. Unfortunately, there is no alternative to will-power in adhering to a diet. Clients should always take as much exercise as possible and try to keep fit. A physiotherapist may help, particularly with breathing exercises and improving controlled breathing during periods of dyspnoea.

Clients who are very dyspnoeic may require additional help/advice from a home help, occupational therapist or social worker. Rehousing on the ground floor may be necessary. Health visitors should ensure that clients understand their medication to establish good compliance. Domiciliary oxygen is not often prescribed since it is potentially dangerous, or may be used as a physiological prop. Room temperatures should be maintained at even levels and sudden changes of temperature avoided, since this can precipitate bouts of coughing.

The stroke patient

The health visitor can do much to relieve the worry, anxiety and/or depression which are not uncommon features after strokes, as when the active member of the household, or the wage earner suddenly finds him/herself dependent on others perhaps for the first time. The health visitor must encourage her client to be optimistic and try to be as independent of others as possible. Patients should be 'stretched' to make the maximum use of his/her capabilities — the specialised advice and help of the physiotherapist, occupational therapists and speech therapists can be of great help in this situation. Clients should be encouraged to express their thoughts and to avoid suppressing feelings which can cause frustration. Relatives, too, will need patience, understanding and encouragement, as well as specialist advice about financial allowances which may be relevant. Both client and relatives may find it helpful to join a local stroke club.

Clients may also worry about a recurrence of a stroke. This is a risk, but then life is generally hazardous. The risk can be reduced if risk factors are reversed — cigarette smoking must cease, weight should be kept within the normal range and hypertension in younger patients controlled (see Table 6.1). Optimism for the future should be maintained and clients encouraged to enjoy life without fear of a possible future event.

The parkinsonian patient

Unfortunately, the cause of this disease is unknown in many cases, although some cases result after the use of phenothiazines (e.g. chlorpromazine or prochlorperazine). The incidence increases with age, with a prevalence in those over 60 years of greater than 1000 per 100 000 population. Since the introduction of L-dopa both the expectation and quality of life for the parkinsonian patient has greatly increased.

The health visitor should be aware that though the clinical features of the disease in the elderly are similar to younger patients, there are two exceptions. Classically patients have an impassive facial expression; a moderately flexed body posture with slowness of movement and absence of arm swinging, leading to a shuffling gait with short steps associated with difficulty in initiating movement. This, together with postural hypotension, due to autonomic dysfunction, can result in frequent falls. However, elderly patients frequently do not have the classical pill-rolling tremor of the hands. In addition, some have impairment of cognitive function, typical of patients with Alzheimer's disease.

Treatment with physiotherapy and drugs is reserved for those with symptoms. Physiotherapy helps to build on improvements made by drugs, and restore confidence, particularly when patients can be taught how to get up unaided following falls. Elderly patients, unlike younger ones, are usually started on L-dopa (usually in combination with a decarboxylase inhibitor). The effect may be supplemented by other drugs such as bromocriptine, amantidine and anticholinergic drugs such as Artane.

Health visitors have a valued role in monitoring drug compliance and recognising adverse drug reactions. L-dopa, for example, can cause nausea, vomiting, postural hypotension, hallucinations and dyskinesia. Anticholingeric drugs frequently cause confusion.

Health visitors must be able to advise on aspects of general health and well-being, and diet. The diet should contain roughage to help combat constipation. Frequent small helpings of food may help overcome chewing and swallowing difficulties. Clients should avoid becoming overweight and should take regular exercise to stretch stiff muscles but avoid becoming over tired. Health visitors must encourage optimism and motivation in order to help ward off depression. They should be prepared to ask the occupational therapist to call and advise where there are problems with the activities of daily living. Writing may become difficult and it can be helpful to suggest the use of felt tipped pens which can be lifted between each letter to make writing more legible. The Parkinson's Disease Society has done most to help those suffering from the disorder. It has established local groups and patients should be advised to make contact with one.

The elderly diabetic

These patients can present many problems for the health visitor such as poor control of the disease due to problems with diet or drug compliance, and the need for special care of the feet due to peripheral vascular disease and neurological disorders. Good diabetic control helps to reduce the risk of complications, particularly those involving the nervous system.

Many elderly people with diabetes can be controlled on diet alone, but this can require considerable self-discipline. An unnecessary large intake of carbohydrate has to be avoided, while adequate amounts of protein, fat, vitamins and fibre in the diet are required. Clients should maintain an ideal body weight and obesity should be controlled or reduced. Adequate exercise is useful to help maintain general health and fitness, reduce weight and improve metabolic control.

Some elderly clients require additional oral anti-diabetic drugs. Health visitors should help to maintain good drug compliance and they should be aware of side-effects. Chlorpropamide, for example, has a long duration of action and can produce prolonged non-specific symptoms of hypoglycaemia such as confusion, disturbed consciousness and drowsiness.

A few elderly people will need to take insulin. The health visitor should ensure that her client knows how, when and where, and in what dose, the injections are to be given. She should ensure that the patient can see and identify marks on the syringe. She and the client must be able to recognise the signs and symptoms of hypo- and hyper-glycaemia.

Health visitors may be involved in monitoring diabetic control. Urine tests are less informative in the elderly due to a raised renal threshold. Consequently blood tests are more reliable, but fortunately these are not often necessary. However, the techniques of using a blood glucose strip, read by eye or meter, is simple, though accurate technique is required to obtain reliable results. The use of glycosylated Hb A, to monitor compliance, and therefore diabetic control over the previous month or so, is not yet widely available.

Elderly diabetics must be warned to take great care of their nails and the skin of the feet, especially if there is evidence of peripheral vascular disease. Comfortable shoes should be worn; the skin kept dry and clean, and any infection treated promptly. Smoking should be discouraged. Sore lesions on the feet may not be noticed until quite late if peripheral neuropathy is present, causing reduction in pain sensation.

The osteo-arthritic client

It is well known that the incidence of osteoarthritis increases with age, but fortunately many of those with radiological evidence of arthritis do not have symptoms.

Osteoarthritis is considered an exaggeration of ageing

changes in the joints, particularly those which take the body weight, i.e. the hips and knees. Severe arthritic changes in the knees can be associated with lateral instability due to disorganisation in the joint and laxity of the knee ligaments. Other joints, such as the shoulders, elbows and wrists may be involved, particularly if a person tends, for long periods, to lean heavily on a walking aid, thus putting much of the body weight through the upper limb joints.

The health visitor can assist in the management of clients with osteoarthritis in three ways. Firstly she can help to ensure that the person gets adequate pain relief. Often analgesic therapy is only taken irregularly with resulting limited effectiveness. What is required is regular therapy to break the vicious cycle of pain — a fact which the health visitor can emphasise. Aspirin and paracetamol are often quite effective for mild pain, but other non-steroid anti-inflammatory drugs, or even indomethacin, may be needed for mild/moderately severe pain. Secondly she might suggest physiotherapy in order to improve joint movement and strength of muscles. Thirdly she may be able to assist the client's motivation to establish a normal weight. Clearly excessive weight can only exacerbate arthritic joint problems and removal of unnecessary pounds or stones cannot but be advantageous. Unfortunately, losing weight is easier said than done — as many know!

If these measures fail and the client is in such pain that it impairs quality of life and mobility, then referral for possible surgery has to be considered. In such cases the health visitor has a supportive role pre-operatively and may be involved in some supervision and aftercare convalescence. Close liaison with district nurses is always necessary.

HOSPITAL TREATMENT AND AFTERCARE

An increasing number of older people are being admitted to hospital for treatment in various specialities. Health visitors, therefore, have an important part to play in pre- and post-hospital visiting. Where an admission is planned, it is helpful if a home visit can be paid to prepare the person, deal with any questions and anxieties and provide them with appropriate information. There is much evidence to suggest that those who receive adequate information beforehand benefit and are more likely to do well. Furthermore a comprehensive assessment of personal and social conditions can often prove helpful to hospital staff, assisting their decision-making about patient care. However, it is post-discharge when the health visitor can often monitor progress and so facilitate client rehabilitation. Not all clients require clinical nursing care, but may benefit from health education, encouragement, guidance and supervision. Through evaluating client and carer needs and taking action to meet these, it is often possible to prevent re-admissions.

A number of geriatric units already have liaison schemes in operation, but the follow-up of older persons from other specialties is less likely to be routine. Expansion of a post-discharge health visiting service is likely dramatically to increase demands, but may well be justified in terms of improved quality of life and the possible reduction in the number of elderly persons re-admitted to hospital. Collaboration within general practice teams can make such a service feasible and can weld hospital and community staffs together in the care of clients.

SUMMARY

This chapter has reviewed the more important ways in which illness can present with the elderly. The differences between disease in the young and old are explained. Keen observation by the health visitor can frequently identify the cause of a non-specific illness. She can also, by early intervention, prevent situations developing into crises.

APPENDiX

Mental test questionnaire

It can be very useful to assess the patient's mental state. Simple tests of memory and orientation can reveal gross impairment in subjects who may superficially pass for normal. An example is shown below (Denham & Jefferys 1972):

What is your name?
What is your age?
What is your address?
What is your marital status?
What was your previous job, or what did you do before marriage?
What year is it now?
I would like you to try to remember an address for me. I'll repeat it twice, and then I'll ask you what it was in about a minute: 74 Columbia Road.
In what years did the Second World War start and finish?
Who were the British Prime Ministers at the beginning and during the war?
What is the name of the present Prime Minister?
What is the Queen's name?
What is the name of the Prince of Wales?
Where is Belfast?
What is happening there?
What was the address I just gave you?

There are 16 questions which do not take long to ask and do not usually lose the patient's concentration. The key questions are the person's name and where he or she lives. If a gentleman is mobile and wanders out of the house, but does not know where he lives, he is very likely to get lost.

The test enables progress of a confusional state to be followed, but it does *not* distinguish a confusional state from a dementing process — it only indicates impairment of cognitive function. Scores correlate well with incontinence/continence and rehabilitation potential. Low scorers tend to be incontinent and take a long time to rehabilitate due to lack of understanding (Denham & Jefferys 1972). False or misleading low scores occur in patients who are deaf, dysphasic or depressed (depressed patients may not even bother to answer). Clearly the questions cannot be usefully applied to those of non-British backgrounds.

REFERENCES

Clarke A N G, Mankakar G D, Gray I 1975 Diogenes syndrome. A clinical study of gross neglect in old age Lancet 1: 366–368

Denham M J, Jefferys P M 1972 Routine mental testing in the elderly. Modern Geriatrics 2: 275

Gilhooley L M 1984 Social dimensions of dementia In: Hanley I, Hodge J (eds) Psychological approaches to the care of the elderly. Croom Helm, London

Gurland B J, Copeland J, Kuriansky, J Kelleher M, Sharpe L, Dean L L 1983 The mind and mood of ageing: mental health problems of the community elderly in New York and London. Croom Helm, London. Haworth, New York.

Hirschfield M J 1978 Families living with senile brain disease. Dissertation submitted in partial satisfaction of the requirements for the degree of Doctor of Nursing Science, University of California, San Francisco

Royal College of Physicians Working Party Report: Medication for the Elderly 1984 Journal of the Royal College of Physicians of London 18: 7–17

Thomas T M, Plymat K R, Blannin J, Meade T W 1980 Prevalence of urinary incontinence. British Medical Journal 281: 1243–1245

FURTHER READING

Chest Heart and Stroke Association, Tavistock House North, Tavistock Square, London WCIH 9JE Very useful leaflets on Asthma, Heart Disease, High Blood Pressure, Reducing the Risk of a Coronary, Coronary After Care, Stroke, Get Thin — Stay Alive, Smoking.

Eastman M 1984 Old age abuse. Age Concern, England

Hamdy R C 1984 Geriatric medicine — a problem — orientated approach. Bailliere Tindall, London

Hodkinson H M 1981 An outline of geriatrics, 2nd edn. Academic Press, London

9

Caring for older people with special needs

All older people experience a degree of loss, either of functional capacity, or social contact, but for some seniors illness, disability, social isolation or deprivation can take a heavy toll, creating particular difficulties and therefore special needs. In this chapter some of these difficulties and needs are explored, in relation to the health visiting role and the services which may be mobilised to help vulnerable clients and their families. The particular groups examined are:

the physically impaired, disabled and handicapped
the sensorily impaired
the psychologically disturbed
the elderly in ethnic minorities.

Although the support of carers is mentioned throughout, the last section of the chapter is devoted particularly to their needs.

THE PHYSICALLY IMPAIRED, DISABLED OR HANDICAPPED ELDERLY

The last 25 years have seen a growing international interest in the welfare of the physically impaired, including the elderly. Three events have particularly fuelled this interest:

1. The Alma-Ata declaration, setting out the goal of 'Health for All by the year 2000' (WHO 1978)

2. The Report of a World Health Organization Working Group on the prevention of disability in the elderly (WHO 1981a)

3. The International Year of the Disabled Person, 1981.

Differences in definition and classification have made it difficult to define the exact number of disabled elderly and to compare data between countries. This has now been partly resolved by the publication of The International Classification of Impairments, Disabilities and Handicaps (ICIDH) (WHO 1980). This defines:

a. *impairment* as any loss or abnormality of psychological, physiological or anatomical structure or function;

b. *disability* as any restriction or lack of ability (resulting from impairment) to perform an activity in the manner, or within the range, considered normal for a human being;

c. *handicap* as a disadvantage for a given individual, resulting from an impairment or a disability, that limits or prevents the fulfilment of a role that is normal (depending on age, social and cultural factors) for that individual.

From this health visitors should note that whilst impairments can arise from several causes, including hereditary disorder, acquired disease or injury, which may or may not be preventable, they need not progress to disability and certainly need not constitute handicap. This is an important concept which allows action to be directed to halt progression at any one stage.

Prevalence studies of physical impairment in the UK

In the UK the most recent national prevalence study of impairment and handicap amongst the adult population was undertaken by Harris (1971). Although using slightly different definitions from the ICIDH, she and her colleagues found that impairment rose steeply in relation to increasing age, with the highest proportion of affected persons being 75 years and over and predominantly female (Table 9.1).

60% of all handicapped people were over 65 (Fig. 9.1), and a higher proportion of them were very severely, severely or

Table 9.1 Proportion per 1000 of adults in different age groups, living in private households in Great Britain and who have some impairment

Age group	Estimated numbers (both sexes)	Proportion per 1000 Men	Women	Total
16–29	(89 000)	10.0	7.9	8.9
30–49	(366 000)	30.2	25.6	27.9
50–64	(833 000)	85.6	84.6	85.0
65–74	(915 000)	211.4	227.1	220.7
75 years and over	(867 000)	316.2	409.0	378.0
All ages	3 070 000	66.7	88.2	78.0

Based upon data supplied in Office of Population Censuses and Surveys, Social Survey Division Report 1971 Handcapped and impaired in Great Britain compiled by A. I. Harris with E. Cox and C. Smith. Table 1 p 4 HMSO, London (Reproduced by kind permission of OPCS.)

appreciably handicapped than were those in younger age groups. Additionally, physical disability was found to be class-related, with a preponderance in the lower socio-economic groups. This is supported by other studies and is believed to be irrespective of downward social mobility as a consequence of impairment.

Health visitors can therefore expect to find approximately 1 in 5 of their elderly clients to be impaired, with approximately 40% of these affected persons also being handicapped. The major causes of impairment were found, in this study, to be:

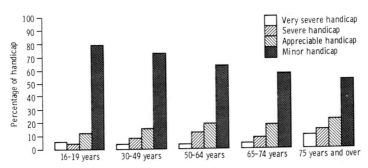

Fig 9.1 The distribution of impairment and handicap amongst the population, aged 16 years and above, in Great Britain, by category of severity. (Based on data derived from Harris A 1971 Handicapped and impaired in Great Britain. HMSO, London and reproduced by kind permission)

- arthritis and rheumatism
- circulatory disorders
- neurological states
- stroke
- respiratory disease
- trauma.

However, whilst 50% of those suffering impairment from arthritis, Parkinson's disease, multiple sclerosis or stroke were considered also to be disabled and handicapped, only 20% of the rest were so classified. With the exception of the respiratory disorders, these impairing and handicapping conditions were higher in females, reflecting the generally earlier male mortality.

All of the disabilities which restrict mobility can cause problems, but clearly they are of most significance for those who do not have mobile persons around them. However, almost 1 in 3 of the elderly impaired were found to live alone; 1 in 20 of those without any resident help were either very severely, or severely handicapped, whilst 1 in 50 were either bed- or chair-fast. Thus, understandably, these sufferers relied heavily upon visiting relatives, friends, and/or the caring services. A more recent, but smaller, survey confirms these findings and shows that families are still heavily involved with their elderly impaired, even though 30% live alone (Charlesworth, et al 1983). What is of particular relevance to health visitors is that approximately one-third of impaired seniors were being cared for by their elderly spouses, often without any supportive help. Furthermore 61% of other carers were close relatives, mostly sons and daughters, and over half of these were over 60 years. In many instances the carer's own health was described as 'poor' or 'very poor', and this was particularly noticeable amongst the 6% of carers who were aged 80 years or more. Not surprisingly, women carried the heaviest share of caring, but amongst couples, elderly men had a substantial role, which may serve to disabuse us of some stereotypes.

Statistics like this sometimes hold little meaning when studied out of context — but used with informed imagination they can tell health visitors a vital story about the potential volume and nature of their work with the elderly impaired, who may not necessarily require clinical nursing care from colleagues, or be greatly involved with other agencies. However, the following case studies may convey something of the all-pervasive effects of disability on the lives of sufferers and carers alike.

Case studies

Peter Day was 66 years old when he developed spastic paralysis and became immobile. Due to an associated arteriosclerotic dementia he gradually became unable to communicate, had great difficulty in swallowing, was doubly incontinent and had bouts of uncontrollable shouting. For 7 years his wife, Louisa, herself of pensionable age, cared devotedly for him with limited help. During this time she had no holidays and rarely went out, apart from shopping at a little store across the road. Finally, worn out by disturbed nights and constant washing, she consented to Peter's hospitalisation. When he died 3 weeks after admission, Louisa was stricken with guilt and suffers from severe depression.

Emily Brown, aged 82, housebound and severely crippled from arthritis, lived alone in a ground-floor flat. She had great difficulty washing herself, cooking, or undertaking domestic work. Her married niece, with five children to care for, travelled 90 miles every fortnight to do Emily's washing, major cleaning and 'stand-by' cooking. A nursing auxiliary came weekly to bath her and a home help visited twice weekly for 1 hour. Between these visits Emily saw no-one; consequently she became apathetic and displayed paranoid tendencies.

The health visiting role

The major part of the health visitor's role with the physically impaired, disabled or handicapped of any age is primary prevention; so the reduction of problems amongst the elderly must begin in the earlier years. By encouraging optimum pre-conceptual care, promoting healthy growth and development in infancy, childhood and adolescence and young adulthood, and by inculcating sound personal health behaviour and environmental hazard control, health visitors help to prevent or mitigate some of the conditions which can cause disability. In this facet of the work the health visiting principles of stimulating an awareness of health needs, and facilitating health-enhancing activities are paramount.

The next important aspect of the role is at the secondary level of prevention. Where primary preventive efforts have failed to eliminate the pre-disposing conditions and impairment has occurred, early detection, prompt treatment and ongoing surveillance are needed. The value of prevalence data is largely that they indicate who is at risk of developing more serious problems, and thus help health visitors to apply the concept of vulnerability, through the exercise of case-finding and screening skills. Considerable health education may have to be undertaken before clients are convinced of the need to take action on pre-symptomatic conditions, or before harmful lifestyles are discarded, but it is only by such teaching, persuasion and continued surveillance that the conditions which cause handicap can be controlled.

The tertiary level of prevention develops when impairment has occurred, especially if it has progressed to disability and possible handicap. To function effectively in this facet of their role health visitors should:

1. Appreciate the effects of disability from their clients' and client-carers' perspectives.
2. Assess needs and offer guidance on ways of meeting these, marshalling services as necessary.
3. Determine clients' and carers' coping strategies and strengthen these, so that optimum functioning is maintained. Where supplementary strategies are required these should be activated.

Appreciating the physical effects of impairment and disability

Whereas minor impairments are frequently well tolerated, and may even act as challenges, the physically disabling states frequently cause immobility. In turn every system is affected. Practitioners will therefore need a comprehensive understanding of pathophysiological processes, in order to advise wisely on the modification of exercise and the nutritional, postural, breathing and hygiene measures necessary to reduce the risks of stasis and infection.

The physical effects of dependency on carers must also be appreciated. Fatigue, and muscular or joint damage from strain and faulty lifting, are common. This calls for skill in teaching and demonstrating, and in locating suitable aids to avoid injury. However, it is important to realise that the physical restrictions create many of the psycho-social difficulties, which cause such distress. Therefore advising on ways of reducing the physical effects of disability, thus maximising movement and independence, will have multiple benefit.

The psycho-social effects of impairment and disability

For many seniors the emotional and social effects of impairment and disability are profound. Chronic pain, altered body-image, restriction of movement and enforced dependency can cause biographic disruption and a sense of loss of self (Bury 1982, Charmaz 1983). Cherished plans may have to be abandoned and notions of reciprocal support reviewed; roles often reversed and lifestyles frequently drastically reconstructed. In consequence, self-esteem may be lowered and ego-identity distorted, depending partly on the nature of the disability and partly on the reaction it provokes in the sufferer and others. Because drives and expectations are altered, and seniors often feel hurt and distressed, emotional responses like grief, anxiety, despair, apathy, regression or hostility are not uncommon. On a social level enforced isolation can generate depression and suspicion, although some individuals have high resilience and regard loss of social contact philosophically. However, almost all research studies support a strong association between physical handicap and psychological morbidity.

Health visitors will realise that, unless affected elderly are given opportunity to ventilate their feelings freely in a safe, confidential relationship, and mourn for the abilities they have lost, they will not be able to apply themselves constructively to problem-solving. Thus the rehabilitative approaches of practitioners will pass unheeded.

Assessment

Sensitive, perceptive assessment of the elderly impaired or disabled, on an initial and ongoing basis, is a most important health visiting activity. Whilst it follows general principles, certain specifics should be noted. Subjective data are highly relevant, as they convey seniors' feelings about their state. Objective data must be environmentally related and are best obtained under unobtrusive conditions, in order to obtain an accurate picture, free from distortions. The model chosen as a framework for thought and action will guide the format of the assessment. For example, as one major goal of care is the maximising of functional ability and independence, the Activities of Living model may be chosen as relevant (see Fig. 5.3). On the other hand, since one purpose of maintaining independence is to promote self-care as far as possible, some practitioners may prefer to use a framework such as Orem's self-care model, thus identifying seniors' abilities to help themselves, determining care deficits and deciding what help is required to bridge the gap (Orem 1980; see Appendix 3). Whichever framework is chosen the following points will be observed:

Gait, posture and locomotion

Practitioners should note the ability of disabled seniors to change position, sit, stand and/or walk with or without help; balance, bend, carry, climb stairs, kneel, stoop or handle prescribed aids. The range of joint movement, the presence of joint crepitus, pain, tremor, gait abnormalities or incoordination should also be determined. Eliciting clients' perceptions of their body-image may reveal how far these are distorted by pain, postural problems, or the use of appliances such as calipers or prostheses. The information gained from the analysis of such data will highlight the type and nature of required teaching and help.

Eating and drinking

In order to meet her client's individual needs and deal with specific problems, the health visitor should assess ability to chew, taste, swallow, and retain substances, cut up food, handle crockery and cutlery, shop for and sensibly and safely prepare meals. In addition the ability of the carer to prepare, serve and supervise meals adequately should be noted.

Eliminating

Problems of elimination met with in ageing are often exacerbated when disability is present. Whilst the focus is always on promoting maximum independence, aids may often be required. It is necessary to ask detailed questions about how clients manage their toilet arrangements, if they experience problems such as constipation, incontinence or retention; what resources they have available to help them deal with these difficulties and how they feel they can best be helped. Carers are often overburdened with washing heavily soiled linen, when clients are incontinent and welcome advice and the provision of protective devices. Where available, laundry services are often invaluable. Assessment on associated skin care is also necessary.

Personal cleansing and dressing

As part of general assessment of the capacity of seniors who have some impairment, attention should be paid to the client's ability to wash, shave and bath, brush and comb hair, cope with oral hygiene, and apply make-up where used. Similarly it is necessary to observe the ability of clients to dress independently, manage fastenings, cope with hosiery and footwear, or put on special appliances such as back supports or prostheses. Frequently benefit is lost because prescribed aids or appliances cannot be fitted, especially where clients live alone.

Maintaining safety

When mobility is restricted, certain safety features are crucial, such as discovering how clients could escape in the event of fire, or similar disaster; how vulnerable they are to criminal attack and what alarm systems are available to attract attention in the case of any accident. Hazard control measures should also be observed in relation to movement about the home, and when travelling away from home, such as by wheelchair, or on foot using aids, or when entering or leaving cars or boarding public transport.

Environmental hygiene

The ability of the disabled elderly to clean their own settings, or manage personal or household laundry, should be judged in the light of available amenities and sources of help. This may be a crucial point when client-carers are also frail elderly.

Communicating

The extent to which disabled seniors can interact and communicate can affect the quality of their entire life, hence it is necessary to determine levels of sight, hearing and speech; seniors' capacity for writing and/or using the telephone or other technical equipment available. Furthermore it is important to assess with whom, and how many people clients interact; the quality and value of such contact and their personal perception of their social support networks, since this appears to be vital in promoting positive attitudes.

Expressing sexuality

Because of the constraints posed by specific impairments there may be particular physical sexual difficulties, which need analysis and help. The Association for Sexual Problems of the Disabled (SPOD) are always willing to give personal advice (see Appendix 6 for address). By appraising gender awareness and relating this to behaviour, health visitor practitioners can determine the ability of the older client to maintain appropriate emotional and social relationships with persons of both sexes and can identify any problem areas.

Sleeping routines

Disordered sleep can be a source of great anxiety to a sufferer and can create considerable problems for carers. It is therefore always necessary to ascertain the type and amount of sleep which disabled seniors obtain, note their preferred sleeping positions and their usual rest routines, particularly whether any aids are used, including medications.

Other aspects

Other points to note include clients' and carers' attitudes to the specific disabilities, what effort is made to overcome difficulties, and the extent to which they are prepared to co-operate in rehabilitation.

After assessment a full report should be made, to establish a base-line from which to work, establish goals and evaluate progress. Others can use this documentation to gain an awareness of client needs and the rationale of care, whilst the records also indicate the extent of the practitioner's accountability.

Recognising and strengthening coping mechanisms

By the time many seniors acquire their impairments they have established coping mechanisms. The strategies displayed will probably reflect their pre-morbid personality. Thus some take impairments in their stride, regarding these as more or less inevitable; a few play down their problems, striving to do everything that their fitter, non-disabled peers achieve. Occasionally some show excessive over-compensation or rationalisation, or attribute inabilities to inappropriate causes. Whilst efforts to achieve 'normalisation' are to be applauded, it is sometimes necessary to discover what lies behind such attempts, in order to ensure that there is not frank denial of obvious difficulties and/or failure to receive required help.

The desirable goal is of course '*re-normalisation*', for this enables seniors to adjust to physical changes, modify their activity, work through their reactions to loss and dependency and accept the help of others. Encouraging every constructive move towards such adaptation, and supporting decisions which give the senior control, will help to reduce further risks to self-esteem.

Sometimes, however, older impaired clients slow their pace inappropriately and become over-dependent. Over-solicitous carers can at times fuel these reactions, so that health visitors have to use tact and skill in communication, guiding these seniors to explore and modify their behaviour. Encouraging an attitude of 'non-acceptance' may halt regressive tendencies and enable seniors to fight back.

Health visiting intervention

Merely assessing need, without acting to ensure that such need is met, is of little value; hence action is required. As always, health visiting intervention is multi-focused, with practitioners working at the individual level to advise and support particular sufferers and their informal carers, activating groups of impaired seniors in self-help, or creating within the community an awareness of the needs of the elderly disabled, so that a caring environment prevails. A wide range of skills is therefore needed and several different roles must be adopted. For example, at the personal level counselling, demonstrating, teaching and motivating will predominate. At group level the practitioner's actions must be more subtle, instigating and stimulating others to action rather than taking overt initiatives. At community level the influence principle is utilised strongly, with practitioners assuming the advocacy role, and seeking to initiate action and marshall resources designed to meet the health needs of the older impaired population. In this socio-political role they share responsibility with all nurses.

Enhancing residual ability

Since enhancement of residual ability, rather than complex substitution, is the main aim of care, very basic help may be required to maximise functional capacity. Seniors can be helped to realise that multi-disciplinary imaginative approaches can offer great benefit. Guidance may be needed with the activities of living, e.g. maintaining independence in dressing through modifications to clothing. Front-opening garments, velcro fasteners, wrap-around skirts or drop-front trousers can enable some seniors to cope alone. Other helpful items include clip-on braces; ready-made ties or bows, on elastic; capes rather than sleeved coats; elastic shoe-laces; dressing sticks; hosiery tongs; long-handled pick-ups and zip aids.

Advice may be offered about washing aids, such as sponges on sticks, suction pads on soap, long-handled bath and hair brushes, long loofahs on straps and long roller-towels, fixed to the walls on flexible rubber rails, to facilitate drying.

Some disabled seniors become very adept at preparing their own food, if provided with raised-edge boards; plates and dishes with suction-cup bases; or spiked boards to anchor vegetables or bread before slicing. Non-slip mats are invaluable under utensils; adapted can openers can be found, and metal sieves or steamers can obviate the need to strain cooked vegetables, and thus reduce the risk of scalding. Other ways of making life easier for the impaired elderly include tea-pot pouring stands; devices on taps to aid turning; guards on cookers; split-level :obs; and the use of oven-to-table ware. For eating and drinking or manipulating tools, thick rubber tubing can build up handles. Velcro straps can attach cutlery to frail wrists; flexible straws and double-handed cups can facilitate drinking. Small walking trolleys, bags on walking-frames or adapted 'shoppers on wheels' can enable some disabled seniors to transport equipment from room to room. Ramps can replace steps; furniture and household goods can be stored in swing-out baskets to make them more accessible; and in some instances stair-lifts may be fitted.

Occupational therapists are skilled in determining the most appropriate aids and gadgets, so their advice should always be sought early. This may mean that assistive equipment is not inappropriately offered. Similarly the family or well-meaning friends and relatives of disabled clients should be included in health teaching about the promotion of independence and self-care; otherwise they may undo rehabilitative measures.

There is a wide-ranging literature on measures for overcoming disability. The British Red Cross Society publish a catalogue of aids and have a permanent exhibition. The Disabled Living Foundation operates a service for professionals which covers an extensive range of information, and has equipment permanently on display. Many self-help groups have 'handy hints' to offer on how to overcome particular difficulties. The Consumers' Association publish a manual on 'Coping with Disablement', and Gray & McKenzie (1980) have a helpful book which is suitable to recommend to clients and carers. The following account may serve to show what can be done.

Case study
Anne King had her left arm amputated for malignancy when she was 69 years old. Living alone, she was fitted out with different gadgets and taught ingenious ways of carrying out daily activities. Ramps, bath rails and tap devices were fitted. Nutrition was maintained through modified cooking equipment and the supplementary use of a near-by luncheon club. Housework was undertaken by using long-handled tools and complemented by a home help twice weekly for 1 hour. Relatives undertook washing, but Anne ironed, using an adapted folding ironing board.

As Anne had a strong liking for card games she was given a device for holding playing cards which enabled her to continue as a champion whist player. Her cheery manner and uncomplaining spirit won the admiration of other players, and indirectly helped others to face up to lesser adversity. Supported by her family and the general practice and social work teams, she remained independent in her own home until her sudden death aged 83 years.

Mobilising services

Mobilising the statutory and voluntary services, in order to supplement self- and lay-care, is a direct health visiting responsibility, hence it is essential to be familiar with these provisions and to know how to contact the various personnel.

Health services

Like other groups, physically impaired elders are entitled to the full range of primary and secondary health care services provided under NHS legislation 1946–1982. Clearly much of the help is channelled through the general practice team, with a major input from the district nursing service. Health visitors and their district nursing colleagues have to determine whom each will visit and when, so that specific skills are most effectively deployed, overlap is avoided, and yet gaps in care are prevented. Additionally, the complex nature of many causative conditions requires elderly impaired clients to receive hospital specialist services. Day Hospitals, short-stay admission, and paramedical services, particularly physio- therapy and speech therapy, are much used. In rare instances night centres may be available.

Personally prescribed aids, like wheelchairs, artificial limbs, or complex equipment such as Patient Operated Selector Mechanisms (Possum) are usually provided through DHSS Appliance Centres, but should not be presented without expert help and advice. Most District Health Authorities operate a loan service for nursing equipment ranging from walking aids, commodes, cradles and back-rests, through to wheelchairs and special beds and mattresses. Incontinence aids are a special feature. Most of the complex items will be recommended by district nurses, who will most probably be carrying out the clinical nursing care required. Nevertheless advice may be needed when families are managing care. In some districts there may be facilities for night-sitting and night-nursing, but these are clearly related to the financial policies operating at national and local levels.

Social services

Just as district nurses and health visitors must collaborate in care, possibly the closest liaison health visitors and social workers achieve comes through their joint concern for the deprived, disabled, or elderly. Hence early referral to and close contact with these colleagues is advised. Local author- ities, through their Social Services Committees (LASS), are empowered to provide a wide range of services for disabled and handicapped persons; however, not all of these services are obligatory, so care tends to vary between authorities:

The relevant legislation comprises:

1. National Assistance Act 1948
2. Health Services and Public Health Act 1968
3. Chronically Sick and Disabled Persons Act 1970

Under the National Assistance Act, 1948, local authorities

were given power to provide for the welfare of persons who are:

> blind, deaf and/or dumb, or substantially or permanently handicapped, by illness, injury or congenital deformity.

Services which were permitted but not made compulsory for the physically impaired include:

> advice on available services and guidance on how to overcome the effects of disability.
>
> the provision of residential homes, hostels or centres where needed
>
> the establishment of workshops for handicapped persons, and help to market any products
>
> recreational and social facilities
>
> maintenance of a register of handicapped persons
>
> ability to contribute to the funds of voluntary organisations and/or use them as agents.

While not all of these provisions would necessarily be required by the elderly, many are applicable if they are available.

The 1968 Health Services and Public Health Act widened the remit for professional workers in that it made it possible for housing to be adapted and gadgets fitted, if these would assist persons to overcome the effects of their disability. It also allowed workers to offer care in settings other than the client's own home.

By 1970, in the wake of the Report of the Seebohm Committee (HMSO 1968) and the efforts of campaigners such as Morris, a complete revision of the social services took place. Revised legislation was contained in the Local Authority Social Services Act, 1970, and the Chronically Sick and Disabled Persons Act, 1970. The latter was intended to become mandatory for all impaired persons, acting as a charter for the handicapped. To date, due largely to economic stringencies, only partial implementation has occurred. The major differences in this Act, which complements the provisions in the National Assistance Act 1948, described above, are:

1. *Mandatory* arrangements for local authorities to ascertain the number of disabled people within their areas and to

determine their needs. However, it should be noted there is no similar obligation on the part of the disabled person to register with the local authority. Furthermore, since no standardised criteria for 'needs' was given, local authorities have imposed their own, with great variation between authorities.

2. *Permissive* power to enable disabled persons to:
   a. obtain practical help in the home
   b. obtain recreational facilities, and travelling help to get to these
   c. adapt their home in order to secure greater safety, comfort and convenience
   d. obtain holidays
   e. obtain meals either in the home, or elsewhere
   f. obtain a telephone and any equipment needed to use this.

In addition local authorities were empowered to require access to be made available, and facilities, including sanitary conveniences, to be provided, for disabled persons in public places. Orange badges are issued for display on motor vehicles which give parking concessions to the disabled. Local authorities may also provide special housing. More comprehensive accounts of these provisions can be found in the relevant Acts and in Donaldson & Donaldson (1983).

However, in practice health visitors may find that whilst most LASS employ occupational therapists, advice on aids and adaptations and run clubs and sometimes day centres for the elderly disabled, for which they provide transport, these facilities rarely keep pace with demands. Whilst all provide home help services, and most have luncheon clubs and meals-on-wheels services, few authorities are expanding these to meet proven increased need. Furthermore, whilst most social workers can arrange holidays for the elderly disabled, few persons can now obtain telephones, even though these might make a substantial contribution to their well-being. This may be a significant point for health visitors who work with the elderly disabled who live alone, since a daily 'check-in' by telephone is an important aspect of surveillance.

Readers will realise that at the time of writing a major review is being undertaken of all welfare services, so considerable change may come about. Meantime, for a critical appraisal of current domiciliary services, readers are referred to Clarke (1984). He notes, as one advance, that a few local authorities have introduced innovatory schemes to help the older disabled. Such schemes include the Crossroads Home Care Attendance Scheme whereby paid attendants, operating on a flexible basis, give domiciliary care to clients, much as a caring relative would do.

Some LASS use Home Aides: personnel who, although unqualified, after some training carry out duties which are a combination of the functions normally undertaken by both home helps and nursing auxiliaries. These cover the preparation and serving of meals; dressing and undressing; getting up and putting back to bed; escorting clients outside the home; cleaning, laundry, shopping and cooking. In most instances assessment is carried out jointly by Home Help Organisers and Community Nursing Staff, the latter prescribing and supervising nusing care. There are controversial points about each of these schemes, but in some localities they are believed to have much improved the quality of life for disabled elderly.

VOLUNTARY ORGANISATIONS

One of the features of the welfare state in Britain has been the continuance of a long tradition of partnership between statutory and voluntary services. This partnership is perhaps most marked in relation to the chronically sick, the disabled and handicapped, and the elderly. There are distinct advantages for voluntary organisations, in that they are often able to respond more flexibly to need than are statutory authorities who are bound by legislation. Staff are dedicated, often unpaid or low-paid, so that costs tend to be lower; also this type of service is frequently locally based, so that it generates community interest. Against this must be set the fact that a plethora of highly specialised, different associations exists, which makes it difficult to co-ordinate care. Clients become confused, effort can be duplicated and some older clients may feel they do not wish local volunteers to find out about their business, so may be reluctant to use services. In many areas a co-ordinating body, such as a Council of Voluntary Service, tries to ensure that overlap is avoided and services are used most effectively. Practitioners will find it most helpful to liaise with organisers of these councils.

It is necessary for health visitors to familiarise themselves with the main organisations in their area, their aims and objectives, and the constraints which may be imposed on them by their own constitution, charter or charitable status. Some bodies are almost entirely concerned with raising and disbursing monies; others promote research into specific conditions; some cover the general field of disablement, whilst others focus on self-help and support. Almost all offer an advisory service; many have excellent publications; and some, such as the St John Ambulance Brigade and the British Red Cross Society, offer practical help. A list of useful addresses is given in Appendix 6.

State Benefits for disabled elderly

Apart from their entitlement to contributory or non-contributory Retirement Benefit and/or Supplementary Benefit, some older people who are disabled may be able to claim other allowances, such as attendance or mobility allowance.

Attendance allowance

> This benefit may be available to persons who require frequent attention throughout the day, and/or prolonged or repeated attention at night, in connection with bodily functions; or if they need continual supervision throughout the day and/or night, in order to avoid substantial danger to themselves or others.

The regulations are stringent. There are residence qualifications, and care must have been required for at least 6 months before the application is made. The latter rules out those many disabled persons who live alone, require help to assist them to function in a number of essential activities, yet by reason of their circumstances cannot receive 'prolonged attention' or 'continual supervision'. Thus they are penalised, and the measure of help they might be able to afford, which could keep them independent, is denied; as a result their condition often deteriorates, making it necessary for them to have greater professional help, sometimes of a long-term nature.

The attendance allowance, which is paid to the disabled person for use as remuneration to the helper, is non-taxable, and is payable in addition to other allowances, except constant attendance allowance. Health visitors may sometimes be asked to supply evidence in support of a claim, or help to prepare an appeal; clients should be advised to contact their local Citizens' Advice Bureau or Welfare Rights Association, or seek guidance from The Disability Alliance.

Mobility allowance

Mobility allowance is a non-means-tested benefit, designed to help severely disabled persons to become more mobile. It is non-taxable, and is disregarded for the purpose of national insurance benefits, attendance allowance, supplementary benefit or war pension.

Older people may be eligible if they claim before they are 66 years old, and provided they could satisfy the criteria before they were 65. After qualifying for the allowance, they may retain it until they are 75 years old. Thus older disabled persons over 75 are not eligible for help, which may render them more vulnerable to social isolation. Qualifying criteria include inability or virtual inability to walk because of a physical condition that is likely to remain so for at least 1 year. There are also residence and other qualifications. This is also true for the new benefit known as Severe Disablement Allowance, which now supersedes Housewives' Non-Contributory Invalidity Pension, and some other benefits. Clients who appear to qualify should be referred to DHSS staff, Citizens' Advice Bureaux, or Welfare Rights Organisations.

What is important is to ensure that disabled clients and their carers are made aware of *all* their entitlements and encouraged to claim these. In this the advocacy role of the health visitor may be employed, as it may be in alerting the community to the needs of those impaired individuals who are borderline in relation to these benefits and for whom refusal would create hardship.

HELP FOR THE SENSORILY IMPAIRED ELDERLY

Visual disability

There are currently about 91 000 elderly persons registered as blind in UK. Amongst these are a predominance of females aged 75 and over, and most are between the ages of 80–89. These figures indicate the areas of greatest need. For the blind there are compulsory legislative provisions, provided they are registered. Such registration is voluntary on the part of the client; it must be made with the LASS department, but is conducted by a registered medical practitioner who is qualified in ophthalmology. Partially-sighted persons may also register; they are included on a separate National Register, which of course represents many more than the number of blind persons. Partially-sighted persons often choose not to register because they receive fewer entitlement than the blind.

Apart from blindness due to congenital causes, or acquired from disease or injury in earlier life, most older people develop their impairment after 65 years of age. Causes are mostly glaucoma; diabetic retinopathy; macular degeneration; or cataract. True prevention of each of these conditions is difficult with the present state of knowledge; however, early detection can sometimes lead to control, thus avoiding complete loss of vision. For these reasons the case-finding and health education functions of the health visitor are all-important.

The physical effects of blindness are seen in its impact on locomotion and balance, the restrictions placed on mobility and the difficulties seniors have in space orientation and hazard control. They therefore need help to manipulate the environmental variables of light, size and contrast to maximum advantage (WHO 1981b). Because visual substitution measures are less easily learned in later life, attention must be paid to enhancing residual vision by every available means. Safety education should receive extra emphasis.

Understandably, psychological reactions are strong, largely because of lack of visual stimulation and the associated social isolation. In a number of studies, depression has been found to be a common concomitant. Although some seniors become aggressive, others withdraw. For these reasons sufferers and their carers need considerable initial support and ongoing help to find compensatory activities and stimulation. The use of Talking Books, radio (sometimes through The Wireless for the Blind Fund), The Braille National Library for the Blind, and specially geared clubs and recreational activities can help some blind seniors find interests and release their emotions. Many partially-sighted persons enjoy the Ulverscroft Large Print Books and there is a range of embossed playing cards and games which some visually impaired clients may enjoy using. Others may benefit from Low-Vision Aids.

Clients should be referred early to the local social services department, so that specially qualified social workers can offer home teaching on the best ways of overcoming their visual impairment. Only a few older people usually manage to read embossed type if their visual impairment occurs late in life, but for those who do, Moon or Braille is available. Social workers can arrange for braille dials to be fitted to watches, cookers and certain other household appliances. There is also a range of specially adapted household items and safety devices available. Furthermore, social workers often act as agents for specific funds for needy blind persons, and can arrange holidays for some visually handicapped elderly and their families.

There are many voluntary organisations for the visually impaired, including such well-known ones as the Royal National Institute for the Blind and the Association for Guide Dogs for the Blind. However, seniors take longer to adapt to changed circumstances, and many of the benefits younger blind persons can utilise, are inappropriate for the elderly, unless they have used them earlier in life.

Other special entitlements include monetary benefits, such as higher rate supplementary benefit, higher income tax allowances and certain postal concessions on embossed literature. The Disabled Living Foundation is currently engaged in the preparation of a pack for community nursing staff, who are caring for the visually impaired, especially older people and this should prove of great value to health visitors.

The deaf-blind

Approximately 2% of those on the Blind Persons Register are elderly deaf-blind. A few have been affected from birth, and are often mute as well. Some may have acquired both handicaps from illness or injury in childhood, or earlier adulthood, but most develop both afflictions in later maturity. They require very special aids and teaching, and need particular support and consideration in order to improve their quality of life. They will, of course, need prompt referral to LASS departments for the care of social workers, and should also be put into touch with the Deaf/Blind Association. They are eligible for the services available to both deaf and blind persons, but sometimes cannot benefit so readily, due to their dual and occasionally triple handicap.

Hearing impairment

The prevalence of hearing impairment amongst the elderly has been variously estimated. Herbst & Humphrey (1981), using audiometric techniques and their community-based sample as reference, assessed the prevalence at 60% of the population over 65 years. This means that over $4\frac{1}{2}$ million older persons have some noticeable hearing loss — far more than the numbers previously ascertained. The implications for health visitors concerning case-finding and specific health teaching are obvious.

The categories of hearing impairment are:

- those deaf without speech
- those deaf with speech
- those who are hard of hearing.

The majority of seniors fall into the last category, with the next highest number being those who are deaf, with speech. Thus most hearing impaired elderly can communicate normally, via lip-reading and oral speech, especially when this is amplified.

As with other groups of disabled seniors, the full range of health and social services is available to the hearing-impaired. Audiometrists and otologists are available through the NHS, and aids are supplied free of charge as needed. Most local authorities employ specialised case-workers to help the older deaf overcome their disabilities, and a number have interpreters. Specific social and recreational facilities are available, such as clubs for the hard of hearing, whilst some colleges and further education centres arrange lip-reading classes. Aids to daily living, such as flashing door bells and telephone or television amplifiers, are available. Spiritual facilities, obtainable through Diocesean Missioners for the Deaf, include counselling for clients and their families and special church services, often using a combination of sign language and speech. In this connection it is helpful if health visitors learn the appropriate sign language.

Although hearing impairment does not necessarily have serious physical effects, some older people do have associated vertigo, tinnitus and attacks of vomiting, as in Menière's disease. These concomitants can prove very handicapping and call for appropriate advice. Nevertheless it is the psychosocial needs of the hearing-impaired which predominate. A number of studies have shown significant relationship between deafness and depression, independent of age or socio-economic status (Herbst & Humphrey, 1980). This points up the area of need which health visitors should explore amongst their elderly deaf clients.

THE NEEDS OF PSYCHOLOGICALLY DISTURBED CLIENTS

Measuring psychological and psychiatric morbidity amongst the elderly is a complex task, for three reasons:

1. difficulties in differentiating normal psychological age changes from pathological ones.
2. difficulties in applying precise diagnostic criteria.
3. the inter-twining of causative events, especially those associated with physical illness and disability, socio-economic problems and/or social isolation and bereavement.

Average prevalence figures show that some 7% of seniors have marked psychiatric disturbance, with a further 10–30% exhibiting moderate to mild symptoms respectively. Contrary to common stereotypes, and in spite of the high bed occupancy by seniors in psycho-geriatric units, 60% of all seniors are without any psychological impairment. Whilst older people can be subject to all forms of mental illness, affecting any age group, they are particularly prone to depression.

Depression

This affective disorder is characterised by sadness of mood, a sense of emptiness and detachment and often raised anxiety levels. Its prevalence has been variously estimated. Murphy (1982) found 29% of her community sample to be frank or borderline depressives, but other researchers have suggested it could be as high as 40%. It is important to be aware of such statistics as unfortunately this condition is often not diagnosed until it is too late. The incidence of successful suicide is high in the elderly, being greater in men and increasing generally in the spring. This is a tragedy, because treatment can be most successful. Such a situation suggests a need for greater health visitor awareness and the deployment of further case-finding skills.

There are two main forms of depression: reactive and endogenous, although they may be difficult to differentiate in the elderly. The majority of cases seen in the older person are reactive. Exact causes are still speculative, ranging across biological and psychosocial dimensions. The most recent theories include:

Constitutional predispositions	
Familial tendencies	Kline 1976
Personality structure	Post 1981
Reaction to illness or disability	
Early life events	Brown & Harris 1978
Disruptive life events	Hall & Zwemer 1979
	Mauksch 1981
Lack of an intimate confidante	Murphy 1982, 1983
Loneliness	Ingham & Miller 1982
Loss: attack: restraint	Hanley &
and/or threat	Baikie, 1984

The depressive mood is patchy in the reactive type, varying with outside influences. The person is tired all day and often worse in the evening, frequently having difficulty getting to sleep. This contrasts with the endogenous type, which appears to be independent of environmental circumstances. In this latter form the depression is markedly worse in the mornings with some improvement later in the evenings. Classically there is early morning waking. Some people may be taking drugs which precipitate a depressive illness, e.g. reserpine.

The features of depression may be specific or non-specific. In addition to the alteration of sleep pattern, there are non-specific features of anorexia, weight loss, constipation, tachycardia, generalised and localised pain particularly back-ache, and a lack of interest and energy frequently attributed to old age. Moreover, because many elderly people often experience low-level wellness, they do not emphasise their lowered spirits and flattened affect. It is important to observe whether older clients are showing an energy loss, lessened interest in personal or environmental hygiene, seem indecisive or vacillating, or are self-absorbed, self-deprecating or self-reproachful. Also to note if there is diffuse pessimism. Sadness and crying may not be admitted by clients unless directly questioned. Additionally clients may be agitated and restless, or retarded and/or confused. They may be hypochondriacal, and sometimes experience delusions (e.g. blocked bowels), as well as harbouring suicidal thoughts. It will be appreciated that the recognition of depression is not easy. Not only are its signs and symptoms frequently 'masked', simulating physical illness, they may be over-laid by the presence of co-existing disease or disability. Frequently they are attributed to old age and hence often accepted as inevitable. However, a personal or family history of depression can be a pointer, indicating how necessary it is to consult past records and to discover significant and recent distressing life-events.

Medical management

The management of depressed patients will clearly depend on the probable cause. In reactive states persons can be helped if the precipitating reason can be alleviated. Admission to hospital can help; indeed relief of the depression can occur before the physical problems are relieved. Restoration of self-respect and non-specific care can do much to help.

The forgetfulness of the elderly depressed client, treated outside hospital, often renders drug compliance difficult, but some psychiatrists feel therapy is of limited value if it does not include an attack on the mood disorder at the central nervous system level. For this reason the tricyclic drugs, such as imipramine, are often prescribed. Care must be taken with dosage, to avoid or reduce such side-effects as dry mouth, postural hypotension, confusion, or retention of urine in men. The tetracyclic anti-depressant drugs, (such as Bolvidon), though having fewer side-effects seem generally less effective. Mono-amine oxidase inhibitors, however, are seldom used, due to hypertensive crises when tyramine-rich foods (cheese, Marmite, broad beans) are taken. Electro-convulsive therapy is sometimes employed, although the ethics of its use and effects are hotly debated. Where it is used, clients and their carers may need support, explanation and encouragement to continue, once they have made an informed decision to accept treatment. Memory is sometimes temporarily disturbed, but longer term benefit is claimed.

Psychological treatment includes both cognitive and behaviour therapy, but the demand for these far exceeds supply, so apart from private treatment one-to-one consultation is rare. Group therapy is more likely to occur, since research suggests that it is less time-consuming and costly than individually based treatment and that it may be more effective. Health visitors may well be involved in such group work, either aimed at reducing the risk of depression following traumatic or disruptive life events incurring loss in any form, or in established cases. They should appreciate that such group work requires skills of organisation and leadership which are distinct and different from work with individuals.

Health visiting intervention

Apart from collaboration in group work and the specific after-care of persons receiving treatment, health visitors can do much to help prevent or reduce the effects of depression. At the personal level intervention consists of an amalgam of preventive, teaching and psycho-social techniques, plus environmental modification where possible and monitoring of prescribed medical regimes. Close collaboration is required with all members of the general practice team, especially the community psychiatric nurse. Co-operation with social workers is essential, especially where there has been hospital admission, or when there is associated physical disability, social need or economic difficulty. Efforts should be made to reinforce non-depressed behaviour, whilst ignoring identified depressive responses. However, affectively disturbed seniors need continued reassurance, supervision and support, to help then regain well-being and preserve their dignity and self-esteem.

Clients should be taught anxiety-reducing mechanisms, such as deep breathing, relaxation techniques, visual imagery and suitably graded physical exercise. They need diversional activities and often respond to therapeutic effects of music, art and drama. Socio-economic measures to relieve any financial distress and environmental manipulation to improve their general circumstances are of course also necessary. Social contact should be tactfully encouraged, using all available and appropriate means, such as day centres, social clubs, leisure interest groups, libraries and voluntary visiting schemes where indicated. Transport often facilitates these ideas. What is important is to encourage reality perception and problem-solving in an empathetic and caring manner, so that through new and personally meaningful activities, older clients become motivated and involved, thus achieving self-help.

At community level the health visiting function is chiefly to create public awareness of the risk of depression amongst seniors, the likely causes and the measures necessary to prevent or ameliorate these. The assumption is that as the public becomes more involved in discussing the cognitive, emotional and social needs of their elderly, they are more likely to promote personal, social and environmental policies which are conducive to improvement. For this reason one important facet of the health visiting role is to discover local organisations who are interested in promoting and safeguarding mental health and in supporting sufferers, and then to liaise with them for the community's good.

CARING FOR THE ELDERLY WITHIN ETHNIC MINORITY GROUPS

Traditionally Britain has accepted a variety of ethnic minority groups within its population, but this process accelerated during and after the Second World War, so that today many different races and cultures are represented within the UK. Some of the elderly within such groups have been here for many years, whilst others have arrived recently, either coming to join families here, or to find refuge. The extent to which they have settled down and integrated within the host country will likely be reflected in the health and social problems they present. As with all other elderly it is important not to regard those from differing ethnic minorities as a homogenous group. The cultural diversity between different immigrants may be as great, or greater than that shown between them and the indigenous population.

Because migration is rarely random it is often helpful to examine the historical associations of each group with Britain. Discovering the reasons why they have come and the circumstances prevailing at and since their arrival, may point up the nature of their actual or potential health and/or social needs. For example, one of the largest groups who have maintained a fairly steady influx to Britain over many years, are the Irish. Their arrivals are usually young and economically active. Whilst many settle in major cities there is also frequent dispersion throughout the country, so that any health visitor may meet with them. Although close contact is usually maintained with Eire, long-term living in Britain is a strong feature, so that a number of Irish elderly may well have been living here many years. Similarities in some customs and lifestyles facilitate assimilation and patterns of health and disease often closely resemble the host nation. Certainly there are particular susceptibilities such as a greater proneness to develop tuberculosis, and, for a few, possibly the risk of alcohol-related conditions; nevertheless, apart from the travelling tinkers who maintain distinctive characteristics, there may be little to differentiate the elderly Irish from the indigenous population. Their health care will therefore follow a similar pattern.

Others who have deliberately chosen migration, usually in order to obtain work, include the Italian and Spanish groups who came to Britain in greater numbers after the Second World War. They have established strong and identifiable communities and have therefore, well-developed social networks for supporting their elderly. Many older persons within these groups cherish the hope that they will return to their country of origin at retirement, but some of pensionable age do remain here. Although they may have some language difficulties, and certain customs and culture patterns differ from British ones, they are usually familiar with the health and social services and are frequently cared for within their extended families. It is important to see that they do not become socially isolated when communication barriers exist.

Later arrivals on a relatively planned basis include Afro-Carribeans, many of whom came in the late 1950s–1960s, frequently seeking work. They were joined in the late 1960s early 1970s by Asians from the Indian sub-continent. It is noteworthy that while these New Commonwealth and Pakistani elderly constitute less than 2% of the total population aged 65 years and over, their actual numbers have increased by 75% between the 1971 and 1981 Censuses. Furthermore the population shape of these ethnic minorities reveals a 'bulge' of those now in their middle years. Thus within the next few years they are likely to make increasing demands on health and social services for older people.

In contrast to these deliberate migration patterns, some other groups have arrived here as refugees, often having to accept that they are unlikely to ever return to their home-lands. Many Jewish immigrants came at the turn of the century, escaping from the persecution in Eastern Europe. They were joined by others before, during and after the Second World War. Their strong sense of community, and corporate concern, is well demonstrated and the Jewish Welfare Board is an example of the formalised help which can be offered to those in need, including the elderly. Whilst certain genetic and early environmental influences are manifest in their patterns of health and disease, as for instance a relatively high incidence of diabetes amongst older people, their health states now tend to resemble national norms. Polish immigrants have possibly fared rather less well. They and the displaced persons from Latvia, Estonia and the Ukraine, have likely seen gradually dwindling numbers of those who have strong cultural ties with their native lands.

Second generation ethnic minorities may be less ready to learn and speak their native tongue, so there may be few available to converse with the elderly in their own language. Consequently such elderly may feel themselves isolated, bereft, prone to anxiety and depression. Such experiences may well have been repeated for successive waves of refugees, notably Hungarians, East African Asians, Turkish and Greek Cypriots and more recently Vietnamese. Because they may have suffered the loss of home and possessions, as well as livelihood and status, they may be particularly vulnerable in their old age.

However, whatever the circumstances surrounding their arrival in this country, all first generation ethnic minority groups are likely to have undergone considerable cultural dislocation: in addition some may have had to face subtle or overt forms of prejudice and discrimination. They, therefore, respond to understanding and supportive help. There is a tendency for specific ethnic minority groups to try to settle in close proximity with one another. Often this means living in inner city areas where, like the indigenous residents, they may share the effects of 'urban decay'. Housing is often substandard; transport and other facilities may be inadequate. Unless they have capital, or have worked in this country long enough to qualify for contributory State Retirement Pension, these ethnic minority elderly may be forced to face long-term living on Supplementary Benefit. The complicated claims procedure which lays much onus on the claimant, may prove very bewildering, so guidance and explanation are frequently required.

Dietary needs

Whilst European and some other ethnic minority elderly may have little difficulty obtaining accustomed foodstuffs, those from the Afro-Carribean and Asian groups may have problems. Although more shops selling their staple foods are now available, the cost of such products, or mobility difficulties may mean older people cannot get them. This can lead to dietary restrictions, superimposed upon the usual taboos. Muslims are forbidden to eat pork or pork products, and may eat only halal meat which has been blessed and killed in a special way. Sikhs, mostly from the Punjab, or East Africa, may be vegetarian, but Hindus almost always are. Some are strict vegans. Where they are unaware of acceptable substitutes for their normal diet, they may have insufficient intakes of calories, protein, iron and vitamin D, to sustain health in this country and climate.

Such dietary difficulties may be exacerbated if older people (who may be less willing to modify their eating habits than younger ones) are admitted to hospital, or require meals-on-wheels or luncheon clubs. Encouraging them to accept much needed services and displaying tact and understanding of their problems, whilst interpreting their needs to others, are all essential health visiting activities.

Dress

Devout Sikh males traditionally wear turbans, which together with the five 'K' signs — uncut hair, a special comb, steel bangle, symbolic dagger and special underpants — are worn constantly, even when washing or ill. Sikh women traditionally wear shalwar kameez, i.e. trousers and shirt suitable for day or night use. They may fear to accept services which may comprise their dress, or cut across strict personal modesty.

Muslim and Hindu women are equally strict, and often need help to arrange examinations by female doctors. Muslim women are clothed from head to toe in garments which do not reveal the shape of the body, and wear items of jewellery which often have social or religious significance, so they may fear their removal. Because they often remain in the home they may be at particular risk of vitamin D deficiency.

There are also, of course, specific religious observances to note, as these may be greatly valued by ethnic minority elderly. Symbolic cleansing and set times for prayer are examples. For those of the Muslim faith, the left hand is usually used for washing and the right hand for eating. This can have important implications in illness and for rehabilitation. Sikhs have no prohibitions against blood transfusions, organ transplants, or post-mortems whereas Muslims do, except for blood transfusions. Specific festivals are celebrated, so it is necessary to discover when these are held and what meaning is attached to attendant customs.

An impression is often given of extended family networks strongly supporting the elderly within ethnic minorities, especially Afro-Caribbean and Asian groups. Whilst undoubtedly older people do command great respect and are often readily helped, not all of them may actually have families living in Britain. This is particularly true for older East African Asians, of whom 25% are thought to be without kin in this country. They are therefore likely to make greater demands on statutory and voluntary services. Taking an accurate and full history can help to identify those most vulnerable.

Health needs

As yet there have been few large-scale research studies, designed to demonstrate the health of the elderly in different ethnic groups, although small-scale projects, usually mounted by local authorities or voluntary organisations, and anecdotal accounts, have provided some information. One future way in which health visitors can contribute to the care of such elderly, is therefore, their willingness to participate in well-designed and ethical research.

Whilst hereditary factors continue to influence morbidity and mortality, (e.g. sickle cell disease in Afro-Caribbean clients), prevailing environmental conditions and the stresses of migration play a strong part. Low incomes may have meant marginal diets over many years, and it should be remembered that many immigrants remit money regularly to their families in their country of origin. Not surprisingly psychiatric disturbance is not uncommon; chiefly anxiety states, depression and psychosomatic conditions, but frank psychotic states do occur. For some cultural groups the stigma of mental illness is very great. This is particularly so where psychiatric disturbance has moral connotations for them. They may hide their problems and/or refuse to accept treatment out of a sense of shame. Conversely when treatment is accepted the patient may be abandoned. Considerable tact and patience, together with sound health teaching, may be required, before families can understand and accept illness-reactions and deal appropriately with them. This may be particularly marked when medico-legal procedures are involved. Close collaboration between general practitioners, district nurses, community psychiatric workers, social workers and health visitors can help to reduce the adverse effects on families.

Some elderly immigrants may suffer from imported infections or infestations, especially when they are new arrivals. They require prompt diagnosis and treatment. In addition they may be highly susceptible to infections endemic in Britain, especially respiratory conditions such as tuberculosis, or gastrointestinal diseases. If they travel back to their homeland for visits, after a long period away, they may find their levels of natural immunity may have fallen. They may therefore benefit from active immunisation before such journeys, and should always be advised to seek guidance beforehand. Those travelling to malaria endemic areas should be advised about necessary protection. Anaemia is another common condition met in elderly members of certain ethnic minority groups. It may be associated with certain infestations, but often relates to insufficient intakes of iron; screening for this condition should therefore be routine, and treatment supervised and encouraged.

Elderly females within such groups may suffer from long-standing gynaecological conditions, or show signs of osteomalacia. They may fear the necessary medical examinations and require explanation and encouragement in order to seek appropriate treatment.

Patterns of consultation

There is some evidence to suggest that while certain groups of elderly may retreat and become withdrawn and isolated, Afro-Carribeans and Asians make considerable use of general practitioner services, more than 90% seeing their family doctor in any one year. Of course such consultations may reflect social as well as medical need, and they provide a great opportunity for supportive contact and health education. Health visitors working within general medical practice settings are thus well placed to identify these vulnerable elderly. However, significantly in one study in Birmingham, less than 3% of those elderly who consulted their General Practitioner actually saw a district nurse or health visitor (Blakemore 1982).

Initiative is thus required to redress such situations. Amongst the needs presented during this study, were difficulties of sight, hearing, walking and dental health; although these tended to occur earlier amongst the Afro-Carribeans and Asians than in the indigenous elderly. Moreover, less than half of those who suffered such problems, had sought remedial help. Such findings suggest great scope for improved collaboration, health education and preventive health care. Whilst Asians showed a 'higher than expected' incidence of heart disease and diabetes, these conditions together with stroke, were significantly greater amongst the Afro-Carribean elderly, especially women. Such findings have been supported by the work of Cruikshank et al (1980) and by Marmot et al (1984).

What is their relevance for health visitors? Surely they indicate that health visitors would be well-employed helping to prevent such conditions, through health education designed to promote stress-control, weight and smoking control, as well as the wise use of screening. Finding ways of making such programmes meaningful to ethnic minority middle-aged and elderly is another exciting health visiting challenge. However, in spite of their high consultation rates in general medical practice, ethnic minority elderly appear considerably to under-utilise advisory and after-care services. There may be many reasons for this such as fear, ignorance, cultural unacceptability, poor comprehension of procedures and communication difficulties. Whatever the reason, there is clearly scope for increasing ethnic minorities' awareness of available services.

Although their health is poorer than that of older indigenous elderly, Asians aged 65 years or more are under-represented in their use of hospital services. This may be because they often resort to Hakims or native healers, as do some Afro-Carribeans. It is always necessary to try to discover if alternative medical systems are being used alongside allo-pathic medicine, as sometimes adverse reactions can occur due to drug interactions or conflicting therapies. Drug compliance is always a sensitive matter when dealing with any elderly; it can become very complex when natural forgetfulness and occasional confusion are compounded by poor comprehension of English. Great care must be exercised to ensure that the basic principles of drug dosage are clearly grasped and that side-effects are promptly noted and reported.

Thus the role of the health visitor with the elderly in ethnic minorities can be said to be highly varied, yet an extension or expansion of her role with indigenous older people. Particular skills are required to elicit information unobtrusively, interpret need and provide culturally acceptable education and help. Positive attitudes towards the different groups and respect for them, together with a readiness to listen to and learn from them, are fundamental points in the developmental process of effective care.

CARING FOR THE INFORMAL CARERS OF THE ELDERLY

The DHSS defines informal carers as:

> persons who are taking primary responsibility in the home, for the care of persons, who because of handicap or illness, need almost continuous care
>
> Social Work Service Development Group (1983)

Many of the elderly who are cared for are not ill or handicapped, but frail. Though the intensity of their care may vary, the constancy of it may be as great as for the disabled and/or sick. Most recent policy documents have emphasised the centrality of community care, both now and in the future, (DHSS 1981a, 1981b) Whilst this is meant to be a humane policy, the reality is that, as yet, resources have not been diverted to this sector in adequate enough amounts, to allow for really caring communities. At present only 30% of the budget of the NHS is directed towards family practitioners and community health services, although 95% of all health care takes place in this sector. Furthermore, at times of financial stringency, preventive work and health education, are often the first to suffer. This means that what could be a praise worthy policy becomes a cheap alternative to institutional care, wherby informal carers bear the burden, without the supportive services they might expect or need.

The burden of caring is currently concentrated on some 1½ million people, mostly middle-aged or older women and elderly men. Only 6% of such carers are officially recognised, since they are entitled to some state benefit because of their caring status. Invalid Care Allowance, paid at a rate which rarely compensates for loss of earnings, is available only to men and single women who have given up work to care for someone for at least 35 hours per week, provided that the person being cared for is already receiving Attendance Allowance. The criteria for qualifying is complex, and married women or divorcees maintained by their husbands are ineligible. Thus the decision to give up work to care may induce great emotional pressure for carer and sufferer alike. This at a time when more women are in the labour market, there is increased geographical mobility, and more divorces and re-marriages are leading to complicated family relationships.

The effects of caring on the carers

The physical effects of caring for an elderly dependent obviously rests upon the nature of the care provided, its intensity and duration. At times the work can be heavy and unremitting. Fatigue, back-ache and ill-defined physical symptoms are common; disturbed sleep may reduce energy levels, especially when the carer is also responsible for various household tasks and is endeavouring to hold down paid employment as well. Carers may have little social life or personal privacy. Insufficient money limits possible diversions, or the employment of occasional paid help, whilst enforced cessation of employment can reduce social contact and later endanger financial security and insurance. If the carer remains at work he or she may find that home responsibilities jeopardise career opportunities. Sometimes when the disabled frail senior lives with the carer there may be housing difficulties, furnishings may be soiled or damaged, and heating and telephone costs may soar. Although many carers derive great emotional reward from caring, they may be very distressed by the nature of their dependent's problems, may fear what will happen if they themselves become ill; they often also experience desperate loneliness.

Help needed and available

Unfortunately there appears at present to be little 'fit' between what carers need and what is available. Many carers say their greatest requirement is for some reliable relief in the home; few social services departments can provide this, and apart from the few Crossroads attendants schemes already described, few voluntary organisations can fill the gap. Many of the statutory services which can be offered merely complement and do not replace what carers do. For example, district nursing and health visiting services currently reach only 1 in 10 of all carers of the elderly. Furthermore, because the help that can often be offered seems so limited in amount for what is needed, research shows that these professional workers are, unfortunately, regarded by many carers as irrelevant (Equal Opportunities Commission 1982, 1983, Nissell & Bonnerjea 1982).

Nevertheless the general practice team is well placed to identify carers and their needs, and to operate a service on their behalf, because at least 50% of elderly dependents will already be in touch with the practice members. For this reason it is essential that good communication exists between team members, and that roles are understood and respected, so that adequate referral and liaison can be made. Furthermore, it is vital that similar good communication exists between team members, social workers and voluntary personnel, so that additional resources can be activated for carers.

Day Centres are helpful, but in woefully short supply, so that the number of times some elderly dependents can attend is curtailed. Short-term admission usually only permits a brief holiday to be taken. Furthermore much help does appear to be discriminatory; women are more often expected to manage than men. When relatives appear to try hard to cope, they are often rewarded by a withdrawal of services! Both district nurses and health visitors acquiesce in such behaviour. Support and self-help groups, notably the Association of Carers and the National Council for Carers and their Elderly Dependants (see addresses in Appendix 6), are beginning to show a higher profile. Through them carers are expressing their requests to have their basic rights considered, their contribution to care acknowledged, and their partnership role taken into account during decision-making. They are actively seeking information, practical assistance, empathetic interest and personal counselling, often related to relationship and attachment problems.

Health visiting help

Within the team the health visitor has a responsibility to promote and preserve the health of carers, although the size of case-loads and the limitations of time profoundly affect how much help can be given. This is why health visitors must highlight the deficiencies in their care and demonstrate the short-falls in their activities. Drawing the attention of health service managers to such shortfalls is as important as recording tasks actually performed. It is only the evidence, based on sensible audit of the potential work-load, as related to the completed workload, that can provide the basis for needed improvements.

At individual level practitioners need the skills of assessment, teaching, counselling and supporting, so that they can safeguard carers' well-being. At family group level they need to be able to recognise and help members to resolve conflicts within the family. At larger group level they should direct particular attention to support groups, stimulating and encouraging self-help and appropriate assertiveness (Drummond 1984). Particular help may need to be offered to those ethnic minorities and cultural groups who exhibit alternative ways of stress management. At community level health visitors need to bring the plight of carers to public attention, focusing concern on policies which are unhelpful towards true community care. In this way the health-enhancing measures which the community offers may be developed. By studying civic affairs, health visitors should also be in a position to use their individual and collective power to influence national policies affecting health.

SUMMARY

In this chapter the needs of specific groups of elderly people and their carers have been explored. The high prevalence of impairment, disability and handicap has been shown and the impact of pain, restriction, immobility and loss of self-respect on elderly people and their significant others has been discussed. The purpose has been to highlight the action needed from health visitors.

Lastly the often invisible, disregarded band of carers has been studied in order that health visiting action in this field could be discussed. The message has been that without these devoted supporters, community care would be a misnomer and the statutory services would be unable to cope.

It is sometimes easy to sound glib about ways of handling these serious, often intractable problems and to be accused of uttering mere platitudes and unrealistic prescriptions for care. The comments made are intended to provoke thought, so that more flexible and imaginative responses can be made towards, and on behalf of, our affected seniors.

REFERENCES

Blakemore K 1982 Health and illness among the elderly of minority groups living in Birmingham: some new findings. Health Trends 14(3) August p 69–72

Briggs A 1983 Who cares? The Association of Carers, Chatham, Kent

Brown G W, Harris T O 1978 Social origins of depression. Tavistock, London

Bury M 1982 Chronic illness as biographic disruption. Sociology of Health and Illness 4 (2): 167–181

Charlesworth A, Wilkin D, Durie A 1983 Carers and services: a comparison of men and women caring for dependent elderly people. Equal Opportunities Commission, Manchester

Charmaz K 1983 Loss of self. Sociology of Health and Illness 5 (2): 168–194

Clarke 1984 Domiciliary services for the elderly. Croom Helm, London

Cruikshank J K, Beevers D G, Verdelle L O, Haynes R A, Corlett J C R, Selby S 1980 Heart attack, stroke, diabetes and hypertension in West Indians, Asians, and whites in Birmingham, England. British Medical Journal 281:1108

Department of Health and Social Security 1981a Growing older. Cmnd 8172. HMSO. London

Department of Health and Social Security 1981b Care in the Community. A consultative document on moving resources in England. 1981 Annex B 5 DHSS, London

Donaldson R J, Donaldson L J 1983 Essential community medicine. MTP Press, Lancaster

Drummond G 1984 Laughter is better than medicine: a support group for caring relatives. Health Visitor July 57: 201–202

Equal Opportunities Commission 1982 Who cares for the carers? Opportunities for those caring for the elderly and handicapped. Equal Opportunities Commission, Manchester

Equal Opportunities Commission 1983 Caring for the elderly and handicapped. Equal Opportunities Commission, Manchester

Gilhooley L M 1984 Social dimensions of dementia. In: Hanley I, Hodge J (eds) Psychological approaches to the care of the elderly. Croom Helm, London

Gray M, McKenzie H 1980 Take care of your elderly relative. Allen and Unwin, London

Hall J H, Zwemer J D 1979 Prospective medicine. Methodist Hospital of Indiana, Indiapolis

Hanley I, Baikie E 1984 Understanding and treating depression in the elderly. In: Hanley I, Hodge I (eds) Psychological approaches to the care of the elderly. Croom Helm, London

Harris A 1971 Handicapped and impaired. OPCS, HMSO, London

Herbst K, Humphrey C 1980 Hearing impairment and mental state in the elderly living at home. British Medical Journal 281 (4th October): 903–905

HMSO 1968 Report of the Committee on Local Authority and Allied Personal Social Services. HMSO, London

Ingham J, Miller P 1982 Consulting with mild symptoms in general practice. Social Psychiatry 17: 77–88

Kline N 1976 Incidence and prevalence and recognition of depressive illness; Diseases of the Nervous System, 37 p 10

Marmot M G, Adelstein A M, Bulusu L 1984 Lessons from the study of immigrant mortality. The Lancet June 30th: 1455–1457

Mauksch I G (ed) 1981 primary care: a contemporary nursing perspective. Grune and Stratton, New York

Murphy E 1982 The social origins of depression in old age. British Journal of Psychiatry 141: 135–42

Murphy E 1983 The prognosis of depression in old age. British Journal of Psychiatry 142: 111–19

Nissell, Bonnerjea 1982 Family care of the handicapped elderly, who pays? Policy Studies Institute, London

Orem D 1980 Nursing: concepts of practice, 2nd edn. McGraw-Hill, New York

Post F 1981 Affective illnesses. In: Arie T (ed) Health care of the elderly. Croom Helm, London, p 89–103

Social Work Service, Development Group 1983 Supporting the informal carers. A project paper and report of a seminar at Oxford, June 1983. DHSS, London

World Health Organization 1978. Alma Ata declaration on primary health care. Report of the International Conference on Primary Health Care, WHO, Geneva

World Health Organization 1980 The International Classification of Impairments, Disabilities and Handicaps. WHO, Geneva

World Health Organization 1981a Preventing disability in the elderly: Report of a WHO working Group: Euro Reports and studies 65. Regional Office for Europe, WHO, Copenhagen

World Health Organization 1981b The use of residual vision by visually disabled persons. Euro Report No. 41, Regional Office, Copenhagen

FURTHER READING

King K (ed) 1985 Long-term care. Churchill Livingstone, Edinburgh

Murray K B, Huelskoetter M M, O'Driscoll D 1980 The nursing process in later maturity. Prentice Hall, Englewood Cliffs, New Jersey

10

What of the future?

The reality of an ageing population is with us. This fact can no longer be ignored, whether we adopt the stance of a professional worker, who will likely face an increased workload; consider it from the view-point of a family, aware of longevity in relatives or family friends; or regard it from a personal angle, with a degree of self-interest as we realise that we too may one day be old. The implications of a rising proportion of older people in the population affect us not only as individuals, but also as citizens, for whilst many of the decisions which affect how we may live active lives in our later years, are our own, it is society which often affords us the chance to do so with dignity and independence.

Throughout this book we have endeavoured to present positive attitudes towards the care of older people, believing that our seniors constitute a great human resource which must be utilised wisely. We reiterate that if older people are to achieve the functional independence, high-level wellness and quality of life, which enables them to participate in family and community affairs to the level they wish, until they attain a dignified and peaceful death, they are unlikely to do so by the dramatic intervention of high-technology. Rather they will depend on a repertoire of self-care competencies; the complementing care of well-informed families, friends and neighbours, and on the perceptive but unobtrusive assessment of practitioners, who are aware of the complex nature of ageing and the specific needs thus generated. Additionally they will require programmes of co-ordinated, progressive and continuing care, often of an innovatory nature, provided by multidisciplinary teams.

An expert technical group looking at services and systems for the elderly world-wide, has outlined a framework which indicates the direction for future research and social policies for older people:

a. services subserving basic vital needs, such as housing and money
b. life-enhancing services, e.g. clubs, education, health education, transport and leisure
c. compensating services when there is difficulty or impairment
d. care services when function is lost

WHO 1980

Within such programmes we believe the health visiting service can play a major part, provided there is a *corporate professional decision to do so*, and a willingness to reappraise methods and techniques used. However, it is also recognised that many practitioners are concerned that they cannot achieve all they would wish for their clients, including the elderly. As one health visitor has put it 'health visitors operate uneasily on the inter-face between what appears to be unlimited need and very limited resources' (Orr 1983). For this reason priorities must be determined. We intimated in our opening chapter that there are great dilemmas facing the profession, which must be collectively debated, so that the role may be clarified and then further developed.

In recent years there is evidence of a greater priority being afforded to older people by some health visitors. The Health Visitor Association set up a special interest group, which is lively and well supported, and is already making its views known to the wider organisation. The Royal College of Nursing, Health Visitors' Advisory Group has drawn attention to the urgent need for the profession to review such matters as 'consultancy' in health visiting as an adjunct to generalist work, and the emphasis given to different groups in the light of demographic trends (RCN 1983, 1984). It is contended that there is a key role in the promotion of health from middle-age onwards, which health visitors should engage in as a corollary to their activities with those in earlier years.

The early health visitors were imbued with pioneer spirit. They initiated and developed child health centres from a hybrid union of schools for mothers and infant welfare centres. There is need for a resurgence of this approach, for individuals in later life. Humanitarian and economic issues dictate that we find relatively low-cost solutions to the problems of ill-health in later years. One way to help in achieving these is to involve people more actively in the control of their own ageing. Therefore health visitors have much to offer if they concentrate their efforts in:

- running well persons health centres
- stimulating older people to run health clubs, in which positive approaches to health in later life receive emphasis, e.g. exercise, weight control, stress control, relaxation, nutrition, self-realisation (see Ch. 7)
- co-operating with health education officers and others to organise health forums, self-health workshops, and study programmes for the carers of older people, both paid and informal
- liaising with occupational health personnel and others in promoting well-designed and client-orientated, pre-retirement programmes.

In these activities many health visitors are already engaged. A few have published descriptions of their work, (Austin 1984, Drummond 1984, Jones 1984, Newell 1984). Their positive experiences indicate the readiness with which many older persons respond to such overtures, and the motivations which can be harnessed when individuals realise that they can play an active part in creating behaviour conducive to their own well-being. Furthermore, personalising risk factors, as indicated in Table 6.1 can, when carefully handled, act as a spur to action.

This is not to decry the importance of individual care for older people, but rather to stress how practitioners might best deploy their unique blend of skills. The early child health centres were developed through a dynamic partnership with voluntary personnel. There is much evidence to suggest that clients of all ages and social groups would welcome such participation, if it were to be tailored to meet their needs. Thus, in re-appraising and further developing their community-based activities, health visitors may well have to re-organise their modes of work. Activities have to be geared to the needs of different groups. This may mean more evening and week-end work, perhaps siting clubs in community centres and shopping precincts, having more 'drop-in' sessions, and making far greater use of local media than perhaps has been the pattern heretofore.

These changes of emphasis for work with those in later life, cannot be achieved only by collective debate and decisions, important though these are. Others have to help health visitors achieve their aims. Professional and statutory bodies have an important part to play, in helping to clarify roles and in making available the resources, especially the educational programmes, which are required to prepare and update practitioners. Other disciplines must recognise health visiting aims, and facilitate these. In this connection the recent research by the Health Education Council, which endorses much of what is given here, is to be welcomed (Phillipson & Strang 1984). In times of financial stringency it is difficult to urge increases in manpower, but steps have to be taken to determine what constitutes a realistic case-load for 'family visitors' and how far additional personnel may be needed to allow for the specific health visiting duties outlined above. Such research can only be commissioned at the highest levels.

Within the profession itself there is a need for practitioners to concern themselves with their own continuing education, but this can only come about if study days and refresher courses, literature and similar media, allow them to do so. This requires a multi-disciplinary interest in providing appropriate means. Most of all enthusiastic members of the health visiting profession have to demonstrate to their colleagues what can be achieved in health care in later life. This will generate the interest which seeks for new initiatives, which provokes research and evaluation, which searches for common denominators in the promotion of well-being, which utilises epidemiological approaches and tests out appropriate and possibly unifying models of care. Such action will help to identify how post-registration basic education must adapt and change, and how management must enable the profession to develop its role. Then it may be possible to represent more fully the dynamic relationship between older people, health visitors and health visiting.

REFERENCES

Austin W 1984 A well man clinic in practice. Health Visitor; 57 (July): 204.
Drummond G 1984 Laughter is better than medicine; a support group for caring relatives. Health Visitor 57 (July): 201–202
Jones L D 1984 A hypertension clinic. Health Visitor 57 (July): 206–207
Newell G 1984 Working in a well woman centre. Health Visitor 57 (July): 207–208
Orr J 1983 Is health visiting meeting today's needs? Health Visitor 56(6):203
Phillipson C, Strang P 1984 Health education and older people; the role of paid carers. Health Education Council, in association with Department of Adult Education, University of Keele, Keele
Royal College of Nursing, Health Visitors' Advisory Group 1983 Thinking about health visiting. Society of Primary Health Care Nursing, RCN, London
Royal College of Nursing 1984: Health Visitors' Advisory Group, Further thinking about health visiting. Society of Primary Health Care Nursing, RCN, London
World Health Organization 1980 Services and systems of care for the elderly. (document ICP/ADR 015) Helsinki

FURTHER READING

Skeet M 1983 Protecting the health of the elderly. Public Health in Europe 18: Regional Office for Europe, WHO, Copenhagen

Appendices

Appendix 1

Extracts from the Mayston Report 1971: Management structure in the local authority nursing services (Appendix 8)

FUNCTIONS OF FIELD WORKERS

THE HEALTH VISITOR

A health visitor is a woman who visits persons in their homes for the purpose of giving advice as to the care of young children, persons suffering from illness and expectant and nursing mothers, and as to the measures necessary to prevent the spread of infection, and who performs such other duties as may be assigned to her; and has the qualifications prescribed for a health visitor. The effect of Section II of the Health Services and Public Health Act 1968 is to widen the areas within which she may work, by removing the statutory limitation conveyed by the words 'in their own homes'. Health visitors may be expected in future to carry out their duties not only in persons' homes but also in doctors' surgeries and health centres, often within attachment schemes.

The general responsibilities of the health visitor

1. Health education and advice to all families or individuals whom she visits in the home, the doctor's surgery, or the clinic or health centre.

2. A regard for the medical, psychological and social needs of the whole family. The health visitor must also be aware of the help given by other workers.

3. A readiness to take account of psychological factors in every case with which she deals. At all times the health visitor should be aware of her role in the promotion of mental health and the prevention of mental illness.

4. Comprehensive counselling services to families in need and the seeking of appropriate help from other agencies.

The health visitor decides how frequently it is necessary for her to visit a family and at all times seeks to discharge the responsibilities described at 2 above. In the following sections particular aspects of her work are dealt with in greater detail.

(Only those duties relating to the care of the elderly are listed here.)

Work undertaken by the health visitor:

In relation to the care of the elderly the health visitor

- identifies old people who require support and help in her area
- gives advice on the maintenance of health and the prevention of ill health
- helps the older person and families to understand the normal physiology of old age
- pays special attention to nutrition
- is fully aware of the predisposing factors of hypothermia in the elderly
- calls on assistance of voluntary agencies as appropriate
- links closely with the social welfare services
- maintains close contact with the family doctor concerned.

In relation to the care of the chronic sick and handicapped the health visitor

- makes herself aware of such patients and visits them as necessary
- gives necessary support to the handicapped
- helps the family with the handicapped person in the home

- ensures that the necessary aids and equipment are provided
- maintains contact with voluntary agencies and the social welfare department.

The health visitor's responsibilities in health education include:

... undertaking health education in old peoples clubs; carrying out health education on the need for prophylaxis, the prevention of accidents, the dangers of smoking, the early detection of cancer ... and any other relevant subjects.

In relation to the care of immigrants the health visitor

- must ascertain immigrant families living in the area
- gives the necessary support and help to these families
- ensures that families understand and make use of the various services available under the National Health Service Act(s)
- gives the care described above for other families.

Screening procedures which the health visitor undertakes include:

... screening the elderly population either in conjunction with general practitioners or health authority staff.

Other duties to be considered

- liaison with appropriate hospital staff
- attendance at co-ordinating committees at field worker levels
- participation in research projects
- membership of committees in the area, such as the old people's welfare committee, after care associations etc.
- record keeping. This is an important aspect of the health visitor's work and involves considerable time. The health visitor holds a case record card for every individual or family she visits.
- preparation of visual aids. It is expected that health visitors

prepare visual aids for their own talks and discussion periods.
- control of infectious disease and follow-up action as required by the medical officer of health.
- supervision of the work of ancillary helpers working with her.

General

The health visitor is concerned with the health of the family as a whole, providing a continuing service to families and individuals in the community.

REFERENCE

DHSS 1971 Management structure in the local authority nursing services. (Mayston Report) DHSS, London

Appendix 2a

Council for the Education and Training of Health Visitors Syllabus (1969)

SYLLABUS

Examination for health visitors in the United Kingdom

Section 1 Development of the individual

This section deals with the range of normal development and significant deviations commonly met in health visiting practice. Its content forms the basis for the recognition and assessment of individual capacities at different ages and in different circumstances.

The influence throughout the life-span of genetic and other prenatal factors.

The physical, emotional, intellectual and social growth of the individual and the factors affecting development, with particular reference to family relationships.

The characteristics of the mature personality.

The biological and psychological effects of ageing.

Section 2 The individual in the group

This section constitutes an introduction to the concepts of sociology. It involves an analysis of the structure of society and the forces that generate social change and influence individual behaviour.

Introduction to the language of sociology and to the concepts of social structure, social institutions and social control.

Formal and informal groups; roles, status and social interaction.

Social stratification and social mobility: their personal and cultural implications.

Socialisation and education.

The nature and patterns of family and kinship groups and their functions in simple and complex societies.

Cultural diversity, social change, deviance and social conflict.

Section 3 Development of social policy

This section is concerned with recent developments and current trends in social policy within the context of its diverse origins and of continuing changes in definitions of social need, in the use of community resources and in public expectations and attitudes.

Factors influencing the development of social policy in an industrialised urban society; the concept of the Welfare State.

An outline of the structure of Central and Local Government.

Current services available to all citizens for employment and income maintenance, environmental and personal health, education and leisure time activity, housing and environmental planning.

Concepts of community care, of family orientated services, of citizen participation; the role of the voluntary organisations and of the volunteer.

Problems of the organisation, financing, administration and staffing of the developing social services.

Section 4 Social aspects of health and disease

The content of this section provides the background for much of the work of the health visitor. It complements previous nursing studies, emphasising the social factors involved in health and disease and the relationship between needs and services.

The use of statistics and of the findings of social research in the identification of health needs and problems.

Health in relation to education, occupation and environment. The impact of disease, disability and mental disorder on the individual, the family and the community. The implications of current health problems for the planning and development of preventive, remedial and supportive care.

An outline of the health services: the organisation in the light of changing needs and resources.

The importance of effective co-ordination and collaboration within the health and social services, for the achievement of personal and community health.

Trends in world health; the work of relevant international agencies.

Section 5 Principles and practice of health visiting

This section is particularly concerned with the development of health visiting as a professional activity, its function in contemporary society, including community medical care and the knowledge and skills essential for its practice. It provides a theoretical foundation for the work of the health visitor and brings together subjects taught in other sections, including her health education activities.

The role of the health visitor in contemporary society.

The development of the health visiting service.

The scope of health visiting and its areas of practice.

The function of the health visitor in relation to different age groups and to members of the community with special needs.

Aims and objectives of the health visiting service

Promotion of good health for individual and community.

Identification of need, primary and secondary prevention.

Care and guidance in cases of breakdown in physical and/or mental health.

Mobilisation of services to meet health and social needs.

Principles underlying effective health visiting

Respect and concern for the individual and recognition of his rights and obligations as a citizen.

A consideration of such concepts as: acceptance, confidentiality, freedom and social control, conflict of interests.

Ethical principles relating to professional practice.
Theories and methods of health visiting practice
The art of looking and listening.
The development and use of understanding and empathy.
The identification and analysis of problems.
The use and methods of recording and communication.
Formal and informal teaching; the aims and scope of health education.
Theories and techniques of organisation and management.
The development of effective inter-professional relationships.

This document is in no way intended to be discriminatory. For convenience the health visitor has been referred to in the feminine gender throughout, but whenever this term is used it includes both men and women.

Appendix 2b

Examination questions

The following are some examination questions which have been set for student health visitors, pertaining to the care of older people. They serve to indicate the scope and range of course content for the elderly but by no means represent an exhaustive list. Not all may be answered in this book.

Section 1 The development of the individual

Part A Psycho-social development

1. Outline the major psychological and social developments in later life.
   How does an understanding of the psychology of ageing affect the work of the health visitor?
2. Retirement . . . crisis point or stepping-stone?
   Discuss this statement, illustrating your answer with special reference to the work of the health visitor with retired persons.
3. 'Retaining and fostering self-esteem is one of the most important aspects of work with older people.' Discuss this statement, with particular reference to health visiting practice.
4. Briefly describe the major theories of learning. What

modifications, if any, are likely to occur in later life? What effect might a knowledge of learning theories and ageing have on the work of the health visitor?

5. Bereavement may be a common experience for the old. Briefly describe the impact of bereavement in later life, showing how health visitors might assist older people to cope with loss, grief and mourning.

6. How are attitudes formed? How may an awareness of attitude formation and change, enable a health visitor to work more effectively with an elderly client, who is overtly hostile regarding her care?

7. Define 'a group' and outline the phases of group development. How might group work with the elderly differ from that with other age groups?

8. Outline the main psycho-social theories of ageing.
How might you, as an health visitor, utilise a knowledge of these various theories to help you in your work with elderly people?

9. Discuss the concept of leadership. How would you utilise knowledge about leadership styles and behaviour when pre-planning group work with older people?

10. Analyse some of the myths and stereotypes related to sexuality in later life. How might these be overcome? What do you see as the main role of a health visitor regarding sexual development in the elderly?

11. What factors influence the development of personality? How would you use a knowledge of personality development when assessing and planning with an elderly client for the first time?

12. What is meant by the term 'individual differences'? How useful is this concept for health visitors and how can it be applied in practice? Illustrate your answer with special reference to the older client.

13. Discuss how health visitors might assist elderly people to achieve the developmental tasks of ageing successfully.

14. Cite some of the characteristics of maturity. What factors are likely to enhance emotional development in the latter years?

15. Define the concept 'emotional health'. Discuss how far physical and socio-cultural factors might influence emotional well-being in the elderly.

16. Briefly describe the cognitive changes that occur in normal ageing. What factors would you take into account when assessing the cognitive state of an elderly client?

17. Define the term 'adaptive behaviour'. Briefly describe the common adaptive mechanisms adopted by older people. What action would you, as an health visitor, take in order to first assess and then strengthen an elderly client's coping ability?

18. Explain how you would approach the task of teaching staff in a Day Centre for the elderly, about cognitive functioning in old age. How would you assist them to promote cognitive well-being in their elderly members?

Part B Physical and physiological aspects of growth and development

1. Describe the main physical changes which normally present in old age. How would you use this knowledge to assess the care an older person might require from a health visitor?

2. Discuss the factors which influence normal ageing. How could you as a health visitor utilise this knowledge to help you promote health in later life?

3. Compare and contrast the normal physical changes that occur in sensory fields in older persons, with those pathological processes which may occur. Why is it important for an health visitor to try to differentiate these?

4. Outline the main principles of locomotor development in human life. What changes may occur in old age? Can the health visitor prevent these? If so, how?

5. You are asked to give a talk to a group of carers of elderly people on 'Ageing skin and how to care for it'. What developmental principles would you seek to impart, and what points would you emphasise during your talk?

6. Describe the nutritional needs of the over-60s. What principles would you use to guide you when checking the diet

of an elderly couple whose sole income is provided by Supplementary Benefit?

7. Trace the process of auditory development during the first 5 years. What changes may occur in hearing with advancing years? How would you, as an health visitor, promote a programme of hearing care during earlier years, so that older persons might enter the last phase of hearing development in an optimal state?

8. Describe the changes which normally occur in the digestive system as a result of ageing. How would you use this knowledge when giving guidance on the nutritional management of a 75-year-old man, who has recently come to live with his daughter?

9. Relate the normal changes of ageing to accident prevention in later life.

10. Of what significance to an health visitor is a knowledge of elimination changes in later life? How would you use this knowledge to promote continence in an older woman who is tending to become socially isolated because of embarassment from stress incontinence?

11. Biological rhythms are an integral part of human life. Discuss how such rhythms may influence the ability of older people to adapt. How would you use knowledge concerning biological rhythms to enable you to **assess** physiological and behavioural responses in a male octogenarian who has been referred to you for follow-up care following a period in hospital? How would you use this information to help you plan his care?

12. 'Chronologic age is a poor marker of the ageing process.' Discuss this statement, with particular reference to the assessment of functional ability in older people.

13. What principles should be adopted in the rehabilitation of the older person?

14. Discuss the psychological aspects of disability, in the light of the incidence of disabling conditions amongst the elderly.

15. Define the concept of 'dependence'. How might a health visitor promote independence in elderly clients?

16. 'Most people prefer to die in familiar surroundings'. Discuss this statement and the role of the health visitor in understanding and meeting the needs of dying elderly people and their families.

17. Discuss the stress caused by such crimes as 'mugging' and 'vandalism' and the effects this can have on the health and well-being of older people. What part can the health visitor play in promoting security in later life?

18. What is meant by 'the quality of life'? Discuss how health visitors can (a) assess and (b) promote the quality of life for their elderly clients.

Section 2 The individual in the group

1. 'In the past when an Eskimo mother became old, her family expected her to wander off into the snow. In contemporary society when an English mother becomes old her family expect her to enter a Home.' Discuss this statement with reference to the role of the family in the care of the elderly today.

2. The number of aged in the United Kingdom population is increasing and is expected to reach 8.3 million by 1991. To what extent, and why, is this increase likely to be of interest to health visitors?

3. Compare and contrast the structure and functions of the ageing family with those of (a) the young adult family (b) the middle-aged family. How might these differences in structure and function affect your work as an health visitor with an ageing family?

4. Discuss the concept of 'the family'. How might health visiting intervention with a family unit differ from that undertaken with an elderly individual?

5. What is meant by the term 'social class'? Discuss how awareness of this concept might affect your work as a health visitor with older people. Illustrate your answer with reference to any recent research findings with which you are familiar.

6. Analyse some of the changing cultural norms and values which may affect older people. How does a knowledge

of culture and change affect health visiting professional activity?

7. Define the term 'an aged subculture'. How might such a subculture develop? Discuss the effect of such a subculture on: (a) the elderly (b) society in general.

8. 'Social and economic trends help to create problems out of normal processes'. Discuss this statement with reference to the changing state of elderly people in our society. Can the health visitor contribute to problem reduction? If so, how?

9. Outline the main points of any *one* community study you have read concerning the elderly. What differences, if any, did/might this research report make to your work as an health visitor?

10. What difficulties, if any, are likely to be encountered by elderly members in ethnic minority families? How can health visitors help?

11. What social problems are health visitors likely to encounter when working with elderly clients in (a) rural communities (b) inner city areas?

12. Why is it necessary for an health visitor to study the discipline of sociology? How is a sociological perspective likely to affect health visiting of elderly client-families?

13. What do you understand by the term 'social health'? How might socio-cultural norms and values influence social well-being in the elderly?

14. Define and differentiate moral and spiritual development. How might cultural differences affect such development? Discuss how an health visitor might foster such development in an elderly client.

15. What characteristics would you look for when assessing the social competence of elderly people? How can health visitors help to promote and maintain social competence in the later years?

16. What is meant by the concept of 'deviance'?. Discuss how an understanding of this concept might help an health visitor when dealing with an elderly client whose neighbours have complained about his 'deviant behaviour'?.

17. Discuss the sociological aspects of housing the elderly. What part can health visitors play in relation to housing and health?

18. What is significant to health visitors in the relationship between epidemiology and sociology? Illustrate your answer with special reference to the care of the elderly.

Section 3 The development of social policy

1. Define and discuss the concept of 'social need', with particular reference to the development of social policy for either the elderly, or the handicapped.

2. Discuss the respective merits of the selectivist and universalist approaches to welfare services, illustrating your answer with reference either to services for the elderly or the mentally disordered.

3. 'The main priority in public sector housing should be to meet the requirements of groups with special needs, such as the elderly or disabled persons.'
   Discuss this statement, in the light of social policy developments on housing over the last two decades.

4. 'Care in the community must increasingly mean care by the community' (DHSS 1981 'Growing Older'). Analyse this statement and comment on it, in the light of current policies for older people.

5. Outline the income maintenance services for older persons in contemporary Britain. What factors may affect elderly persons utilising these benefits? How can they best be helped to do so?

5. Define the term 'retirement'. Discuss the advantages and/or disadvantages of a policy of mandatory retirement for women at 60 years and men at 65 years.

6. Discuss the notion that partnership between statutory and voluntary services is a vital ingredient in the provision of services for the elderly.

7. 'Poverty is the giant from which our elderly would feign escape.' Discuss this statement with reference to social policy developments to combat poverty since 1970.

8. What is meant by social policy?. How can an understanding of this discipline help health visitors in their care of the elderly?

9. Discuss the role of (a) the home help service (b) the chiropody service in the care of older people. How can health visitors improve their liaison with members of these services?

10. How far do demographic trends affect demands made upon the National Health Service? Illustrate your answer with special reference to the demands currently being made on the psycho-geriatric services.

11. Explore the idea that a major social policy need is to develop leisure resources. How might this notion affect the health visiting care of elderly clients?

12. Discuss the notion that poverty or inequality are less likely to concern the elderly than ageism and dependence are.

13. Trace the developments in social policy concerning the Mental Health Services. What is the significance to health visitors of an awareness that elderly people currently form the largest single group of in-patients under the care of the psychiatric hospital service?

14. 'Public authorities need to support and encourage all those involved in providing care for elderly people, and to develop local networks of provision'. Analyse this statement and outline the provision you would wish to see developing through such local networks.

15. How far do gender-stereotypes affect the development of social policies for lay-carers of elderly persons? Is this issue of any consequence to health visitors? Why?

16. Trace the developments in adult education throughout this century. How would you wish to see education services for the multi-cultural elderly develop in the next 10 years? What part can health visitors play in relation to such policies?

17. Discuss the following statement: 'Don't grow old gracefully, grow old rebelliously.' (Kleyman P 1974 Senior power. Glide Publications, San Francisco.) What is the

significance to the health visiting service of effective efforts to raise the collective consciousness of older people?

18. Discuss the concept of voluntary service in relation to the elderly (a) as recipients of such service (b) as volunteers. What part might health visitors play in relation to such voluntary service?

Section 4 Social aspects of health and disease

Part A Epidemiology, social aspects of health and disease and health service administration

1. What is food poisoning? Differentiate briefly between the main types. What guidance would you give to the staff of a Day Centre for elderly people concerning the prevention of food poisoning?

2. What sources of health information are there? Discuss the sources you might use, including specific publications, to enable you to offer a health visiting service to elderly people in your community.

3. Briefly explain the principles of vaccination and immunisation. What routine vaccination and immunisation procedures are available to: (a) children? (b) the elderly? Explain how you would encourage acceptance of such procedures.

4. State briefly the provisions of The Social Services Act 1970 and the Chronically Sick and Disabled Persons Act, 1970. How would you aim to utilise these provisions when providing care for elderly disabled clients?

5. Discuss the components of a comprehensive geriatric service. How far do you consider the structure and function of the National Health Service meets these requirements?

6. 'Society gets the diseases it deserves.' Discuss this statement with particular reference to the elderly population.

7. Of what use to an health visitor is a knowledge of Epidemiology? Explain how you would apply an understanding of this discipline in practice, when working with

(a) the elderly in a specific locality (b) a population of children in a special school.

8. Differentiate descriptive epidemiology from analytic epidemiology. What problems beset epidemiologists when endeavouring to identify possible causal relations in disease states amongst an elderly population?

9. Differentiate between the incidence rate and the prevalence rate in community assessments of diseases. Discuss the relative merits of each of these two rates in (a) evaluating preventive efforts and exploring the natural history of disease amongst older people (b) planning services to meet needs, met with in the elderly population.

10. Discuss the usefulness of the host-agent-environment model, to health visitors working with elderly persons in a community.

11. What is the relationship between the epidemiological process and the health visiting process? Show how you would use your awareness of this inter-relationship to help you assess the health needs of an elderly practice population and plan and deliver care to them.

12. What is the significance to a health visitor of an understanding of the natural history of disease processes? How would you use this knowledge to enable you to plan a health education programme for the members of an 'Over-60s Club' in your area?

13. Discuss the role of the Health Visitor in the Primary Health Care Team. How would you organise her activities to make the best use of her services in (a) the care of the 75-year-old group and upwards, within the practice (b) the care of those aged 45–60 years?

14. Using examples to support your answer, discuss the advantages of health screening (a) a population of school children (b) a population of elderly people.

15. Discuss the respective roles of health visitors and community psychiatric nurses in the care of the mentally frail elderly.

16. You have the opportunity to give a series of talks on accidents and their prevention to a group of older people.

Using the epidemiological approach show how you would deal with this and the emphases you would make.

17. 'Chronic bronchitis ... the English disease that should *not* happen!' Examine and discuss this statement in the light of current epidemiological knowledge. How would you use such knowledge to help you plan either to give health education to an adult group, or to work with a specific family, where the household head is a 64-year-old male suffering from chronic bronchitis?

18. You are moving to a new locality to work as an health visitor, and find you are working in a general practice team where the overall practice population is 9000. You discover there are 1350 persons aged 65 years and over, registered with the practice. You are the second health visitor of 2, and the other members of the team are 3 district nurses and 3 general practitioners. What information would you seek and how would you set about planning your work with this elderly population?

Part B Current health problems

1. Mr H, aged 64 years, is disabled by chronic bronchitis and emphysema. His wife, 70 years, suffers from generalised osteoarthritis and congestive cardiac failure. Neighbours and friends appear unable or unwilling to help. Can the health visitor do so, and if so how?

2. Discuss, with examples, the different ways in which disease can present in the very old as compared with younger persons, and suggest possible causes.

3. Discuss the investigation and management of dementing illnesses in the elderly.

4. What are the problems faced by elderly diabetics, and how may they be overcome?

5. Discuss the *physical* causes of anti-social behaviour in an older person.

6. Discuss the advantages and disadvantages of both home and hospital care for a person who has sustained a myocardial infarction. Outline the role of the health

visitor in the care of older people who have had a myocardial infarction.

7. Discuss the management role of the health visitor in cases of self-neglect (Diogenes syndrome).

8. How would you, as an health visitor, try to sort out and then remedy, the main causes of confused behaviour in older people?

9. 'Depression is different from unhappiness'. Discuss this statement and outline the health visiting care of a person who has been diagnosed as depressed, 6 months after retirement.

10. Discuss the role of the health visitor where it is suspected that an elderly grandfather has been abused, (battered).

11. At 3.00 p.m. on a Friday afternoon before a Bank Holiday, you discover that an 81-year-old woman, living alone, has just returned home from the casualty department of the local district general hospital, having had her fractured right humerus reduced and splinted. Discuss the problems which may arise and how they can best be coped with.

12. Discuss the value of routine screening in the elderly. What, in your opinion, are the most important features of a screening programme for the elderly?

13. Discuss the possible causes of urinary incontinence in elderly women. What is the role of the health visitor in the prevention and management of urinary incontinence in later life?

14. A 67-year-old woman who lives with her 74-year-old husband has recently been hospitalised for a moderately severe cerebrovascular accident. You are the liaison health visitor for follow-up care. What enquiries would you make prior to her discharge and how would you ensure she received effective follow-up care?

15. What are the common psychiatric problems met with in later life? Discuss the role and function of the health visitor in the prevention and control of such disorders. How would you support a family caring for an elderly person with just one such a problem?

16. State the causes of transient confusion in the elderly. How can this state be differentiated from Alzheimer's disease? Discuss the treatment of transient confusion, stressing the part health visitors might play in this.

17. An elderly couple, whom you visit, appear distressed when you next call. The wife complains of deteriorating vision and instability, whilst the husband has a severe hearing incapacity. How would you handle this situation? What could be done to alleviate some of their distress?

18. Discuss the respective roles of health visitor, district nurse and social worker, in the care of an elderly couple, where the wife is suffering from Parkinson's disease and the 80-year-old husband has maturity-onset diabetes and a history of three myocardial infarctions in the past 5 years. How can the couple be assisted to function as independently as possible, without feeling either unsupported or over-visited?

Section 5 Principles and practice of health visiting including health education

Part A Principles and practice of health visiting

1. Describe an age-sex register and discuss its uses and limitations. What are the implications of such a register in terms of: (a) identification of vulnerable groups, including the elderly (b) general health visiting practice?

2. A 72-year-old man who has been a widower for 2 years is found to be suffering from diabetes mellitus. Discuss the dietary advice which might be required in his case and the methods you might adopt to ensure satisfactory nutritional management.

3. What are the *common* nutritional problems which may be met with amongst the elderly? Discuss how you would carry out nutritional assessment for older people and the emphases you would seek to give when discussing nutritional status.

4. Discuss the principles of interviewing. How would you apply these principles when visiting an elderly couple for the first time?

5. 'Records are a vital part of health visiting practice.'
   Discuss this statement with particular reference to responsibility, authority and accountability in health visiting.

6. Outline the process of communication. Discuss some of the problems which may be encountered in (a) verbal communication (b) non-verbal communication with elderly people. How would you endeavour to prevent these problems arising as far as possible? How would you cope with them if prevention had not occurred?

7. State the objectives of health visiting care for the elderly. How far do you consider the present preparation of practitioners fits them for effective work with elderly people?

8. Explain the role and function of the health visitor to either a group of social work students or a group of lay carers of the elderly.

9. Define and explain the three levels of prevention, namely primary prevention, secondary prevention and tertiary prevention. What is the value of this concept to health visitors? Illustrate your answer with particular reference either to the care of children 0–1 year or to the care of the elderly.

10. What are the identified principles of health visiting? Illustrate how they may each be applied to the practice of health visiting (a) school children (b) old people. Are they?

11. A 64-year-old woman, who has had a right mastectomy, for malignant disease, seeks your help about her subsequent care. How would you handle this situation and plan care with her?

12. Discuss the principles of good record-keeping. What changes, if any, would you wish to see in the format, storage, completion and use of health visiting records (a) in the pre-school period (b) for those aged 65 years or more.

13. Discuss the view that health visitors use 'lack of time' as an excuse for avoiding work with the elderly, when in fact it is because they have no appropriate 'frame of reference' (Luker 1981).

14. What do you understand by the term 'anticipatory guidance'? Describe the use of this technique in relation to **three** of the following:
    1. Persons in a pre-retirement stage.
    2. A family coping with terminal illness in a grandmother.
    3. An elderly couple contemplating a move into sheltered accommodation.
    4. A 62-year-old woman awaiting admission for an eye operation.
    5. A family planning to have their elderly father come to live with them.
15. Define the term 'effective health'. How might a health visitor employ this concept in her work with older people?
16. Discuss the implications of a declining proportion of 'younger elderly' (60–74) compared with a rising proportion of 'older elderly' (aged 75 years or more), in the United Kingdom population. How is this likely to affect the health visiting service?
17. Discuss the notion that care of the elderly has a lower priority amongst members of the caring professions than some other age groups.
18. Discuss the problem of abuse of the elderly.
    What is the role of the health visitor in relation to the prevention and/or control of such abuse?

Part B Health education

1. Since the quality of life in old age rests largely on effective health promotion in earlier life, how do we set about educating those in their middle years for retirement and subsequent old age? State the likely benefits to be derived for the individual and the community.
2. 'The 75 year old is at risk in the community.' How do you see the health educational role of the health visitor operating in this sphere?
3. Discuss imaginative and effective ways of presenting budgeting knowledge and nutritional guidance to a group of older people whose incomes are limited.

4. You have been asked to participate in the planning and conducting of a Cancer Education Programme in your area. Your particular responsibility relates to health education for persons in later life. What factors would you take into account when establishing your objectives? Outline the principles and practice you would adopt in designing and carrying out the programme.

5. What advice would you give to a 40-year-old factory worker about retirement?

6. You have been asked by the leader of an Over-60s Club to conduct a series of health education sessions on 'health promotion in later life.' What objectives would you set and how would you design the overall syllabus? Select **one** topic, giving a topic web and indicating how you would design, deliver and evaluate the session.

7. Discuss the relative merits of one-to-one education and group health education. What specific points would you bear in mind when using each of these methods?

8. Discuss the purpose and content of a short course for wardens of sheltered accommodation for the elderly, on 'Our seniors and how to care for them'.
   How far would you consider health visitors should be involved in such courses?

9. Describe how you would prepare and present an health education session for older people on *one* of the following topics: (a) dental health (b) foot care (c) eye care (d) leisure activities.
   What steps would you take to see that your session had been effective?

10. You are asked to participate in a support group for lay-carers of elderly people. What are the important principles you would consider regarding group work? What emphases would you encourage and how would you see the group developing?

11. Accidents are a major cause of mortality and morbidity in the elderly. What knowledge would you utilise to enable you to plan a relevant programme of accident prevention for the elderly in your area? How would you design and execute such a programme?

12. Team work is of vital importance in the care of elderly

people. How would you prepare a group of health visitor students to appreciate the multi-disciplinary approach that is needed in this sphere?

13. Discuss the causes of hypothermia. How can health visitors help to prevent this problem? Outline the health education you would give (a) to an elderly housebound couple living in a large house. (b) the members of a 'Good Neighbour Scheme' who are participating in a local surveillance scheme.

14. What factors concerning learning would you take into account when working with a group of older people on 'Creative contributing by older people'? What methods would you adopt in order to help these seniors realise what they can give to the community?

15. How would you assess the health education needs of a family unit where the elderly grandfather has been discharged from hospital with carcinomatosis? He and his wife live near to their middle-aged daughter, who is married to a business executive whose firm is facing difficulties. They have a 25-year-old unmarried daughter, who has recently taken up a new teaching post and tells you she is very fearful of seeing someone die.

16. Discuss the health education needs of a group of elderly residents in accommodation provided by a voluntary organisation. How far does the health visitor have a responsibility to consider such needs? What role might a health visitor play in meeting any identified needs?

17. You are working as an health visitor in an inner city area. A student nurse is seconded to you for her community experience. Show how you would plan a programme for her that would help her to grasp the purpose and scope of community care for the elderly. What steps would you take to confirm that learning had taken place?

18. Identify the likely health education needs of a 62-year-old woman who has recently retired from an exacting professional post and finds herself caring for a 76-year-old former colleague who lives with her and a frail, handicapped uncle who is a widower and lives nearby. How would you attempt to meet these needs in a supportive and effective manner?

Appendix 3

Models and frameworks used in nursing and health visiting practice

MODELS RELATED TO THE CONCEPT OF HEALTH AS ADAPTATION,

1. Crisis intervention model

Caplan (1964, 1974) proposed a model, based on adaptation theory, which he felt had particular application to community health personnel, in that it was intended to be used as a preventive measure, but chiefly at primary prevention level. He perceived this model as a crisis-intervention device. The model assumes that:

    a. Individuals are holistic beings who throughout life react to environmental stress in a total-person fashion. Since through the life-span persons encounter constant internal or external stressors, they are constantly engaged in a struggle to achieve homeostasis and meet their energy needs. Such adaptation is brought about by a series of inborn and learned coping strategies.

    b. At certain times in individuals' lives they encounter events which constitute overwhelming stress. Such experiences constitute 'crisis'. The labelling of an event as a 'crisis' is, however, highly personal; since it is the *significance* of the experience for the individual and the *impact* it makes upon them, that causes them to regard an event so. Thus what constitutes 'crisis' for one person, may appear relatively trivial to another person. However there are certain events which appear to be regarded as crisis by many people, these include death of a loved person, pet or object; loss of health or functional ability; loss of home and valued personal possessions.

c. Crises constitute 'turning points' in people's lives. They can cause such adaptation and change that it is possible for individuals to emerge from them stronger and enriched. This is considered a healthy outcome and hence becomes the overall goal of interventionist-care.

d. Certain events, such as developmental transitions, can also come to be regarded as crises, e.g. retirement. It is possible to anticipate such events, and sometimes to predict the probability of others. Where practitioners can invoke probability, they have a clear role in primary prevention. They can assist the individual to take 'avoidance action', as in advocating prophylaxis to reduce the chance of encountering the crisis of infectious disease, or to become a non-smoker to prevent smoking-related disease or disability. When the event cannot be avoided, it is possible through the technique of *anticipatory guidance*, so to prepare persons that they are able to cope with the experience in a healthy manner.

e. Where an event has occurred and the use of primary preventive techniques has proved unsuccessful, secondary or tertiary level prevention can be practised, depending on the stage of the reaction. Such intervention depends upon practitioners being able to recognise specific stress-reactions and the characteristic pattern of reaction to crisis is thought to be shown as: shock; disbelief and numbness; defensive retreat; sad acknowledgement of reality; adaptation and change; integration and enrichment. The aim of the intervening practitioner is to enable the person to move through these stages in a healthy fashion and complete the last one satisfactorily.

f. Thus during the acute phase of shock the practitioner aims to nourish, protect, sustain and comfort.

During the time of defensive retreat the practitioner aims to promote healthy grieving and 'worry-work', within a supportive relationship. As the individual moves into an acknowledgement of reality the practitioner assists the person to problem-solve and gradually withdraws intensive support as the person implements his/her decisions, adapts and changes. Finally through supportive discussion, the practitioner helps them to discover meaning in their experience and integrate this realisation into their life.

The model is thought to have value for older people as they are susceptible to potential and actual crises, some of which can be predicted. For this reason it has been used in this book in connection with intervention during bereavement (see Ch. 7).

The relationship between the model and the health visiting process may thus be seen as follows:

Crisis intervention model	Health visiting process
Rests on adaptation theory	*Assessment* Collects data pertinent to stress events and identifies client perception of their significance.
Takes account of Crisis theory Probability theory	Identifies client's normal coping patterns and any variation in present state. Determines phase of reaction and associated needs and problems, sets out these in priority order and decides direction of care required, in order to achieve positive adaptation.
Perceives interventionist as assuming roles as supporter; protector; helper; motivator; counsellor	*Planning* Assists client to identify goals. Selects actions to support and care for client whilst he is in state of disequilibrium. Plans with client for eventual self-help and autonomy, following healthy grieving, for loss of any kind.
Perceives intervention as following a distinct pattern, intensive at first then tapering off as balance is regained	*Implementing* Executes care plan to help client cope with crisis and regain balance.
	Evaluating Monitors progress; judges outcomes against goals and relevant criteria.
	Reorganising Re-plans and implements as needed.

2. The Roy adaptation model

The Roy adaptation model is primarily a systems model with interactionist elements. It is based on adaptation theory, derived from Helson (1964). It is applied to nursing (Roy 1970, Riehl & Roy 1980). The model assumes:

a. People are bio-psycho-social beings, in constant inter-action with matching environments. They respond to internal and external stimuli by a process of adaptation and change. The innate and acquired mechanisms of response constitute a unique pattern for each individual, which Roy suggests constitutes an *'adaptive zone'*. Stimuli falling within this 'adaptive zone' will be responded to positively, those by reason of amount or strength, which fall outside this 'adaptive zone' cannot be responded to positively and therefore the 'steady state' will be lost. Individuals will then likely require help to assist them to achieve homeostasis, whenever possible.

b. Roy classifies the types of stimuli individuals encounter as *focal*, *contextual* and *residual*.

Focal stimuli are immediate and confronting events/experiences, and include any which cause physiologic or psycho-social disturbance.

Contextual stimuli are regarded as background events which occur alongside the novel focal stimuli and can affect these.

Residual stimuli are those which relate to the beliefs, attitudes and traits held and the emotions culled from earlier experiences, which may affect the way an individual responds to current stimuli.

For example, an elderly man may fall whilst visiting the toilet during the night. He is unable to rise or contact help, and lies there feeling pain in his right leg and hip (focal stimuli). Whilst on the floor he is affected by the lowered environmental temperature (contextual stimuli). He may, or may not, be aware that the latter is partly related to his socio-economic state (also contextual stimuli) as well as to to his attitudes towards economy and habits of thrift, which cause him to turn off his heating at night, even during very severe weather conditions (residual stimuli).

c. Roy sees the individual as reacting in four ways to these three different forms of stimuli. These ways or modes she classifies as:

1. Physiologic mode
encompassing changes in temperature; oxygen exchange; electrolyte balance; or sensori-motor response.

2. Self-concept mode
whereby adjustments are made in the way an individual sees and conducts himself, as he interpretes the way others perceive him.

3. Role function
alterations in the way an individual fulfils specific roles, as a result of changes in the role behaviour of others with whom he is in a role-relationship.

4. Interdependence mode
behavioural adjustments in light of changing circumstances, in order to maintain relative balance in interpersonal relationships.

Roy sees intervention by the practitioner as therefore occurring whenever a need or deficit exists in client or client-resources, in any one of these four modes. Such intervention is two-pronged and demands the exercise of professional judgment. It is directed towards manipulating the stimuli, to prevent stress encounters, or to minimise their effect. Stimuli may be singly manipulated, or in combination. The other action is directed towards strengthening and extending the client's 'zone of adaptation'. For example, returning to our earlier example of the elderly man who sustains a fall. Health visiting intervention would aim to determine the probability of falling; prevent the risk by advising a commode near the bed at night; would point out the need to maintain an even temperature during the day and night and would discuss with and educate client on the need to temper thrift during periods of excess cold, in favour of survival. This manipulation of stimuli would be accompanied by efforts to extend the client's adaptive level, by helping him to work out an emergency plan to cope with such an eventuality, so that help could be promptly summoned.

Although, as with other conceptual models, there are distinct differences between the framework used and the health visiting process, the link between them might appear as follows:

Stress-adaptation model

This model was described by its authors, Saxton & Hyland

Roy adaptation model	Health visiting process Data collected on personal and social level
Theory of adaptation	*Assessment* Identify risk of encountering stimuli. Classify stimuli and decide on forms of client reaction and adaptation.
Postulates of client bio-psycho-social response to stress	*Planning* Identify client goals. Select behaviour which will achieve goals; then clarify actions which meet goals, modify stimuli and increase client coping ability.
Goals to care	*Intervention/Implementing* Execute plan and alter stimuli of fall within client adaptive zone. Extend client adaptive zone to cope with stimuli. *Evaluating* Scrutinize client and practitioner action in terms of outcome against desired goals and process used. *Reorganising* Review plan and reorganise in light of evaluation.

(1979) as based on adaptation theory. The model assumes that:

a. Throughout life an individual must constantly face stressors, to which he must adaptively respond as a total person. Such stresses may be environmental, namely physical, chemical, micro-biological or social, or may be personal physical, developmental, or emotional stressors. Whilst the normal adaptive responses to stress can cause an individual to grow and develop, extra stress such as that arising from accident, illness, infection or loss, can overwhelm and impair balance.

b. Whilst adaptations are usually appropriate, there are times when individuals act inappropriately, and these maladaptations are not only ineffective, but can themselves impose further stress so compounding the original disturbance. An example of this might be when an elderly widow reacts to the death of her husband by refusing to eat or make any social contact.

c. This chain reaction of primary stress-reaction→secondary

stress-reaction can be repeated, so that the person is increasingly pre-occupied with endeavours to cope with cumulative stress.

Saxton and Hyland (1979) describe 5 levels of adaptive behaviour:

  (i) normal responses to stress including reflex action

 (ii) more conscious adaptation; individual aware of attempts to change and cope

(iii) individual reacts and displays adaptive signs and symptoms

(iv) secondary-level stress adaptive reactions appear

 (v) life-threatening stress reaction takes place.

   d. Practitioners are therefore seen as intervening:

  (i) to reduce the extent and intensity of the stress encountered

 (ii) to limit the individual's attempt to restrict compensatory responses

(iii) to deal with the symptoms of response

(iv) to interrupt and re-direct secondary stress reactions.

 (v) to supplement individual responses to maintain life-function.

Thus in the example of the elderly woman, recently bereaved of her husband, a health visitor practitioner might try, where possible, to prepare her beforehand for the inevitability of such a loss, would encourage anticipatory grieving and limit the individual's efforts to deny the likelihood of such an event. When the death actually occurred, the practitioner would deal with the ensuing symptoms of shock, through comforting and sustaining the individual and limiting the client's attempt to ignore hunger needs, by arranging for light appetising food and drink to be unobtrusively served to her frequently during the shock-phase. Furthermore she would subtly circumvent her client's attempts to withdraw totally from social contact, by allowing some time for solitude and respecting the client's need to be alone, yet paying short visits to her, to support and supervise her, and encouraging suitable others to do so. Additionally the practitioner would marshall resources to see that shopping, cooking, and personal care activities which sustain life, could be suitably continued on the client's behalf, until the widow could reassert adequate personal control. The practitioner would then gradually withdraw help as the client's coping mechanism improved.

The link between the model and the processes of care are shown below

Stress-adaptation model	Health visiting process
Based on adaptation theory, taking account of physiological and psychological theories.	*Assessment* Collects personal, family and community data to enable identification of causal stress-agents and client reaction patterns.
Postulates innate and acquired adaptive responses	Recognises adaptive needs and sets these out in priority order.
Emphasises the dynamic relationship between organism and environment and personal coping behaviour.	*Planning* Determines care goals with client as far as possible. Selects actions designed to strengthen adaptive responses and prevent or modify maladaptive ones.
Sets out indicators related to 5 levels of stress-reaction.	*Implementing* Acts to modify stressors and execute plan. Actively seeks to improve client coping ability through involving client in responsibility for care.
	Evaluating Estimates progress with client, assessing outcome against desired goals and judging process against valid criteria for efficiency and effectiveness.
	Re-organising Re-arranges intervention in accordance with evaluation and continues to scrutinise and re-plan as needed.

Orem's self-care model

This is a systems model, designed specifically for nursing and based on Orem's conceptualisation of man as an independent and self-governing individual (Orem 1971). It is based on the values of self-help and service to others. The model assumes that:

a. All persons function in bio-psycho-social-spiritual dimensions, and initiate and perform activities on their own behalf, in order to sustain life and health in each of these realms.

b. Self-care is learned behaviour, developed through curiosity, instruction and spaced repetition. The successful performance of self-care activities rests on an individual's level of cognitive awareness; their degree of maturity and the extent of their knowledge and skill concerning what constitutes suitable activities to sustain life and health.

c. To engage in effective self-care the individual must be able to initiate and maintain actions which will sustain life processes: regulate hazards and promote normal growth and development.

Additionally Orem sees self-care as divided into two categories:

- universal self-care needs
- health-deviation self-care needs.

Universal self-care needs require concern about the common elements we all need to sustain life, such as air, food, fluid, activity, rest, solitude and social inter-action. They also relate to the promotion of normal age-phase behaviour through conformity. On the other hand health-deviation needs only require attention when changes have occured as a result of injury, illness, disability, deprivation or loss and/or through the changes brought about by any medical diagnosis and treatment.

Intervention is, therefore, seen as identifying an individual's self-care needs, through the exercise of professional judgment. Determining any deficit in an individual's capacity to meet such needs it also seeks to design action to help persons bridge this self-care deficit, either through teaching the person new coping mechanisms and self-care techniques, where this is possible, or in teaching and supporting lay-carers, who may meet the self-care deficit for the person. Where these two courses of action are inappropriate, the practitioner may actively supply the self-care deficit by doing for the person what he cannot do for himself, or arranging for some other agency to do this and then monitoring its fulfilment. Other intervention includes structuring the environment in such a way as to support the fulfilment of identified self-care needs and so guiding, supporting and helping the individual as to lead them to assume that level of self-care which is appropriate for them.

The link between the model and the health visiting process is possibly as follows:

Orem's self-care model	Health visiting process
Self-maintenance and self-care are basic values, needed for effective functioning in human society.	*Assessment* The practitioner identifies the extent to which the client *does* practice self-care activities normally, and the ways in which present circumstances cause *deficit* in his self-care ability. Furthermore practitioner identifies what potential for self-care the client possesses; how far any deficit could be met by other lay-carers; what knowledge and skill person requires in order to meet the client's self-care needs and if they are unable to do this at present what action the practitioner needs to take to enable them to learn to do so.
The individual who is normal will wish to engage in self-care, and in all circumstances will strive to do this.	*Planning* Specifies care measures, resources and co-ordinating activities. With client and other carers determines different responsibilities for action, allocating these, in line with the goals of care. Monitors each stage.
Perceives care goals as related to autonomy through self-care activities. Regards practitioners as identifying self-care deficits and remedying these.	*Implementing* Initiating, controlling and delivering care according to the detailed plan. *Evaluating* Determining the results of action taken, against the desired goals of personal independence in self-care. *Reorganising* Scrutinises evaluation data, decides how to redesign the care given and then adjusts same.

Goal-attainment model

The goal attainment model can be said to be a systems model with interactional elements. It is concerned with evaluation and its conceptual advantages are seen to lie in its action-setting. For the elderly its significance is that it focuses on short-term services to a community-based group, rather than to the institutionalised or severely mentally impaired aged. It is based on personal and social values, including the belief that people should have the opportunity to assess their own capacities, needs, and interests, and should make the decisions that affect their well-being.

Assumptions underlying the model are:

a. Most people, including the elderly, are able to determine what they need, can make decisions about how best to achieve these needs, and want to make such decisions for themselves. Furthermore they need to make such decisions if they are to remain functional in contemporary society.

b. Persons who have the decision-making power taken away from them stagnate, become apathetic and eventually lose touch with reality.

c. Professional intervention is of value since it is seen as facilitating the individual to achieve his/her goals, and not perceived as imposing goals on individuals.

d. Such professional intervention is likely to be most effective if concentrated on helping clients achieve specific and limited goals of their own choosing, within brief bounded periods of service'.

e. It is possible to determine the success or failure of such intervention, because outcomes can be related to predetermined objectives.

Thus such a model emphasises the strengths of an elderly client as well as taking account of his/her limitations. Furthermore by causing the worker to be tuned in to the client's definitions of his/her problems, through the use of a framework which stresses the client't ability to cope with these, and to work towards solutions within a limited time-period, engenders a more positive view of the client-system (Cormican 1977). Where an older person has a positive self-image and perceives himself/herself to be positively viewed by others, and seen to be self-directing, he or she is likely to use their potential to achieve satisfactory outcomes. In societies where ageism is a constant risk, such positive elements are highly constructive.

Although the model is not synonymous with the health visiting process it may be operationalised through the latter, as Luker (1982), was able to show. The links between them are shown below.

Goal-attainment model	Health visiting process
Recognises personal and social values, including those of the organisation of which the practitioner forms part.	Recognises underlying values. *Assessment* Collects relevant data in effort to identify client goals, values and problems. Analyses steps needed to be fulfilled in order to achieve goals. Helps client prioritise goals.
Recognises desire for independence present in individuals and asserts their ability to make and follow through on decisions, despite age.	*Planning* Structures tasks, so that the primary responsibility for reaching goals rest with the client and not the worker, thus promoting independence.
Respects the right of the older individual to cope with life-activities, test out action and make other plans, should initial actions fail to meet desired objectives.	*Implementing* Describes and explains the action taken and by whom
Supports evaluation as a highly complex activity, which seeks to determine observed change, and relationship to actions taken and/or other causes.	*Evaluating* Measures the degree of change which has taken place, relating these to the action taken. Determines both process and outcome.

The most marked differences between the model and the operational tool which seeks to utilise it, lie in the fact that the model assumes evaluation research against set goals for a pre-defined population, whereas the health visiting process describes care given to one individual, for the express purpose of helping that one person; hence the measurement of the effectiveness of that care becomes a secondary activity, albeit a very important one. However, the use of the model has been said to increase client motivation (Kastenbaum 1973).

REFERENCES

Caplan G 1964 Principles of preventive psychiatry. Basic Books, New York
Caplan G 1974 Support systems and community. Mental Health Behavioural Publications, New York
Cormican E J 1977 Task-centred model for work with the aged In: Social Casework October: 490–494
Helson H 1964 Adaptation Level Theory. Harper and Row, New York

Kastenbaum 1973 The foreshortened life perspective. In: Brantl V M, Raymond-Brown 1973 Readings in gerontology. Mosby, St Louis

Luker K 1982 Evaluating health visiting practice. Royal College of Nursing, London

Orem D E 1971 Nursing: Concepts of practice. McGraw-Hill, New York

Riehl J P, Roy C 1980 Conceptual models for nursing practice, 2nd edn. Appleton-Century-Crofts, New York

Roy C 1970 Adaptation: a conceptual framework for nursing. Nursing Outlook 18(3):42

Saxton D F, Hyland P A 1979 Planning and implementing nursing intervention: stress and adaptation applied to patient care, 2nd edn. Mosby, St Louis

Appendix 4

Guide to Family Assessment, with special reference to the elderly

ASSESSMENT

Family characteristics

Composition of family:
Name: Address: Date of birth: Sex:
Occupation:
Relationship to household head. Ethnic group. Socio-economic group.

Health status of family members

Describe the current health status of each member, identifying any deviation from the norm regarding growth, development and health.

List significant past accidents or illnesses affecting members: state current ones.

Describe family history of allergies: use of prostheses or appliances, including spectacles and hearing aids; state patterns of specific therapy, including medications taken by family members.

Obtain current immunisation state of members: habits in relation to eating, drinking, smoking and any other addictions. Describe nutritional status, outlining levels of family

343

nutritional knowledge; group eating patterns; facilities for the preparation and storage of food; cooking facilities and significant shopping behaviour.

Ascertain family patterns of consultation with health services personnel, and levels of use of services. Relationship with personnel.

Family housing

Describe the type of home and its size in relation to family needs, particularly the needs of older members. Note if rented/owner occupied. Describe standards of domestic hygiene and home management: note if facilities such as heating, ventilation, lighting, toilet arrangements, hot water supply, bathroom and laundry provisions are adequate for family needs. Can elderly persons utilise these facilities appropriately?

Check if there are specific accident hazards such as unlighted passageways, halls, steps: unprotected windows: unguarded fires, stoves and similar appliances: unsafe steps/stairs or walkways: loose floor coverings; inappropriately sited shelves, cupboards, hooks and so on? Ascertain what aids, gadgets and/or adaptations have been utilised to assist family with care of older person in home; identify shortfall in order to meet need.

Describe housing location in relation to civic amenities, including shops, markets, post office, banks, places of worship, public libraries, telephones, public transport, leisure facilities, educational establishments, ambulance services, health centres, hospitals, social services, police and fire services and voluntary organisation centres.

Family transport

Describe forms of family transport, including whether family owns a car, cycle or other vehicle. If public transport used, identify frequency and adequacy of service; suitability/accessibility/for elderly people. Identify any specific transport needs.

Family income

Describe major sources, relating income to family needs and determining adequacy/inadequacy. Identify standards of family budgeting, noting any specific financial need. Are all entitlements to benefit being received? Note relative socio-economic status against family peer-group; is there evidence of relative financial deprivation?

Pattern of family activities

Describe family work and leisure patterns; sleeping patterns and other significant activities. Are home and community facilities adequate to fulfil these activities or desired family activities? Identify how far family show interest in, and facilitate the activities of older family members.

Describe family values and goals, including religious activities and levels of involvement. How far can/do family resources permit expression of family values?

Family resources

Briefly describe family physical, psychological, social and economic resources. How far can family meet present demands? How far are family likely to be able to meet foreseeable future demands? Identify family coping resources: how far can family be described as an effective family, in relation to stage of family development and the tasks it has to meet to supply the needs of each member?

Family dynamics

Identify levels of family care for each other, especially elderly members.

Describe levels of family stability and interaction and the pattern of family decision making. Are family members flexible? Able to interchange roles as required? What are family attitudes towards elderly member(s)? Are there aspects of family care and understanding which give rise to concern? How can family be assisted to achieve greater growth?

Family relationship with the community

Describe how family members interact with others within the community. Are members active in civic affairs? Are they involved with specific groups; clubs; voluntary service? Outline the particular involvement family have with activities designed for older people.

Family perception of the present health and social needs

How do the family perceive their present health and social needs? What priorities in care can be set, in the light of family goals? Specify particularly those priorities which directly impinge on older members. How far can family meet these needs? Are they willing to do so? Of remaining needs, which are amenable to health visitor intervention? Which needs require referral? Has family consent to referral been obtained?

SUMMARY OF FAMILY HEALTH CARE PLAN

Summarise the main goals of family health care, if possible in behavioural terms. Specify the actions to be taken, allocating responsibility to various members and to practitioners. State the criteria for determining action-outcomes. In subsequent visits evaluate action and re-organise care with family as desired.

REFERENCES

This guide was formulated after reference to the following:

CETHV Guide to the health visiting syllabus and Guide to health visiting studies. CETHV, London
Helvie C O 1981 Community health nursing: theory and process. Harper and Row, Philadelphia, p 299–303
Murray R, Huelskoetter M M, O'Driscoll D 1980 The nursing process in later maturity. Prentice-Hall, Englewood Cliffs, p 33–50, 294–317

Appendix 5

Guide to Community Assessment, with special reference to the elderly

In depth studies are not always possible, although student health visitors are expected to produce neighbourhood studies as part of their background assessment material. However, whenever practitioners move to new areas, and at periodic intervals in areas where they have already been working for some time, it is wise to review the existing structure and services, within communities.

Familiarisation with the epidemiological patterns of health and disease and the community dynamics can prove invaluable to health visitors, helping them to take a population perspective and enabling them to slot work with individuals and family groups, into context.

Thus the following guide is provided to assist readers to think about those aspects of community life which impinge on members, and which can profoundly affect the quality of living.

The framework is not claimed to be exhaustive and can be adapted to meet individual need.

Acknowledgement is freely made to other publications which have helped to guide thinking including:

CETHV Guide to the preparation of health visiting studies. CETHV, London
Helvie C O 1981 Community health nursing: theory and process. Harper
and Row, Philadelphia, p 304–322

Murray R B, Huelskoetter M M, O'Driscoll D 1980 The nursing process in later maturity. Prentice Hall, Englewood Cliffs, p 33–36.

ASSESSMENT

Name of community. Boundaries as defined geographically or administratively: size, shape and demarcating characteristics.

Community characteristics

Brief description of main geographic and topographic features. Main climate, rainfall, mean temperature and seasonal variations. Brief reference to major historical features, especially those that have a direct bearing on current care for the elderly.

Demographic features

Note population size and structure; trends in population growth and change, especially identifying the proportion of elderly persons within the population over the past 20 years and forward projections. Identify the likely implications of these population trends for the health and social services in general and the health visiting services in particular.

Identify the main mortality and morbidity statistics, noting the general trends and the age specific death rates; major causes of death; trends in morbidity patterns, with particular reference to the major causes of morbidity amongst the elderly population. Specify what programmes, if any, have been started to deal with these major causes of death and disease amongst the general population, and especially amongst the elderly.

Community health services

Analyse the major health services in terms of stated criteria. Are the bed ratios, especially for the elderly, adequately met in local hospital and residential provision? Identify the manpower establishments in terms of any available and valid criteria, indicating funded and filled posts in hospital and domiciliary services. Discover staff-population ratios for medical, nursing and paramedical staffs in hospital and domiciliary services. Note how the Community Health Council and other similar local 'watchdog organisations' view the adequacy/inadequacy of services. Specify any areas of unmet need. Collect data relevant to the pattern of hospital admissions and discharges especially relating to older people. Examine the use of accident and emergency departments, again identifying, where possible, the specific local problems which cause elderly persons to use these services.

Community nursing services

Review the data pertaining to the number of visits paid by (a) District Nurses and (b) Health Visitors to different sections of the population. Draw the inferences from these patterns of service as set against the age-specific population groups. Identify the percentage of persons served and not served, particularly noting the short-fall in service for elderly persons.

Where possible relate the service given to the various settings, viz home visits: consultations in clinics, surgeries and health centres: visits to day centres, residential establishments, sheltered housing and other places where care may be given. Obtain the 'feel' of the distribution of activities, noting where inadequacies appear. Note the formal (recorded) health education activities designed especially for the elderly, and the approx proportion of the elderly population so contacted.

List out the major goals of the health visiting service for (a) the next year, (b) the next 5 years, **for this community**, particularly noting goals set for the elderly.

Environmental health services

Note standards of environmental health care, with specific reference to water supplies: sewage and refuse disposal: food hygiene and supervision: housing: nuisance abatement: public lighting, street cleaning, supervision of shops, markets and restaurants: particular attention paid to the needs of elderly persons within the environment, especially related to the incidence of infectious disease, food poisoning and accidents amongst elderly people.

Social services

Briefly describe the services available, identifying adequacy/inadequacy in relation to community needs. Note staff-population ratios in relation to recommended establishments and identify any short-fall. Identify the lines of communication between health and social services personnel and the existence of any arrangements for improving these, such as regular liaison groups.

Briefly describe the services specific to the elderly, including the provision of clubs, leisure facilities; services for the handicapped elderly; provision of day centres: proportion of service allocated to the elderly by the home help service: meals on wheels service: laundry services, if available, and any specific home aides scheme.

Discover the details of short-term admission facilities for the elderly, within the social services sector: numbers of places in residential accommodation in relation to need: the existence of special programmes designed to facilitate rehabilitation in the case of disability. Discover any specific social problems affecting the community which call for particular action.

Educational services

Briefly describe the services available in relation to population need. Are educational establishments easily accessible to the elderly? Are there any specific programmes available for the elderly population? Discover if older persons use the educational facilities available in this community.

Details of local government

State the composition of the local council and note the electoral machinery. Note the sources of local authority finance and the disbursement of funds against stated community needs. What proportion of available monies are used for services affecting the elderly?

Are there specific policies affecting the elderly being pursued by the civic authority?

Identify the key figures in public life and community affairs.

Does the community show a keen interest in electing and lobbying its leaders? What degree of interest and support is shown by these key persons, especially in relation to the care of older persons?

Communication measures

State the local newspapers and any local radio station or other measure for communicating; how far do health visitors use these forms of communication? To what extent does the media appear to influence policies affecting the elderly? What scope, if any, does the media offer to health visitors to promote health education issues?

Housing and associated amenities

Briefly examine the general housing layout, noting the overall design in terms of accessibility, structure, personal convenience and aesthetic appeal. Does housing overall enhance the quality of community living? Describe the major types of dwelling, noting the proportion of home owners to public and private tenants. Identify the pattern of living for the elderly population.

What is the overall percentage of sub-standard housing? What proportion of elderly persons live in such substandard housing? Outline the proposed programmes for dealing with local housing problems, noting the adequacy/inadequacy of such. Examine trends in waiting lists. Are there specific provisions for elderly persons within this community's housing programmes? Do these provisions meet the needs of the elderly population? What avenues of communication exist between housing department personnel and health service personnel? Are these channels well used? Can communication be improved and if so, how?

Note the distribution of shops, markets, post offices, public libraries and places of worship. Is there adequate neighbourhood provision, especially for elderly persons who may be unable to travel to a town centre? Is public transport available, accessible and suitable for older people? Are there concessionary fares for senior citizens? Are leisure facilities accessible to older persons and can they easily avail themselves of these? Do they do so? Is the range of recreation clubs and peer-group interests appropriate for older people? Can elderly housebound be transported easily and regularly to these facilities? What action if any is being taken to improve any inadequacies in common amenities for community members, especially the aged?

Protective services

Briefly describe the availability of fire, ambulance and police services. Note lines of communication. Consider the distribution of services in relation to community needs. Are there specific schemes for protecting older persons?

Employment facilities

Briefly review the major types of employment available in the community. Is there a broad diversification of employment? What is the percentage of unemployed persons? How does the trend compare with 5 years ago? With the national average?

Is there specific provision for the employment of older persons in this community? If so briefly describe scheme(s) noting the lines of communication and system of referral of elderly people who may wish to work.

Are there particular problems presented by industry within the community, viz problems of air pollution? Of distribution of toxic wastes? Specific chemical hazards?

Voluntary services

Is there a directory of voluntary services available in the community? Identify particularly those societies with interest in the elderly and note how to contact them. Are services well-staffed? Are there arrangements for older persons who wish to perform some voluntary service? Are there specific gaps in the service? Is there any co-ordinating body? What contact do health services personnel have with specific organisations? With the co-ordinating body?

Community dynamics

Identify the levels of interest shown by community members in community affairs. Can 'key individuals' be identified? How far can the community be described as a caring community? Why is this so? Identify particularly the degree of community interest and support for programmes and policies affecting the care of older people.

SUMMARY OF HEALTH AND SOCIAL NEEDS WITHIN THE COMMUNITY

Summarise the main unmet health needs of the community arising from:

a. community composition and structure
b. community resources
c. community dynamics.

Identify the major unmet health needs of the elderly population. Set out the priorities for meeting

- general community health problems
- the health problems of the elderly in this community.

List out which of these problems are amenable to health visiting intervention. Outline the action proposed to deal with these health visiting concerns. State with which of the other problems health visitors may be able to assist. Which of these main health problems should be referred to other health or social agencies? Outline how this has been done. State the evaluation criteria being used to ascertain if action taken is proving effective.

Appendix 6

List of useful addresses for those caring for elderly persons

Abbeyfield Society, 186/192 Darkes Lane, Potters Bar, Herts EN6 1AB — Offers housing, usually bed-sitting rooms to older persons.

Across Trust, Crown House, Morden, Surrey SM4 5EW (01-540 3897) — Operates transport scheme for chronically sick or handicapped elderly going on holiday.

Action for Dysphasic Adults, Northcote House, 37a Royal Street, London SE1 7LL (01-261 9572) — Acts to facilitate the rehabilitation of adults with speech impairments, usually following strokes or associated neurological conditions.

Age Concern (England), Bernard Sunley House, 60 Pitcairn Road, Mitcham, Surrey CR4 3LL (01-640 5431) *see also* telephone directory for local branch. — Operates an advisory and welfare service for the elderly; has a wide range of useful publications; instigates research.

Ageing, The Centre for Policy on, Nuffield Lodge Studio, Regents Park, London NW1 4RS (01-586 9844) — Has a reference library and information service

Alzheimer's Disease Society, Bank Buildings, Fulham Broadway, London SW6 1EP (01-381 3177) — Has very useful publications; gives advice and support to those caring for persons with dementia.

Arthritis Care, 6 Grosvenor Crescent London, SW1X 7ER (01-235 0902)

Arthritis and Rheumatism Council, 41 Eagle Street, London WC1 4AR (01-405 8572) — Gives information and conducts research into these diseases.

British Association of the Hard of Hearing, 7–11 Armstrong Road, London W3 7JL (01-743 1110) — Publishes the magazine *Hark* quarterly: offers advice; runs clubs; encourages self-help groups.

British Association for Service to the Elderly (BASE) 3 Keele Farmhouse, Keele, Staffordshire (0782 627280) — A registered charity which provides opportunities for those who care for the elderly to meet together informally to exchange ideas and experience in order to further better care for the elderly.

British Diabetic Association, 10 Queen Anne Street, London WIM OBD
(01-323 1531)

British Geriatrics Society, 1, ST Andrew's Place, Regents Park, London NW1,
4LB 01-935-4004 An organisation of medical personnel, who are interested
in research, and the prevention and treatment of diseases of elderly
persons.

British Red Cross Society, National Headquarters, 9 Grosvenor Crescent,
London SWIX 7EJ (01-235 5454) *see also* telephone directory for local
branch. — An advisory, instructional and welfare society.

Blind, Guide Dogs for the, Alexandra House, 9–11 Park Street, Windsor,
Berks (0753-55711) — Some elderly blind may benefit from a guide dog,
especially if blinded earlier in life.

Blind, National Library for, Cromwell Road, Bredbury, Stockport SK6 2SG
(061-491 0217) — Offers advice on services for blind: publications, aids
and access to some welfare funds.

Blind, Royal National Institute for the, 224 Great Portland Street, London
WIN 6AA (01-388 1266) — Offers an advisory service; gives guidance on
welfare provisions.

Blind, Telephones for the, Fund, A Chudley, Mynthurst, Leigh Surrey (0923
862546) — May provide grants towards the cost of telephone installation
and rental for the elderly blind.

Blind, Wireless for the, 224 Great Portland Street, London W1 (01-388 1266)
— May help towards the provision of wireless sets for elderly blind
persons.

British Legion, The Royal, 48 Pall Mall, London SW1Y 5JY (01-930-8131) *see
also* telephone directory for local branch — Offers information, social
and supportive contact; and has limited accommodation available to
elderly persons who have served in H M Forces or been enaged in work
of national importance.

Cancer Relief, The National Society for, Michael Sobell House, 30 Dorset
Square London NW1 (01-402 8125) — Provides grants for needy sufferers.

Carers and their Elderly Dependants, National Council for, 29 Chilworth
Mews, London W2 3RG (01-262 1451/2) — Offers advice and support to
carers and cared for.

Carers Association of, Medway Homes, Balfour Road, Rochester, Kent
(Medway 813981) — Offers an advisory service to carers of all ages.
Publications: research.

Chest, Heart and Stroke Association, Tavistock House North, Tavistock
Square, London WC1H 9JE (01-387 3012) — Offers an advisory service
and publishes a wide range of helpful literature.

Citizens Advice Bureaux, National Association of, Myddleton House,
115–123 Pentonville Road, London N1 9LZ (01-833 2181) *see also*
telephone directory for local bureau — Offer an advisory and legal
service, comprehensive information on care of elderly.

Colostomy Welfare Group, 38/39 Eccleston Square, London SW1V 1PB (01-
828 5175) — Offers advice and help to professional staff and sufferers.
Encourages rehabilitation and self-help. useful literature.

Community Health Councils for England and Wales, Association of, Top
Floor, Barclays Bank Chambers, 254 Seven Sisters Road, London N4 2HZ
(01-272 5459) *see also* telephone directory for local branch — Monitors
health services; will investigate concerns referred to them.

Community Service Volunteers, 237 Pentonville Road, London N1 (01-278-
6601) Contacts reached on Ext. 68/or 58–Provides a limited but one-to-
one service.

Consumer Association, 14 Buckingham Street London WC2N 6DS (01-222-9501) — Acts as the consumer's watchdog. Useful range of publications.

Contact, 15 Henrietta Street, Covent Garden, London WC2E 8QH (01-240-0630) — Offers friendship and outings to elderly housebound persons.

Crossroads Care Attendant Scheme Trust, 94 Coton Road, Rugby, Warwickshire (0788 73653) — Sets up schemes nationwide to care for elderly and handicapped persons in their own homes.

Cruse, The National Organisation for widows and widowers, 126 Sheen Road, Richmond, Surrey, TW9 1UR (01-940 4818)

Counsel and Care for the Elderly, 131 Middlesex Street, London E1 7JF (01-621 1624) — Offers information on private and voluntary residential accommodation nationwide and on changes and grants which may be available.

Deaf Association, The British, 38 Victoria Place, Carlisle CA1 1HU (0228 48844)

Deaf-Blind Helpers' League, 18 Rainbow Court, Paston Ridings, Peterborough PE4 6UP (0733 73511) — Publishes a newsletter and offers an advisory service for deaf-blind persons and their carers, including elderly persons.

Department of Health and Social Security, Alexander Fleming House, Elephant and Castle, London SE1 6BY (01-407 5522) *see also* telephone directory for local offices.

Depressives Associates, 19 Merley Ways, Wimbourne Minster Dorset BH21 1QN — A self-help group for sufferers and their carers.

Disability Alliance, 25 Denmark Street, London WC2H 9NJ (01-240 0806) — Offers a wide range of information on benefits and services for disabled persons and their families. Produces a helpful Disability Rights Handbook annually.

Disabled Living Foundation, 380/384 Harrow Road, London W9 2HU (01-289 6111) Gives an extensive information service on aids for the handicapped. Permanent exhibition viewed by appointment. Range of very useful literature.

Elderly and Gentlefolks, Friends of, 42 Ebury St, London SW1W 0LZ (01-730 8263) — Runs some residential homes: makes grants for elderly at home.

Employment Fellowship, Wensley House, Bell Common Epping, Essex CM16 DY (78 77047) — Encourages employment opportunities for retired elderly.

Epilepsy, British Association for, Crowthorne House, New Wokingham Road, Wokingham, Berks RG11 3AY (0344 773122)

Extend, 5 Conway Road, Sheringham, Norfolk NR26 8DD (0263 822479) — Encourages exercises for the elderly. Plan available but send S.A.E.

Forum on the Rights of Elderly People to Education (FREE) 60 Pitcairn Road, Mitcham, Surrey, CR4 3LL (01-640 5431) — Promotes learning in all aspects for older people.

Friends by Post, 6 Bollin Court, Macclesfield Road, Wilmslow, Cheshire (0625 527044) — Encourages pen-friends for the elderly housebound.

Health Education Council, 78 New Oxford Street, London WC1A 1AH — Offers a range of useful leaflets, suitable for older people.

Health Visitors' Association, 36 Eccleston Square, London SW1 (01-834 9523)

Help the Aged, 1–7 Sekforde Street, London EC1R 0BE (01-253-0253) *see also* telephone directory for local branch — Offers a range of supportive services and information for older people.

Housing Aid Trust, 157 Waterloo Road, London SE1 8XF (01-633 9277) — Will give advice to elderly persons with housing problems.

Invalids at Home Trust, 17 Lapstone Gardens, Kenton, Harrow HA3 0EB (01-

907 1706) — Provides some financial help for handicapped persons living at home, including their older handicapped.

MIND (National Association of Mental Health,) 22 Harley St, London WIN 2E

Marie Curie Memorial Foundation, 28 Belgrave Square, London SW1X 8QG — Assists in the provision of night nursing services for older persons suffering from malignancy.

National Sounds, Contact House, 6 Castletown Road, London W14 9HE (01-385 4211) — Circulates a national magazine for the blind on tape.

National Association of Widows, Chell Road, Stafford ST16 2QA

Old Age Pensions Associations, National Federation of, Melling House, 91 Preston New Road, Blackburn, Lancs BB2 6BD (0254 52606)

Open University, Walton Hall, Milton Keynes MK7 6AA — Offers home study courses for persons of all ages: has many older students.

Parkinson's Disease Society, 36 Portland Place, London WC2H 0HR — Offers useful publications and support for sufferers.

Partially Sighted Society, 40 Wordsworth Street, Hove, Sussex (Brighton 736053)

Pre-Retirement Association, Greenfield House, 19 Undine Street, London SW17 8PP — Range of useful publications.

REACH (Retired Executives Action Clearing House), Victoria House, Southampton Row, London WC1B 4DH (01-404 0940)

Royal College of Nursing, 20 Cavendish Square, London WIM 0AB — Has an active Geriatric Nursing Society: also an extensive library.

Royal Society for the Prevention of Accidents, Cannon House, The Priory, Queensway, Birmingham B4 6BS — Useful publications.

Rukba, 6 Avonmore Road, London W14 8RL (01-602 6274) — Makes grants and offers annuities to some professional persons who are in need, infirm or old.

SAGA, Embrook House, Sandgate, Folkestone, Kent CT20 3AY — Arranges holidays on a commercial basis for older people. Runs clubs and offers a pen-friend service to members of these clubs only.

Samaritans, 39 Walbrook London EC4 *see* telephone directory for local number.

Sexual and Personal Relationships of the Disabled (SPOD) 286 Camden Road London

Social Services Departments *see* telephone directory for local office.

Social Workers, British Association of (BASW), 16 Kent Street, Birmingham B5 6RD (021-622 3911)

St John Ambulance Brigade *see* telephone directory for local number.

Talking Books for the Handicapped, National Listening Library, 12 Lant Street, London SE1 1QR (01-407 9117) — Provides cassettes by post: book catalogue available.

Task Force (also known as Pensioners Link), 17 Balfe Street, London N1 9EB (01-278 5501/4)

Tinnitus Association, 105 Gower Street, London WC1E 6AH

University of the Third Age (U3A) c/o D. Norton, 6 Parkside Gardens, London SW19 5EW (01-947 0401) — Based on a European idea of helping people to learn in their later years.

Women's Royal Voluntary Service, 17 Old Park Lane, London W1Y 4AJ (01-499 6040) *see also* telephone directory for local number.

Workers Educational Association (WEA), 9 Upper Berkeley Street, London W1 (01-402 5608/9) — Provides a range of courses for all age groups but often relevant to the local community and aspects of its life: caters for older people in any field for which there is a local demand.

There are of course many other national and local organisations concerned with the care of the elderly. Further details and addresses may be obtained from:

The Charities Digest (to be found in most reference libraries)
The Disability Alliance, 25 Denmark Street, London WC2H 8NJ
Knight S, Help! ... I need help. Kimpton Press — contain useful annotated details of most voluntary organisations.

Social Services Departments are usually able to supply details of local branches of organisation.

Appendix 7

Checklist for health visitors working with elderly clients

Background data

How aware am I of the number and distribution of older people within the community in which I work.?

How familiar am I with pertinent epidemiological data affecting the elderly population in the community in which I work?

Do I know the major causes of mortality and morbidity amongst the elderly population and can I describe the trends? What steps, if any, have I taken to ensure that health visiting programmes relate to these needs. Do I participate in overall health care programmes designed to reduce these specific health problems? How effective are the measures taken?

Data related to specific settings

If I am undertaking geographic-based health visiting, what steps have I taken to effect liaison with others involved in the care of older persons? How far have we been able to agree joint goals and work towards meeting these?

If I am working in general-practice based health visiting am I aware of the distribution of elderly persons within the practice population? Have I a systematic and efficient method for identifying them and determining their level of vulnerability?

What steps, if any, have I taken to ensure that the general practice team, of which I am a member, studies the overall needs of the elderly within the practice population and sets joint goals in care?

How frequently do I attend meetings designed to evaluate action taken to meet such goals? How often do I participate in re-planning and re-organisation of joint-care programmes?

How ready am I to initiate and maintain contact with elderly clients when the onus is left to me?

How frequently do I liaise with other team members, particularly social workers and para-medical personnel such as chiropodists, dentists, occupational therapists, physiotherapists and speech therapists, opticians and pharmacists?

Do I have clear lines of communication with hospital personnel and am I familiar with the various policies for admission, discharge and follow up of elderly patients? Do I have close contact with staff in accident, emergency and outpatient departments and with dieticians and other consultative personnel?

Do I clearly understand the policies of my employing authority concerning the care of the elderly?

Am I aware of the community facilities which exist for older people and do I attend co-ordinating meetings, care conferences and public meetings as necessary?

Preparation for visits

Before undertaking visits to the elderly, whether at their homes, in clinics, health centres, residential accommodation, day centres, clubs or other settings, how well do I prepare myself by scrutinising available data and checking out related material from colleagues and other agencies?

Ensuring that advice and information I plan to give is based on sound scientific principles and is feasible for elderly client(s) or their carer(s) to implement?

How carefully do I structure the plan of my visit, in order to cover relevant problems of which I am aware? Do I use a clear model/framework? How ready am I to allow the agenda to be flexible, should the client wish to introduce new issues into the situation?

During visits

How carefully do I study the sociocultural background of my client(s) and their family(ies), in order to set them at ease? Work within their value system? Afford them dignity?

How thoughtful am I in ensuring that the language I use and the modes of approach I adopt are comprehensible and suitable for them? What steps do I take to gain and hold their confidence and respect? How ready am I to allow the client to take the initiative in identifying their needs, problems and goals? Am I an active listener and do I direct conversation into productive channels when necessary?

How ready am I to pay attention to both verbal and non-verbal communication from client(s) and carer(s)?

Do I give high priority to maintaining functional independence amongst my elderly clients?

How careful am I to ensure that I have collected data in all the realms of living, before making an assessment of situations?

Do I take advantage of the many opportunities I have for teaching, whether by example, demonstration or precept? Do I take time to study the learning style of individual client(s) being aware of the emotional factors which influence learning, and taking time to evaluate if learning has occurred?

Do I elicit client(s) coping abilities and build on and strengthen these, so that I utilise every resource the client has for his/her benefit?

Am I careful to place the client into the context of his/her family?

Do I study the family as a unit, recognising the needs of family members and perceiving the family in totality?

Do I recognise the contribution client makes to the family and the demands they place upon it?

Do I take into account the special needs that may be posed by the illness or disability of the elderly member?

Am I aware of family dynamics and of the environmental stresses they encounter? Is the advice and help I am able to give, adequate for the family's needs?

Do I perceive the relationship of client-family and community?

Am I able to interpret community policies and programmes

for the benefit of client and family? Do I take full account of all the community influences that operate on the client and family?

At the close of the visit

Do I allow time for recapping on salient points? Do I ensure that the client is fully aware of what has been discussed and decided between us? That the client and/or carer is quite clear about the responsibilities they have for putting any jointly-prepared plans into operation? That client and/or carer know what action I have agreed to take and approve same? That both client, carer and myself are clear about evaluation criteria? That I have written down all relevant material and left it in an accessible place for the benefit of client, carer and any professional personnel who may be involved?

Do I make sure that the client knows when to expect me again?

After the visit

Do I ensure a systematic format for recording significant data?

Do I check that the format is clear, concise, accurate and suitable for use within the health visiting organisation and amongst other colleagues?

Do my records make explict the basis of my assessments and demonstrate my rationale in care?

Do I ensure that the documents are treated correctly, respecting confidentiality?

Within the team

Do I seek to facilitate the work of other team members, especially in the care of the elderly? Do I try to understand their problems and support them as appropriate? Do I work constructively with them to improve our services, especially to the elderly population?

Do I respect the health visiting management and co-operate with them?

Index

363